RECENT ADVANCES
IN PAEDIATRICS

DAVID HULL

BSc FRCP(Lond) DObstRCOG DCH(Eng)
Professor of Child Health
Medical School, University of Nottingham

RECENT ADVANCES IN PAEDIATRICS

EDITED BY

DAVID HULL

NUMBER FIVE

CHURCHILL LIVINGSTONE

Edinburgh London and New York

1976

CHURCHILL LIVINGSTONE
Medical Division of Longman Group Limited

Distributed in the United States of America by
Longman Inc., 19 West 44th Street New York,
N.Y. 10036, and by associated companies,
branches and representatives throughout
the world

© LONGMAN GROUP LIMITED 1976

ISBN 0 443 01488 4
Library of Congress Cataloging in Publication Data
Main entry under under title:
Recent advances in paediatrics.
  Earlier eds. edited by D. Gairdner and D. Hull.
  Includes bibliographies and index.
  1. Pediatrics. I. Hull, David. II. Gairdner, Douglas.
Recent advances in paediatrics.
RJ45.G25 1976   618.9′2   76–19054

Printed in Great Britain

PREFACE

This edition, like the previous ones, is written to help busy doctors keep abreast of developments in paediatrics.

In the last few years obstetricians have developed a wide range of tests in an attempt to identify the sick fetus and since the last edition fetal intensive care during labour has come of age (Malcolm Symonds, Chapter 1). Notwithstanding, the vulnerable fetal brain is still at risk of damage in the last days of gestation; considerable clinical judgement and attention to detail is required to minimise the long term effects (Keith Brown, Chapters 2 and 3). The pre-term infant's chances of survival continue to improve, sometimes despite, but mainly because of, major developments in neonatal care (Pamela Davies, Chapter 4). But we tend to assess the success of our artificial hospital environments by immediate results and to ignore the more subtle and complex and long term social aspects which we are unable to measure, but which are of equal, if not of more, importance (Marshall Klaus and John Kennell, Chapter 5). On the other hand, improvements in hospital care have made little impact on infant mortality and we are left with the question posed by John Emery (Chapter 8) that if unexpected death in infancy is shown to be due to non-utilisation of the health service, what then?

In North American and many European countries preventive medicine is given the same sort of lip-service as Christianity. Surely a much higher percentage of our limited resources must be invested in preventive or anticipatory medicine. To date, the most effective preventive measure has been immunisation and further advances might be anticipated (Alistair Dudgeon, Chapter 7). But preventive measures involving identification by screening have much wider implications and in some instances the necessary intrusion into the community may be unacceptable. Various aspects of these problems are considered by Barbara Clayton (Chapter 6), Otto Wolff and June Lloyd (Chapters 12 and 13). But prevention can also be achieved by modifying the environment. John Colley (Chapter 9) reviews the evidence for the influence of the environment on respiratory disorders, the commonest diseases of children. Finally, a sick adult might be avoided by adequate and thorough medical care of the child. This is particularly so for renal diseases, which are the subject of two fine chapters by Cyril Chantler (Chapters 10 and 11).

After careful consideration, I decided not to change all the units in the text to SI units because these have not, as yet, been accepted internationally and conversion tables are readily available in those countries that are adopting the new system.

The authors are all busy clinicians themselves and they were invited not only to review their topics, but also to describe their own personal views and practice. I am most grateful to them for making the time to write their chapters and for their kindly tolerance during the preparation of their texts for publication.

Dr Douglas Gairdner introduced this series and edited the early editions. It was a privilege for me to work with him on the fourth edition. I hope this edition has maintained the standard he set.

Finally, it is a pleasure to acknowledge the help of Shelagh Roberts, my secretary, and of the publishers, Churchill Livingstone. I must also apologise to my wife and G., J. and J. for using some of 'our' time.

Nottingham, 1976   DAVID HULL

CONTRIBUTORS

J. K. BROWN MRCP(Edin) DCH(Eng)
Consultant Paediatric Nephrologist, Royal Hospital for Sick Children
and Simpson Memorial Maternity Pavilion, Edinburgh; Senior Lecturer,
Department of Child Life and Health, University of Edinburgh

C. CHANTLER MD MA MRCP
Consultant Paediatric Nephrologist, Department of Paediatrics, Guy's
Hospital, London

BARBARA E. CLAYTON MD PhD FRCPath FRCP
Professor of Chemical Pathology, Institute of Child Health, University
of London; Honorary Consultant in Chemical Pathology, The Hospital for
Sick Children, Great Ormond Street, London

J. R. T. COLLEY MD BSc MFCM
Professor of Community Health, University of Bristol, Canynge Hall,
Whiteladies Road, Bristol.

PAMELA A. DAVIES MD FRCP DCH
Senior Lecturer, Institute of Child Health; Honorary Consultant and
Children's Physician, Department of Paediatrics and Neonatal Medicine,
Hammersmith Hospital, London

J. A. DUDGEON MD FRCP FRCPath
Professor of Microbiology and Dean of the Institute of Child Health,
University of London; Consultant Microbiologist to The Hospital for
Sick Children, Great Ormond Street, London

J. L. EMERY MD FRCPath DCH
Professor in Paediatric Pathology, The Medical School, University of
Sheffield

JOHN H. KENNELL BS MD
Professor of Pediatrics, Case Western Reserve University School of Medicine, University Circle, Cleveland, Ohio, USA

MARSHALL H. KLAUS BS MD
Professor of Pediatrics, Case Western Reserve University School of Medicine, University Circle, Cleveland, Ohio, USA

JUNE K. LLOYD MD FRCP
Professor of Child Health, St George's Hospital Medical School, Blackshaw Road, London

E. M. SYMONDS MD FRCOG
Professor of Obstetrics and Gynaecology, University of Nottingham, City Hospital, Hucknall Road, Nottingham

OTTO H. WOLFF MD FRCP
Nuffield Professor of Child Health, Institute of Child Health, University of London, Guilford Street, London

CONTENTS

1
THE EVALUATION OF FETAL WELL-BEING IN PREGNANCY AND LABOUR

E. M. Symonds

FACTORS INFLUENCING PERINATAL MORTALITY AND MORBIDITY

Perinatal mortality ratios are known to vary widely in different parts of the world. For example, the 1970 WHO report on 'The prevention of perinatal mortality and morbidity', shows perinatal mortality ratios for 1965 to vary from 82.0/1000 live births in Mauritius to 19.3/1000 live births in Bulgaria. The characteristic features of those countries with high perinatal mortality rates include widespread malnutrition, poor social environment, high parity and inadequate medical services: these factors are associated with high infant mortality ratios as well. It has been estimated that 30 per cent of the children born in deprived communities will die before the age of five years.

Within the same community the rates of perinatal and infant mortality vary with social status, but other factors such as maternal age, preconceptional and interconceptional malnutrition and anaemia, specific protein and vitamin deficiencies, cigarette smoking and a history of previous abortions or stillbirths, are all important in the identification of a high-risk group (Butler and Alberman, 1969).

Nesbitt and Aubry (1969) developed a grading system by which anticipated perinatal vulnerability was expressed as a numerical value derived from the history at the first visit to clinic. In general, the risk of antenatal and intrapartum complications as well as a poor perinatal outcome was twice as high among the low scoring patients. The exercise is important, if potential problem pregnancies can be identified early, then medical resources can be concentrated on women at risk.

Complications arising during pregnancy also affect the outcome. For example, haemorrhage occurring at any stage of pregnancy is associated with a high risk of damage to the placenta and a high risk to the fetus. Maternal hypertension puts the infant at risk and factors such as multiple pregnancy, rhesus isoimmunisation and haemoglobinopathies, such as sickle cell anaemia, are associated with increased perinatal mortality ratios. Conditions which impair uterine blood flow and lead to placental damage such as pre-eclampsia, chronic renal disease and antepartum haemorrhage commonly result in intrauterine growth retardation. However, it may occur in apparently normal women with none of these complications.

Factors which result in increased fetal hypoxia in the antenatal period will be particularly hazardous during parturition. Any pregnancy complicated by these factors should be subjected to careful scrutiny and monitoring during labour.

Of the 16994 deaths surveyed in the British Perinatal Mortality Survey, necropsy was performed on 14873 infants. The commonest cause of perinatal mortality was fetal asphyxia: 2519 deaths resulted from fetal distress. A total of 1051 of these deaths occurred during labour and a further 509 deaths occurred in the first week after delivery; 909 occurred before the onset of labour (Gruenwald, 1969).

It is in this group that there is the greatest potential for fetal salvage. Already, the availability of placental function tests and fetal monitoring techniques have made significant inroads into the mortality rate from fetal distress.

The question of fetal and neonatal morbidity carries far more serious implications than mortality. For example, in severe fetal growth retardation, there is evidence to show that brain and intellectual development may be permanently impaired (Dobbing and Smart, 1973), although it now seems likely that modern neonatal care can prevent many of these problems. Lovell (1973) has shown that there is a significant increase in pulmonary infections and sleep rhythm disorders in the first year of life in infants born with evidence of placental insufficiency and dysmaturity where the gestational length was prolonged. There is no doubt that severe brain damage may result from prolonged fetal asphyxia, but what does remain in doubt is the degree to which more subtle forms of cerebral and intellectual impairment result from severe asphyxia either antepartum or during parturition (see Chapters 2 and 3).

It seems reasonable to work on the premise that if mortality rates can be reduced by an active policy of antenatal and neonatal scrutiny and therapy, then a corresponding reduction in neonatal morbidity can be achieved with improvement in the subsequent intellectual and physical development of the newborn child. The last 10 years have seen a progressive fall in perinatal mortality in the United Kingdom. At least part of this improvement must be attributed to the identification of problem areas in Health Care Services, and in the sophistication of antenatal and neonatal care. The economic and emotional demands of the intellectually and physically handicapped child on the community and the parents are enormous. It is these factors which designate the continuing need for directing resources into both research and good health care delivery for the fetus and newborn child.

PLACENTAL FUNCTION TESTS

There is no doubt that a great deal can be learnt by identifying the 'at risk' fetus from the medical, social and obstetric history and examination of the pregnant woman. Placental function tests have been introduced into obstetric practice in an attempt to quantify the degree of impaired function in the feto-placental unit, and thus to improve the decision-making process in relation to therapy or induction of labour.

The placenta is known to be an active site of steroidogenesis and of enzyme production. Some of the enzymes are specific to the placenta. The increase in production of these compounds during pregnancy forms the basis of most biochemical methods of assessing the function of the feto-placental unit.

Progesterone and its metabolites

In 1936, Venning and Browne demonstrated that the administration of progesterone to the pregnant woman resulted in an increased excretion of pregnanediol in urine. It has subsequently been shown that as pregnancy advances, increasing amounts of pregnanediol are excreted in the urine. Progesterone has been conclusively shown by Morrison, Meigs and Ryan (1965) to be formed by mitochondria from human placental tissue, and Zander (1959) has calculated that up to 250 mg of progesterone are produced daily by the full-term placenta. The measurement of urinary pregnanediol concentration in 24-h urine samples formed the basis of one of the most widely used placental function tests in the 1960s. Unfortunately, urinary pregnanediol measurements proved to be of little use in the assessment of the feto-placental unit. In the first instance, the fetal contribution to the maternal excretion of pregnanediol is small (MacNaughton, 1969). It has been shown that pregnanediol levels may not change after fetal death in utero. Secondly, despite the early finding by Shearman (1959) that preg-nanediol excretion reflected growth and development of the placenta, there is great variation between normal patients. Thirdly, Klopper and Billewicz (1963) has shown a day-to-day coefficient of variation of 24 per cent within individual women.

All of these factors led to the conclusion that pregnanediol measure-ment is of limited value as a placental function test, although in cases where oestriol excretion is low because of suppression of fetal adrenal function, it may still be a worthwhile observation. In general terms, pregnanediol measurement has now been largely replaced by other placental function tests.

The levels of progesterone in peripheral venous plasma increase from about 2 μg/100 ml at 10 weeks gestation to about 25 μg/100 ml at term (Short and Eton, 1959). Until recently, it seems unlikely that for technical reasons the measurement of plasma progesterone levels could be employed as a placental function test. With the development of competitive protein binding assays and radioimmunoassay methods, progesterone can now be measured rapidly with a high degree of precision and at very low cost. Although the levels of plasma progesterone appear to bear some relationship to fetal size, the levels do not necessarily fall either prior to or after fetal death. Tulchinsky and Okada (1975) have shown that in 11 patients with pre-eclampsia where the fetus died, only in four did the levels become subnormal, whereas plasma oestriol fell prior to fetal death in all of these patients. Clearly, plasma progesterone is unlikely to prove useful in the management of impaired placental function.

Oestrogen measurements in the assessment of the feto-placental unit

It has been known for many years that oestrogens are produced by the placenta. This was first demonstrated by Halban in 1905. Over 20 different oestrogens have been identified in the urine of pregnant women. The oestrogens found in maternal blood and urine, which have been most extensively investigated, are oestrone, oestradiol-17β and oestriol.

In pregnancy, the most important oestrogens are the C_{16}-substituted oestrogens, and of these, oestriol is the most important. Oestriol production in pregnancy is particularly important because it involves metabolism within both the placenta and the fetus. Siiteri and MacDonald (1966) have shown that the major precursor of oestriol is dehydroepiandrosterone (DHEA) produced by the fetal adrenal. 16-Hydroxylation of this compound occurs in the fetal liver and the formation of free oestriol from 16-OH DHEA takes place in the placenta.

Only 10 per cent of the precursors come from maternal sources. Free oestriol released by the placenta is conjugated with a glucuronide or sulphate moiety in the maternal liver. Thus, oestrogens occur in human urine as conjugates in the form of oestriol glucosidurate or oestriol sulphate. The ratio of oestriol:oestrone:oestradiol becomes 30:2:1, instead of 3:3:1 as in non-pregnant women (Brown, 1957). Because oestriol constitutes such a large fraction of the total oestrogen levels in pregnancy, there is good reason to simplify methodology and measure total oestrogens rather than oestriol. Brown et al introduced such a method in 1968 and showed a close correlation between the total oestrogen measurement and urinary oestriol. The method is suitable for automation and takes only 3.5 h to complete. Hainsworth and Hall (1971) have introduced modifications which have further reduced the assay time to 1 h. Thus, the measurement of urinary oestrogens has become established as a simple and economic placental function test.

The groups of most concern to the clinician are the complications that result in placental damage and intrauterine growth retardation. Earlier mention has been made of the conditions which are associated with an increased risk of feto-placental insufficiency and serial urinary oestrogen measurements are particularly useful both in terms of absolute values and in terms of the rate of increment in the assessment of placental function.

Numerous studies have now established the predictive value of these measurements. MacLeod et al (1967) showed a mortality rate of 23 per cent in patients with pregnancies complicated by various forms of hypertension, and showing abnormal oestriol levels. One hundred and three women were included in this study and in the 73 women who showed normal oestriol excretion, no deaths occurred.

Similar findings have been demonstrated in pregnancies complicated by proteinuria (Reid et al, 1968), and in pregnancies complicated by antepartum haemorrhage (Beischer et al, 1970). Thus, where pregnancy is complicated by conditions associated with placental damage, and low oestriol excretion is found, a high risk of fetal or neonatal death exists.

It has also been shown that low oestriol levels are associated with a high incidence of fetal acidosis in labour (Fliegner et al, 1969), and this emphasises the importance of carefully monitoring these infants during labour.

Not all low oestriol levels result from feto-placental insufficiency. There are certain artefacts which are particularly important and should always be remembered when low oestriol levels are detected.

Oestriol formation by the placenta is dependent on precursors supplied by the fetal and maternal adrenal glands.

The administration of cortisone and its analogues can therefore depress oestriol excretion. The effect appears to be variable and the work of Oakey (1970) has shown that this, in part, appears to be dose related. The mean depression achieved by these drugs is probably about 60 per cent so that grossly abnormal oestriol values are still significant even in patients on large doses of corticosteroids.

Ampicillin has been shown to suppress oestriol excretion by 57 per cent in dosages of 2 g/day but the mechanism by which this occurs is not understood (Willman and Pulkkinen, 1971).

Certain drugs interfere specifically with the assay methods and therefore produce spurious results without actually interfering with oestriol production.

Methenamine mandelate produces a marked fall in oestriol values by hydrolysis of the methenamine to formaldehyde with destruction of the phenolic oestrogens. Valid oestriol results can be obtained two days after discontinuing the drug (Touchstone, Stojkewycz and Smith, 1965).

The use of laxatives containing dihydroxy anthraquinone produces bright yellow discoloration in the phenolic extracts, and interferes in the Kober colour reaction in the assay method. Whilst this problem is easily recognised, it is sensible to avoid the use of laxatives such as Danthron and Doxiden, where urinary oestrogen measurements are to be undertaken.

Placental sulphatase deficiency. In 1969, France and Liggins described a patient with persistently low oestriol excretion due to a specific deficiency of sulphatase activity in the placenta. Normally, deconjugation of oestrogen precursors presented to the placenta is necessary before aromatisation to oestrogens can occur. Although the condition is rare, several further cases have now been reported in the literature and there is some evidence to suggest that this condition is associated with a failure to establish normal labour.

Fetal malformations. Anencephaly is commonly associated with adrenal hypoplasia, and is now well recognised as a cause of low oestriol production.

There is, however, evidence to suggest that the range of excretion even in this condition is variable (Fransden and Stakemann, 1964), and this is probably related quantitatively to the amount of adrenal tissue present.

The fact that other congenital malformations also result in low oestriol values is not as widely recognised, but it is a particularly important consideration where fetal growth retardation is suspected to consider the possibility of fetal malformation. Macafee et al (1971) have shown that low oestriol excretion occurs in 45 per cent of pregnancies with fetal cardiac malformations. Low oestriol excretion has been demonstrated in association with conditions such as achrondroplasia, Potter's syndrome, trachea-oesophageal fistula (Macafee et al, 1972), and Down's syndrome. Many of these conditions are associated with growth retardation and it is likely that this accounts for the low oestriol values.

In the management of pregnancies complicated by diabetes mellitus or rhesus isoimmunisation, it is particularly important to have a safe index of fetal condition, in order to assist in deciding the time of induction. Various studies have given rise to conflicting data in diabetes mellitus. It can generally be said that low oestriol values in diabetes are associated with high fetal risk whereas normal values do not ensure fetal safety. Beischer, Holsman and Kitchen (1968) have shown that intrauterine death occurred in association with large-for-dates infants, as well as in small-for-dates infants. In fact, small-for-dates infants are less common than in the overall obstetric population. Klebe, Winkel and Lyngbye (1974) have recently reported the results of serial measurements of oestriol levels of 159 pregnant diabetic women. In pregnancies not complicated by hypertension or renal disease, the urinary oestriol estimations fell within the normal pregnant range up to 35 weeks gestation. After 35 weeks, the increase in urinary oestriol excretion in diabetics is greater than the normal range—in other words, pregnant diabetics have their own normal range of oestriol excretion.

In rhesus isoimmunisation, a similar situation occurs. Some authors have found abnormally high oestriol excretion in the presence of severe rhesus isoimmunisation (Klopper and Stephenson, 1966), but there is evidence to show that whilst low oestriol values indicate fetal risk, normal high levels do not indicate fetal safety.

Plasma measurements of oestriol are performed by radioimmunoassay and have certain advantages relative to the use of 24-h urinary measurements. Plasma oestrogen measurements can be performed on small samples of plasma and the assay result can be made available on the day of collection. There is some evidence that diurnal variation of oestriol occurs (Selinger and Levitz, 1969). However, this finding has not been consistently shown in other studies. Furthermore, renal disease may cause a fall in renal clearance and this may produce an increase in plasma oestriol. Despite these potential disadvantages, patients with toxaemia, diabetes or intrauterine fetal death have been shown to have low plasma oestriol values (Ratanasopa et al, 1967). Masson (1973a) has shown that single plasma oestriol measurements are as reliable in the assessment of feto-placental function as single urinary estimations. Further data have also confirmed that plasma oestriol measurements provide a reliable index of placental function in severe pre-eclampsia (Masson, 1973b). Oestriol is not the only oestrogen that can be measured in plasma as a placental function test. The measurement of unconjugated 17β-oestradiol has been employed as a placental function test (Tulchinsky and Korenman, 1971). Chard and Klopper (1974) have shown that whilst there is some fluctuation in plasma oestradiol-17β in late pregnancy, the coefficient of variation is only 7.2 per cent as compared with plasma oestriol measurement (14 per cent). It seems likely that plasma measurements of oestriol-17β or plasma oestetrol may replace urinary oestrogen measurements as standard placental function tests within the next few years.

Human placental lactogen

Human placental lactogen (HPL) or human chorionic somatomammotrophin was first described in 1962 by Ito and Higashi and in the same year by Josimovich and MacLaren, and was originally described as a substance produced by the placenta with the biological activity of both growth hormone and prolactin. HPL is a peptide hormone consisting of 191 amino acids. Radioimmunofluorescence studies have shown that the hormone is localised in the placenta (Sciarra, Kaplan and Grumbach, 1963), and synthesis within the placenta has subsequently been confirmed by uptake studies with labelled amino acids in vitro (Suwa and Friesen, 1969). HPL has been detected as early as the fifth week of gestation in maternal serum and the levels increase steadily throughout pregnancy until the thirty-eighth week when they tend to remain constant or decrease. Figure 1.1 shows the results of serial HPL measurements in 40 normal pregnancies in a prospective study performed at the City Hospital, Nottingham (results provided by courtesy of Dr J. B. Foote). Only a trace of HPL is found in maternal urine and whilst amniotic fluid levels are approximately 10 per cent of maternal serum levels (Singer, Desjardins and Friesen, 1970), cord serum HPL is only about 1 per cent of the maternal serum concentration (Grumbach et al, 1968).

The biological function of HPL in the human species remains obscure. There is evidence that the injection of the hormone into non-pregnant individuals results in a decrease in blood glucose levels and an increase in free fatty acids and insulin—changes which are observed in normal pregnancy. A growth-promoting effect could not be demonstrated when HPL was administered to hypopituitary preadolescent patients (Schutt-Aine and Drash, 1972). The lactogenic effect of HPL in early animal studies (Josimovich and MacLaren, 1962) has not been demonstrated in the human species.

In practical terms, HPL has become widely used as a marker index for placental function. Measurement is made by radioimmunoassay and requires only 0.1 ml of serum. No separation procedure is required before immunoassay as the assay relies on the specificity of the antiserum. Whilst some cross-reaction with growth hormone may occur, the difference in concentration of the two hormones in pregnancy is so large that growth hormone does not significantly interfere with the assay. As HPL is labelled with radioiodine counting efficiency is high, and the assay time is short. The method also lends itself well to automation. There is evidence of considerable variation in levels between laboratories which appear to mainly result from lack of suitable reference standards and it is therefore advisable for laboratories to establish their own range of normal values.

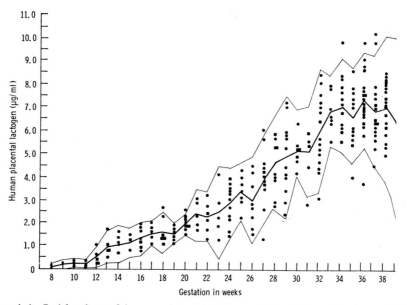

Figure 1.1 Serial values of human placental lactogen obtained from 40 women during normal pregnancies. The mean is shown by the solid line and the tenth and ninety percentiles shown by the lighter lines. (By courtesy of Dr J. B. Foote, Department of Chemical Pathology, City Hospital, Nottingham)

It must be remembered that the measurement of placental lactogen in clinical practice measures specifically enzyme production from trophoblastic tissue, and it is not dependent on fetal precursors. It is therefore important that several studies have now established a correlation between HPL and placental weight (Seppala and Ruoslahti, 1970; Spellacy et al, 1971), both in the lower and upper range of weight and similar relationship has been established between HPL and birth weight (Letchworth and Chard, 1972).

Letchworth and Chard (1972) have shown that a significant increase in the incidence of fetal distress in labour is associated with the recurrence of low serum HPL levels. A single measurement in the last six weeks of pregnancy below 4 μg/ml is associated with a 30 per cent risk of fetal distress and/or neonatal asphyxia, and three or more measurements below 4 μg/ml indicates a 71 per cent risk. This fact alone is useful in the identification of patients who require fetal monitoring in labour if intrapartum deaths are to be avoided.

Several studies have now established that HPL levels fall in association with pre-eclampsia (Spellacy et al, 1971; Kelly et al, 1975), and there is sufficient evidence to recommend serial measurements in all pregnancies complicated by pre-eclampsia on the basis that these measurements will provide a useful guide to the timing of surgical induction of labour when a decision based on the fetal risk in utero and the risks of prematurity has to be taken.

The value of HPL measurements in diabetes, rhesus isoimmunisation and multiple pregnancies involves the same restrictions as the case of oestriol measurements in these conditions. For example, Ursell, Brudenell and Chard (1973) and Ylikorkala (1973) have shown that the range of values for diabetic pregnancies which are normal apart from the diabetes, is higher than corresponding normal non-diabetic population, and in interpreting results in a diabetic it is important to take this fact into consideration.

In rhesus isoimmunisation, severe disease is associated with elevated levels of HPL—the reverse of the usual situation in the presence of fetal jeopardy (Ward et al, 1974).

Multiple pregnancies are associated with high levels of HPL, but again, a true assessment of the value of HPL measurements in multiple pregnancy is dependent on the description of a normal range of levels specifically for multiple pregnancy.

Enzyme measurements as placental function tests

A large number of enzymes have now been identified in the human placenta and many have now been explored as placental function tests. However, many of these enzymes are not specific to the placenta and therefore only two of these enzymes have received detailed investigation and application as placental function tests.

Serum oxytocinase (cystine-aminopeptidase). The plasma of pregnant women contains an enzyme known as oxytocinase, which splits the oxytocin molecule at the cystinyl–tyrosilpeptide bond. The major source of this enzyme in pregnancy appears to be the trophoblast and it is known that the concentration of the enzyme increases progressively throughout pregnancy and provides an index of placental function.

The methodology has a great deal to recommend it as it is relatively simple and inexpensive. Using L-cystine di-beta-naphthylamine as a substrate, hydrolysis by oxytocinase or cystine-aminopeptidase leads to the formation of beta-naphthylamide. This substance is then converted to an azo dye producing a blue colour which can be measured spectrophotometrically. The method is quick, does not require expensive equipment and can be performed on a small sample of serum.

Tovey (1969) and Blunt (1971) have studied cystine-aminopeptidase (CAP) levels in relation to urinary oestrogen levels and have shown a significant correlation in both normal and complicated pregnancies. The increase in CAP levels in pregnancy follows an S-shaped curve with the rate of increase diminishing in the last trimester of pregnancy. The range of values seen in normal pregnancies with normal birth weight infants is wide and the method would appear to suffer from the same difficulties in interpretation as the earlier use of pregnanediol measurements. However, it now seems likely that it is particularly important to assess the discriminant function of any placental function test on the rate of increase over a given time interval rather than single measurements in late pregnancy.

On this basis, Petrucco, Cellier and Fishtail (1973) have shown that the discriminant function of serial measurements of CAP in relation to the prediction of birth weight is superior to urinary oestrogen or serum heat stable alkaline phosphatase measurements. Despite these observations CAP has not been widely used as a placental function test and the data are still too limited to draw any final conclusions as to its value.

Heat stable alkaline phosphatase (HSAP). The term alkaline phosphatase refers to a series of enzymes that catalyse the splitting of phosphoric acid from monophosphoric esters in an alkaline medium. It is known that a rise occurs in serum concentrations of alkaline phosphatase during pregnancy and the rise is progressive with advancing gestation.

The discovery that the rise in this enzyme was due to the increase in heat stable alkaline phosphatase led to the suggestion that this enzyme could be used as the basis of a placental function test. Furthermore, the discovery that alkaline phosphatase produced by the placenta was heat stable, whereas alkaline phosphatase from other sources was heat labile suggested that the placental contribution to the circulation could be specifically defined. The enzyme in fetal serum is inactivated by heat and EDTA and does not travel in the same electrophoretic zone as the placental enzyme.

The critical temperature for differentiating between the heat stable and heat labile alkaline phosphatase is 60°C (Ylikorkala, 1973) and the use of lower incubation temperature in the measurement of alkaline phosphatase has led to substantial errors with widely scattered results.

Studies using HSAP in high-risk pregnancies have shown variable results (Curzen and Morris, 1965) and placental failure has been related to low values, high values, abrupt rises and abrupt falls in serum levels. Even within studies on pregnancies known to be normal, the variation in values is enormous. For example, Shane and Suzuki (1974) recently studied a group of 330 normal pregnancies in an attempt to establish a normal range of values for HSAP, but they concluded that there was no reliable range, no usable trend of values and no correlation with birth weight.

The measurement of HSAP cannot be considered to make any useful contribution to assessment of the feto-placental unit.

Alpha feto-protein and placental function

Certain proteins can be identified in maternal and fetal serum, which are not usually found in non-pregnant animals. Alpha feto-protein is one of these proteins, and it can be measured in blood or amniotic fluid by radioimmuno-assay. The use of these measurements is rapidly assuming significance in the detection of central nervous system abnormalities, but the value in assessment of feto-placental function has not yet been fully explored. Serum alpha feto-protein is present in high concentrations in early pregnancy and low levels in late pregnancy (Bergstrand et al, 1972). Maternal serum levels have been shown to be significantly elevated above the normal range preceding fetal death (Seppala and Ruoslahti, 1972), and abnormal levels are associated with a high incidence of fetal distress in labour.

Thus, unlike most placental function tests where depressed levels are significant, studies so far suggest that elevated serum levels of alpha feto-protein indicate incipient fetal risk.

PHYSICAL METHODS OF ANTENATAL MONITORING

A variety of physical methods for monitoring fetal growth and placental function are now available and are widely used in antenatal care.

Ultrasonography and fetal growth

Feto-placental insufficiency results in fetal growth retardation. The clinical signs of such a disorder are oligohydramnios, poor maternal weight gain and failure of increase in fetal size.

The clinical assessment of fetal size is notoriously inaccurate. Willocks et al (1967) showed that only 25 per cent of babies thought clinically to be small-for-dates were below the tenth percentile and Beard and Roberts (1970) showed that only 15 per cent of suspected small-for-dates babies were below the fifth percentile. Loeffler (1967) has shown that inaccuracy in predicting birth weight increases markedly where birth weight is less than 2.27 kg and greater than 4.54 kg. Because of the difficulties in assessing fetal size, there has been a need to introduce a precise method of measuring fetal growth.

In 1958 Donald, MacVicar and Brown first introduced diagnostic ultra-sound into clinical obstetrics. The method consists of directing pulsed sound waves of very high frequency from a piezo-electric crystal through the maternal abdomen and fetal head. Echoes are reflected from the different tissue interfaces and are detected by the same crystal. These echoes are displayed as vertical deflections and this is known as an A scan. The interval between any two spikes represents the time taken for the sound waves to pass between the two tissue interfaces. If the velocity of sound in human tissue is known, the actual distances between the tissue interfaces can be detected.

By moving the crystal at different angles to the surface of the skin, a two-dimensional scan can be obtained and this is known as a B scan. With a combination of both A and B scans and by identification of the falx cerebri in the midline, it is possible to measure the biparietal diameter of the fetal skull with a high degree of precision.

Whilst earlier studies by Willocks et al (1967) showed a high degree of error in the assessment of skull size with 57 per cent of babies, who exhibited low ultrasonic growth rate, of normal birth weight, Campbell (1968) showed that the accuracy of measurement of biparietal diameter could be markedly improved using the combination of A and B scan. The mean error in this study was less than 1 mm. The growth rate of the fetal biparietal diameter is linear until 30 weeks gestation, but then the rate of increase diminishes gradually until term.

Single measurements of biparietal diameter are of limited value in the assessment of birth weight and, indeed, have little to offer over routine clinical examination. On the other hand, there seems little doubt that serial measurements of biparietal diameter can provide accurate information concerning fetal growth.

Campbell (1974) has emphasised that it is possible to make assessment of fetal growth from two measurements separated by one week, but more numerous measurements—particularly in early pregnancy—will improve diagnostic precision. In a study of 406 'at risk' pregnancies, Campbell and Dewhurst (1971) showed that of 140 infants exhibiting growth retardation in this study as assessed by ultrasound cephalometry, 68 per cent were below the fifth percentile weight for gestation. This group of fetuses exhibited a significant increase in the incidence of low Apgar scores, perinatal deaths and fetal abnormality compared with the normal group. Ultrasound cephalometry is now being widely used in the assessment of fetal growth.

Two points should be made about this method in general. Firstly, the equipment required is expensive. Secondly, results in the hands of those expert in the technique are good, but these results do not necessarily reflect the general applicability of the method.

Various authors have reported measurement of transverse sections of the fetal trunk and thorax, but so far, none of these methods have been shown to be better than cephalometry.

Ultrasonic measurement of fetal breathing

The fact that some respiratory movements occur in the fetal animal in utero has been known for many years. It is only recently that this pheno- menon has received intensive investigation and now promises to offer a useful clinical tool in the assessment of fetal condition. Boddy, Dawes and Robinson (1973) have shown that respiratory movements in the fetal lamb are associated with rapid eye-movement sleep and occur in an episodic fashion. Furthermore, these movements are inhibited by hypoxaemia, hypoglycaemia or infection. Boddy and Robinson (1971) have devised a method for detecting human fetal respiratory movements and further studies (Boddy and Mantell, 1972) have established similar patterns of episodic respiration in the human fetus as compared with the fetal lamb. Studies have so far shown that fetal respiration is reduced in pregnancies complicated by diabetes, hypertension and pre-eclampsia. Both the practicability and precision of this method in the assessment of fetal welfare remain to be established.

Stress tests in the assessment of placental function

Stress tests are based on the concept that some form of stress applied to the mother may affect the fetal circulatory system in a differential manner in the presence of placental impairment. The two major methods used to induce stress have been maternal inhalation of low oxygen tension gas mixtures or by the intravenous infusion of oxytocin. These tests have not received general acceptance, firstly, because the tests are not without risk in themselves and secondly, because the results of most investigations have not made a significant contribution in the differential assessment of placental function.

Essentially, oxytocin infusion tests consist of studying the effect on fetal heart rate of graduated infusions of oxytocin into the mother. Kubli, Kaeser and Hinselmann (1969) showed that oxytocin infusions used to induce uterine contractions antenatally produced specific changes in fetal heart rate in the 'at risk' pregnancy. Of the infants who developed persistent tachycardia, loss of the normal beat-to-beat variation or deceleration of the fetal heart following uterine contraction, 50 per cent had low Apgar scores at delivery.

The studies of Baillie (1974) have suggested that the only clear prediction of fetal condition is late deceleration of the fetal heart rate during and following a prolonged uterine contraction and it is clear that this type of procedure may carry some inherent risk.

It has therefore been concluded that there is probably little future—both in relation to safety or practicability—for the oxytocin stress test in the assessment of placental function.

The oxygen stress test consists of the administration of low oxygen gas mixtures to the mother and observing changes. Early studies in this method by Hellman et al (1961) showed that whilst abnormal changes in heart rate could be demonstrated in some infants, the changes were too inconstant to constitute the basis of a reliable clinical test. Baillie (1974) has shown that when a 12 per cent oxygen mixture is administered to pregnant women in late pregnancy, the condition of the infant at birth can be predicted by the time taken for the fetal heart rate to return to normal after discontinuation of the gas mixture.

Despite these positive findings, the reliability of these tests is not widely accepted and the stress tests generally seem unlikely to pass into general usage in the assessment of placental function.

ASSESSMENT OF THE FETUS IN LABOUR

Parturition is associated with a reduction in utero-placental blood flow during uterine contractions. Approximately 40 per cent of all perinatal deaths resulting from asphyxia occur during parturition, and yet this is a group of deaths which, with the development of modern techniques, must be considered as avoidable. It is the time during which the fetus is most accessible for study and observation.

The clinical signs of fetal distress include fetal tachycardia, bradycardia, the presence of meconium in amniotic fluid and excessive fetal movements. One or more of these signs occurs during 14 per cent of all labour, and whilst there is ample evidence to show that the perinatal mortality rate is higher in association with clinical signs of fetal distress, the signs frequently occur where there is no evidence of fetal asphyxia and therefore, do not form a satisfactory basis for clinical decision on the method of delivery.

The difficulties encountered in accurate identification of the presence and severity of fetal asphyxia has led in the past to either excessively high fetal wastage or excessive use of Caesarean section. Over the last 20 years, an intensive search has been made to identify methods by which the diagnosis of fetal asphyxia can be improved. These methods are biophysical or biochemical. The biophysical methods involve recording fetal heart rate by electrocardiography, phonocardiography or ultrasonography. The biochemical methods are based on the measurement of acid–base status of the fetus by obtaining blood samples from the fetal scalp or buttocks, and the method is only practicable during labour and once dilatation of the cervix has begun.

Fetal electrocardiography

The first successful recording of the fetal electrocardiogram was made in 1906 by Cremer. Using a string galvanometer, Cremer placed electrodes on the abdomen and in the vagina and obtained a recording of both maternal and fetal electrocardiographs. Over the next 24 years, only four further papers were written on this subject, although at the same time some excellent work appeared on neonatal electrocardiography. For example, Krumbhaar (1916) produced an excellent description of the changes that occur in the electrocardiogram in the first 12 years of life and showed that there is a right ventricular preponderance at birth.

Subsequent developments can be entirely related to the development of suitable amplifying techniques and the application of electrodes directly to the fetus. The introduction of valve amplifiers such as those employed by Bell (1938) produced a threefold increase in sensitivity over previous machines, but the presence of background noise imposed severe limitations on the interpretation of recordings obtained from the maternal abdomen. In 1952, Vara and Halminen obtained considerable improvement in recording the fetal electrocardiograph by using electrodes inserted into the vagina and by placing their patients in an earthed cage of wire. However, the most significant advance occurred in 1953, when Smyth introduced a silver wire into the amniotic sac and into contact with the fetal head. The signal obtained was free of maternal interference and clearly showed the various features of the wave form.

Modifications of electrode design introduced in 1961 (Hon, Bradfield and Hess) have provided the basis for scalp electrodes used in modern obstetric practice. Indeed, electrode design is critical to the development of the clinical use of fetal electrocardiography. The design must incorporate a good conducting contact with fetal tissue but must exclude contact with maternal tissue. The indifferent electrode is now built into the neck of the electrode so that it lies in the vagina. The two electrodes most widely used at present are the 'Michel' clip type of electrode which can be placed on to the scalp using specially designed forceps, and the spiral electrode which can be easily screwed into normal scalp tissue.

Both electrodes have a high retention rate and yield consistently good recordings. The spiral electrode has the advantage of being applicable when cervical dilatation is minimal. These techniques all necessitate application to the fetal scalp after the fetal membranes have been ruptured. Signals obtained from the presenting part are used to trigger a cardiotachometer to present a continuous recording of fetal heart rate.

Using these techniques it soon became apparent that the interpretation of changes in fetal heart rate was dependent on relating these changes to uterine contractions. All recordings during labour should include the measurement of the intensity, and duration and frequency of uterine contractions and these measurements are made by inserting an open-ended cavity through the cervical canal into the amniotic sac and attaching the catheter to a pressure transducer.

The difficulty in identifying the significance of the changes in fetal heart rate can be related to the problem of describing satisfactory criteria of fetal asphyxia. Fetal or neonatal death constitute a very crude index of the most severe form of fetal asphyxia and the use of the Apgar score has limitations as not all low scores are associated with fetal hypoxia.

The measurement of fetal acid–base balance during labour or at the time of delivery is now recognised as the most reliable index and a comparison between patterns of fetal heart rate variability and fetal acid–base status have led to the identification of 'risk' patterns.

Fetal heart rate patterns

Hon (1963) described a series of heart rate patterns in labour. The development of bradycardia during uterine contractions but associated with the return to normal heart rate by the end of the contraction, did not appear to indicate hypoxia. However, artificially induced maternal hypoxia resulting in fetal hypoxia was associated with fetal bradycardia which developed during contractions and did not return to the normal base line until well after completion of the contraction. Lee and Hon (1963) also described the development of prompt and profound bradycardia following cord compression.

Newman (1963) showed that bradycardia was a common finding during delivery. In cases of placental insufficiency, tachycardia was found to precede the contraction followed by late onset of bradycardia in the contraction phase. In 1967, Mendez-Bauer et al presented a report of the first joint study of fetal acid–base status, and fetal heart rate obtained during labour. Their findings showed that a low scalp pH was associated with typical fetal heart rate patterns characterised by a high basal heart rate and transient falls of heart rate occurring towards the end and following contractions.

In normal labours where the scalp blood pH remained higher than 7.20, these changes in heart rate did not occur and the rate varied between 130 and 150 beats/min. Wood et al (1967) performed an extensive study of fetal heart rate patterns and fetal acid–base status during labour. The mean Apgar score at 2 min was 3.6 in those subjects where the fetal scalp blood pH was less than 7.2, and 6.4 in those subjects with scalp blood pH greater than 7.2. There appeared to be no obvious risk to the fetus where heart rate remained constant in relationship to uterine contractions, even if bradycardia or tachycardia occurred during resting phases. Fetal acidosis was associated with marked slowing of the heart rate during contractions and with a heart rate greater than 160 beats/min during the resting phase. Slowing of the heart rate at the end of contractions was also associated with asphyxia.

Beard et al presented a similar study in 1971 and confirmed many of these findings. They also suggested that loss of beat-to-beat variation in fetal heart rate was associated with fetal acidosis, particularly where late decelerations of heart rate occurred.

In an attempt to quantify heart rate changes, Shelley and Tipton (1971) studied the total number of dropped beats in the hour prior to delivery and found a high negative correlation with the Apgar score.

Whilst these and many other studies have shown that none of the methods available provide an infallible guide to fetal condition, a reasonable consensus of opinion has now been achieved in interpreting heart rate patterns, and until further information is available, should provide a modus operandi in fetal monitoring. The basic terminology and pattern of heart rate change are therefore described as follows:

The baseline fetal heart rate. This is the rate between uterine contractions and normally varies from 120 to 160 beats/min. Beat-to-beat variation of the fetal heart rate is a characteristic of a normal recording and usually varies about ± 8 beats/min. A variability of less than 5 beats/min is defined as loss of beat-to-beat variation (Fig. 1.2).

Baseline tachycardia is defined as a fetal heart rate greater than 160 beats/min between contractions. Whilst fetal tachycardia is often associated with fetal hypoxia, it may also be related to other factors which cause tachycardia in the mother.

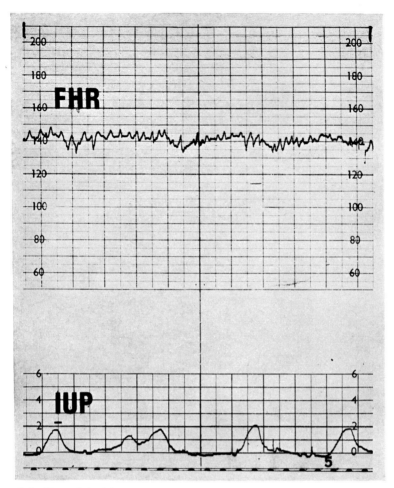

Figure 1.2 Normal fetal heart rate showing normal beat-to-beat variation in the uterine resting phase and during contractions. FHR—fetal heart rate, beats per minute; IUP—intrauterine pressure, arbitrary units

Baseline bradycardia is defined as a fetal heart rate of less than 120 beats/min between uterine contractions. It may occur in the normal fetus, and like tachycardia, is not a particularly reliable sign of fetal asphyxia.

The most significant changes occur during uterine contractions and may also be associated with bradycardia or tachycardia.

Transient acceleration that occurs at the onset of a contraction is known as an acceleration pattern and may sometimes indicate early asphyxial change.

The early deceleration pattern or type I dip is a deceleration in heart rate which occurs during uterine contractions and recovers to the baseline before the end of the contraction (Fig. 1.3). The fall in heart rate does not usually

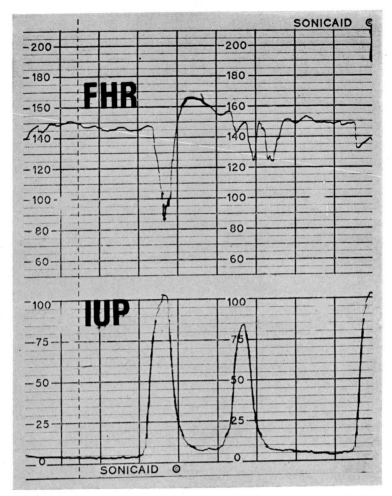

Figure 1.3   Type I dips in fetal heart rate with the fall in heart rate occurring during uterine contractions and returning to normal by the end of the contraction. IUP (mmHg)

exceed 40 beats/min. This type of heart rate change commonly results from head or cord compression. Although it is not generally associated with fetal acidosis, profound early deceleration must be viewed with concern and fetal condition ascertained by scalp blood sampling.

Late decelerations (type II dip) describe a deceleration in heart rate which exhibit a lag time in relation to uterine contractions. Thus, the nadir of the fetal heart rate follows the zenith of the uterine pressure by 18 s or more and recovery to a baseline rate occurs after the uterine contraction is completed. The degree of slowing rarely exceeds 20 beats/min and should be considered significant if it exceeds 5 beats/min (Fig. 1.4).

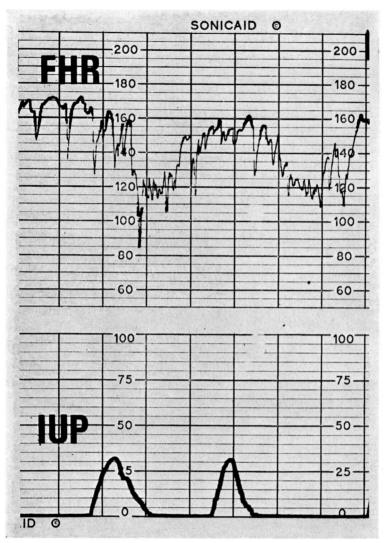

Figure 1.4 Type II dips in fetal heart rate with the fall in heart rate following zenith of the uterine contractions and returning to the previous rate following the contraction

The only way in which it has been possible to assess the significance of any particular heart rate change has been to relate such changes to clinical condition of the infant at birth or acid–base balance during labour or at the time of delivery. Whilst there is a general consensus of opinion on the significant patterns of heart rate change, these changes are not in any sense absolute and can still only be considered as a useful guide of fetal asphyxia. Heart rate changes provide an indication for scalp blood sampling and fetal acid–base assessment.

Several different types of fetal monitors are now available and widely used. These instruments provide a continuous display of fetal heart rate and uterine contractions (Fig. 1.5).

Fetal phonocardiography and ultrasonic monitoring

The direct application of electrodes to the fetal presenting part provides the most reliable method of monitoring fetal heart rate. However, this method is only applicable during labour. Fetal heart rate can also be determined from fetal heart sounds detected through the maternal abdominal wall. Fetal phonocardiography was initially used as the principal method for monitoring the fetal heart rate, either before or during labour. There are serious technical disadvantages to phonocardiography which have limited its usefulness. Movement and descent of the fetus during labour may lead to alteration of

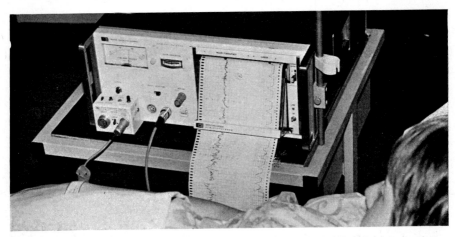

Figure 1.5   Fetal monitor used to record intrauterine pressure and fetal heart rate during labour

signal strength and extraneous noise may also affect the quality of the signal. Some of these problems have been overcome by using ultrasound monitoring. By directing an ultrasound beam through the maternal abdominal wall, movements in the fetal heart or great vessels can be detected by alterations in the frequency of the ultrasound beam as it is reflected from these structures. Despite the introduction of wide-angle multiple crystal transducers, it is still necessary to readjust the position of the recorder to allow for fetal movement. The ultrasound method does obviate the problem of extraneous noise, and certainly reduces the frequency of readjustment usually required with phono-cardiography.

For successful implementation, both methods require a minimum of both fetal and maternal movement—conditions which are not generally applicable in the late stages of labour.

The fetal electrocardiogram

Most investigations have concentrated attention on heart rate as the most significant parameter in the detection of fetal asphyxia, and this approach to the problem is likely to achieve its ultimate function by the application of computer analysis techniques to cardiotocography as recently described by Crawford (1975). Studies on the configuration of the electrocardiogram have, therefore, been rather limited—partly because of the difficulty in obtaining consistently high-quality electrocardiograms sufficiently free of background noise to allow consistent interpretation of subtle changes in wave form, and partly because interpretation is more difficult than the analysis of changes in heart rate.

Nevertheless, several investigators have produced evidence that there are significant changes in the electrocardiogram which may well be of practical use, provided that the interpretation and display of this data can be presented in a readily understandable format.

Southern (1957) reported the first extensive study of the prenatal fetal electrocardiogram in relation to fetal anoxia. In this study, he showed that low oxygen saturations at birth were associated with prolongation of PR intervals, and the QRS and ST segment duration. T waves were also noted to be isoelectric or inverted in 35 per cent of the anoxic cases. Hon and Lee (1963a) described the fetal electrocardiogram from nine fetuses that diet during or shortly after parturition. The changes described consisted of high, peaked, biphasic or inverted P waves and shortened PR intervals. Widened QRS complexes and ST segment depression were also noted. Several studies (Figueroa-Longo et al, 1966; Kaplan and Toyama, 1958; Hon and Lee, 1963a) have attempted to define normal time constants for the fetal electrocardiogram and these constants were defined in relation to acid–base balance by Symonds (1971). This last study also showed that prolongation of electrical systole occurs in the presence of fetal acidosis and this is associated with T-wave flattening and inversion. The prolongation of QT intervals cannot be explained on the basis of heart rate changes as it still occurs when rate compensation is included in the analysis. In 1949, Gruenwald showed that coronary lesions can be demonstrated in the anoxic stillborn infant resulting in damage to the media and amounting, in severe cases, to complete destruction of the vessel walls. However, it seems rather more likely that changes in configuration related to asphyxia are due to electrolyte shifts rather than morphological damage. Symonds (1972) has shown that hyperkaliaemia occurs in the acidotic fetus, and has suggested that the alteration in potassium gradient from fetal to maternal circulation may lead to intracellular potassium depletion, and hence changes in the fetal electrocardiogram. The work by Singh and Symonds (1972) has lent substance to this hypothesis by showing that red cell potassium depletion occurs in severely asphyxic infants.

The real difficulty in using the wave form as a clinical tool has been in obtaining a rapid and consistent method of analysis. In 1963, Hon and Lee

described a method of averaging fetal complexes obtained from scalp electrodes. Signals were recorded on magnetic tape with an Ampex FR1100
recorder. This was subsequently played back and further amplified to raise
the voltage to the required peak to peak level of 6 V for a CAT computer. The
filtered ECG was used as an input to a pulse generator which provided a pulse
of 1.5 V to act as a trigger to instruct the computer to begin averaging. Since
this time, considerable advances have occurred in computing techniques so

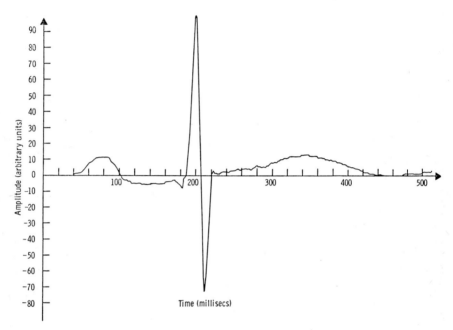

Figure 1.6 Fetal electrocardiogram obtained by the use of signal filtering and processing
programmes on a digital computer. The amplitude is expressed in arbitrary units. (By courtesy
of Mr J. E. A. Sheild, Department of Electronic Engineering, University of Nottingham)

that it is now possible to develop a system of real time analysis of the fetal
electrocardiogram which can provide continuous monitoring of a series of
parameters from the fetal electrocardiogram, rather than just heart rate
(Sheild, J., personal communication). An example of such a computer analysis
is shown in Figure 1.6.

Various attempts have also been made to develop a system of vector cardio-
graphy by studying the ratio of the R wave to the S wave of the fetal ECG.
Clearly, there are difficulties in drawing conclusions from data derived from a
single lead system. However, there is some evidence that the fetal cardiac
axis can be estimated from the fetal electrocardiogram obtained by leads
applied to the maternal abdomen (Larks, 1965) and also from scalp electrode
recordings.

Studies on the effect of changes in acid–base status on the fetal cardiac axis have shown that a significant shift to the left can be demonstrated, both in the fetal and neonatal electrocardiogram in relation to fetal acidosis (Symonds, 1972) and it is possible that this measurement may provide an index of fetal condition, provided quantification and interpretation can be simplified.

Fetal cardiac arrhythmias

Whilst the main emphasis in studies on the fetal heart have been directed towards heart rate, one of the problems that sometimes confronts the obstetrician is the presence of fetal cardiac arrhythmias. The question that faces the clinician in these circumstances is whether the abnormality of rhythm is related to fetal asphyxia or congenital cardiac malformation, or whether it is of no clinical significance and will revert to normal after delivery.

Irregularity of the fetal heart beat has for many years been considered as one of the signs of fetal distress but evidence which has now accumulated since the introduction of fetal electrocardiography suggests that most of the arrhythmias are of little clinical significance.

Larks (1963) described a series of 10 abnormal fetal ECGs from a group of 1500 recordings using leads applied externally to the maternal abdomen. The changes described included widening and flattening of the QRS complex, pulsus bigeminus and other cardiac arrhythmias. It was observed that seven of these patients exhibited complications of cord compression. Kendall (1967) reported a series of 19 patients in whom abnormal fetal arrhythmias were recorded also using abdominal fetal electrocardiography. The abnormalities observed included atrial extrasystoles, sinus tachycardia, bigeminal rhythm and heart block. Although the study did not include any measurements of the acid base system, it was concluded that arrhythmias did not necessarily indicate fetal asphyxia.

Hon and Huang (1962) reported a series of 25 patients with fetal cardiac arrhythmias during labour using scalp electrodes. The cases were characterised by premature and missed beats. In 22 patients the arrhythmias disappeared almost immediately after birth, and in two patients, it persisted for 48 h. All infants in this series were delivered in good condition and it was suggested that vagotonia possibly associated with mild hypoxia was the main cause of the arrhythmias.

In 1967, Komaromy et al reported a study on five pregnancies in which the fetus exhibited extrasystoles in labour. Acid–base studies on all five infants showed no evidence of fetal acidosis.

Symonds (1972) reported three cases of different arrhythmias in which acid–base studies were performed both during labour and at the time of delivery. In the first case, changes in the shape and direction of the P wave denoted a wandering pacemaker and missed beats were demonstrated depending on the refractory state of the atria and ventricles. The same changes were demonstrated in the neonatal electrocardiogram 5 h after delivery. The scalp blood pH was 7.2 and the cord arterial blood pH 7.11. The infant subsequently made an uneventful recovery and the electrocardiogram reverted to normal.

In the second case, gross changes in the fetal electrocardiogram were consistent with a nodal tachycardia. The changes were seen to persist after delivery. The scalp blood pH was 7.20 and the cord arterial pH 7.16. The infant showed obvious signs of cardiac failure following delivery and finally responded to digitalis therapy. In the third case, the fetal electrocardiogram recorded with a scalp electrode showed the appearances of auricular flutter with a variable 2:1:3:1 block. The neonatal electrocardiogram 4 h after delivery was normal. The cord arterial pH was 7.11.

Various authors have commented on the possibility of artefacts producing misleading tracings under certain conditions which produce the appearances of gross tachycardia or auricular fibrillation (Sureau, 1962; Kantor, Bowman and Abbott, 1966; Whitfield, 1966), but most of these artefacts have been recorded from abdominal leads.

Whilst it appears that the most commonly observed arrhythmias appear to be atrial extrasystoles, and there is little evidence that these disorders are associated with asphyxia, it is advisable at the present time, unless the observer of the electrocardiogram can be certain of the nature of the arrhythmia, to assess all cases in labour with scalp blood samples.

Fetal acid–base balance and fetal blood sampling

In 1932, Eastman showed that, under conditions of severe asphyxia, the oxygen content of fetal blood was low, large amounts of lactic acid accumulated in the blood and carbon dioxide tension rose. These findings were confirmed by Noguchi in 1937, but in this study, Noguchi pointed out that 'a low pH can be regarded as one of the characteristic changes in the blood properties of asphyxiated newborns—a poor oxygen content of the fetal blood cannot be regarded as one of such characteristics'.

By 1953, the specific nature of fetal biochemical adaption to hypoxia was being realised. Villee studied the metabolism of fetal liver and placental tissue in vitro. The glycogen content of fetal liver was shown to increase as gestation proceeded. Placental glycogen decreased as pregnancy advanced. The ability of the placenta to produce glucose was shown to increase during gestation. It was also recognised at about this time that the fetus has the ability to exist for long periods without oxygen and that the considerable powers of anaerobiosis are dependent on glycolysis. This process leads to the accumulation of fixed acids such as lactate and pyruvate. However, fetal asphyxia is not the only cause of fetal acidosis. Goodlin and Kaiser (1957) showed that the administration of ammonium chloride to mothers resulted in a fall in fetal blood pH, an increase in partial carbon dioxide pressure and a reduction in oxygen saturation. These findings suggested that maternal acidosis could result in fetal acidosis. Various workers (Spackman, Fuchs and

Assali, 1963; Low, 1963) have shown that the normal fetus exists in a state of metabolic acidosis as compared with maternal acid–base status. However, it has been established that fetal distress and fetal hypoxia are the most common causes of fetal acidaemia and may be associated with a profound fall in fetal blood pH (Vermelin, Dellestable and Muller, 1962; James, 1960; Macrae and Palavradji, 1965).

Whilst it was soon realised that the association between fetal acidosis and fetal asphyxia had clinical importance in management of the depressed neonate, it was not until 1964 that the potential clinical value of these observations for the fetus became a practical reality.

At this time, Saling described a method for obtaining capillary blood directly from the fetus during labour. The method involved introducing a conical tube described as an amnioscope through the dilated cervix during labour and directly exposing the presenting part of the fetus. The skin was sprayed with chlorethylene to induce hyperaemia and arterialisation of the capillary blood. A small drop of silicone grease was wiped on to the skin to prevent smearing of blood and the skin was incised to a depth of 2 mm and a width of 1.5 mm. Blood was aspirated into heparinised tubing and oxygen saturation, carbon dioxide tension, actual pH, buffer base and standard bicarbonate measured. The influence of caput formation of the fetal scalp on these various parameters did not appear to be significant. Because the blood sample was not obtained in a strictly anaerobic manner, the influence of exposure to air on blood gases was studied using an experimental model. Oxygen content of blood did not appear to be significantly affected by exposure to air within the time range of the study, but carbon dioxide tension was diminished marginally. This resulted in a small increase in pH which was corrected by subtracting 0.024 pH unit and adding 9 per cent to P_{CO_2} values. The range of pH values in the first 77 deliveries reported varied from 7.209 to 7.415. This work provided the basis for a new approach to the management of the 'at-risk' fetus.

The potential advantages were twofold. Firstly, it provided a method which gave more reliable information concerning the actual condition of the fetus, enabling appropriate intervention to be instituted when a severe degree of acidosis occurred. Secondly, and perhaps more important, it provided information which enabled the obstetrician to defer intervention if acid–base status was within normal limits, even in the presence of clinical signs of asphyxia.

Beard and Morris (1965) studied 26 normal pregnant women in labour and showed that the normal scalp blood pH in the late first stage of labour tended to be higher than early in labour. Thus, the pH in early labour was 7.29 ± 0.05 (s.d.), in late first stage 7.30 ± 0.05 and a fall to 7.28 occurred in the second stage. Beard, Morris and Clayton (1966) also showed on a study of 220 patients that a scalp blood pH of less than 7.20 was associated with asphyxial depression of the fetus and the difference between maternal and fetal base deficit also provided an index of the severity of asphyxial depression in the newborn child. The same workers (Beard et al, 1967) presented a further study of 250 patients with clinical signs of fetal distress and showed that a scalp blood pH greater than 7.25 in a sample taken within 30 min of delivery was associated with an Apgar score of 7 to 10 in 92 per cent of infants, and a fetal scalp sample of less than 7.15 was associated with an Apgar score of less than 6 in 80 per cent.

Bretscher and Saling (1967) defined the basic limits of pH for clinical practice, and there is general agreement that these limits are valid from a large number of studies in this field. The lower limit of normal pH values in the first stage of labour is 7.20 and values between 7.20 and 7.25 should be regarded as prepathologic and an indication for a further sample to be taken within 30 min.

It is interesting to note that Newman et al (1967) using Saling's technique to study oxygen transfer from mother to fetus during labour, demonstrated that the inhalation of oxygen-enriched gaseous mixtures in the mother increased both maternal and fetal partial oxygen pressure in both normal subjects and subjects with known placental insufficiency. Partial oxygen pressures per se cannot be considered to reliably indicate fetal asphyxia.

Complications of fetal blood sampling

Not all investigators have been convinced of the reliability of fetal blood sampling methods and there are clearly technical difficulties in the successful implementation of fetal scalp sampling at a clinical level. MacDonald and Kelman (1967) demonstrated the difficulties of heparinisation and sample clotting. Initially, PVC tubing was used for sample collection, and this tubing was shown to be permeable to carbon dioxide. This has now been replaced by heparinised glass tubing. Paul, Gare and Whetham (1967) described the results obtained in 146 patients followed by means of fetal scalp samples. Of these patients, 56 showed clinical signs of fetal distress but no difference could be demonstrated in the acid–base values of this group as compared with the clinically normal group. The scope of this study was insufficient to constitute a significant criticism of the method. Hon and Khazin (1969) studied 199 patients with scalp sampling techniques and suggested that the variation in pH measurements was such that samples needed to be collected at no longer than 10 min intervals if a true measure of fetal acidaemia was to be obtained. However, it seems likely that the frequency of sampling in this study interfered with the measurements of pH values. Nevertheless, in a review of data collected from 14 different workers, Lumley, McKinnon and Wood (1971) showed that the range of lower and upper limits of the parameters of acid–base balance established by investigators in this field showed widely variable values. Factors which may produce a low fetal pH and which are not associated with a basis of hypoxia in the fetus are maternal acidosis, hyperventilation during anaesthesia (Morishima et al, 1964; Moya et al, 1965) and vena caval occlusion associated with supine hypotension in late pregnancy (Crawford, 1972). Complications of the procedure of scalp blood sampling are surprisingly uncommon but problems such as wound infection, persistent bleeding and bleeding associated with a consumptive coagulopathy with a prolongation of the thrombin clotting time (Hull, 1972) have been reported.

Clinical results

Saling and Schneider (1967) reported the results of a study of 850 labours selected out of 4396 deliveries and showed that the incidence of significant acidosis in the 850 clinically 'at risk' labours was 14.4 per cent. Wood et al (1968) measured scalp blood pH, Pco_2 and Po_2 in 147 patients with hypertension in pregnancy. Sixty-nine of these women exhibited hypertension and proteinuria and in this group, the pH was significantly lower than in normal subjects and in hypertensive subjects without proteinuria.

Beard (1968) reviewed the clinical application of scalp sampling over a 40-month period at Queen Charlotte's Hospital and showed that the Caesarean section rate for fetal distress fell during this period. Twenty-six stillbirths occurred in 10400 deliveries, and 13 of these were due to placental insufficiency. Blood samples were collected in only three of these patients, and two of these values were abnormally low.

Coltart, Trickey and Beard (1969) investigated 295 out of 1668 patients in a six-month period who developed clinical signs of fetal distress, and showed that 45 of these patients showed a scalp blood pH of 7.25 or less. Fetal acidaemia in association with clinical signs of fetal distress occurred with twice the frequency in patients who had existing complications of pregnancy before the onset of labour. It was also of interest and importance that no cases of acidaemia were detected in any of the fetal blood samples performed on 'at risk' patients in the absence of clinical signs of fetal distress.

These studies have in general confirmed the clinical value of fetal scalp sampling and established its role in the clinical management of labour.

Monitoring by direct application of oxygen electrodes

Various attempts have been made to introduce other continuous methods of monitoring.

In 1967, Althabe et al inserted oxygen electrodes into the fetus percutaneously and through the uterine wall. Administration of oxygen to the mother produced a rise in fetal muscular partial oxygen pressure. A rise in fetal muscular Po_2 did not produce any alteration in fetal heart rate. However, in patients showing type II dips in heart rate during labour, oxygen administration corrected the fetal heart rate—thus providing additional evidence for an anoxic basis for these heart rate patterns. The method employed in this study was unlikely to be suitable for clinical application.

Walker et al (1968) developed an oxygen electrode which could be attached directly to the fetal presenting part, and showed that marked changes in tissue oxygen tension occurred during contractions in normal labour. This method appeared to have more potential for a continuous monitoring technique. However, considerable technical difficulties arise in the development of these techniques. Calibration for absolute values is virtually impossible. The elec- trodes tend to be pressure sensitive, and are relatively easily 'poisoned'. Also, there is little evidence that transient changes in oxygen tension have any clinical significance, as they can be easily compensated by the fetal acid–base system, unless severe and prolonged.

CONCLUSIONS

Placental function tests provide a quantifiable index of fetal growth and placental efficiency. These tests cannot be used in isolation as their effective- ness is dependent on careful consideration of each problem in its clinical context. The range of normal values and the coefficient of variation at any given gestation provide the criteria for a satisfactory placental function test. There is clearly a need to continue searching for greater precision in these tests as none can be considered ideal at the present time. Furthermore, future developments also need to be directed towards cost reduction and ease of applicability if tests are to be used on the basis of total population screening. The same factors also apply to monitoring procedures during labour. Placental function tests certainly help to identify those pateints in whom there is a significant risk to the fetus of asphyxial deaths or damage during parturition. It is still not clear whether multiple tests used during the antenatal period have any advantage over a single test used at the appropriate time intervals. It is certain that serial studies during pregnancy give better results than single tests.

Fetal heart rate monitoring is now the most widely used method of fetal observation during parturition, but the patterns of heart rate change which have been identified as asphyxial sometimes occur in a fetus which is apparently perfectly normal at birth. Conversely, apparently normal heart rate patterns with minimal abnormality of pattern may occasionally be associated with intrauterine death. Heart rate is a relatively crude index and there is a need to expand the parameters that can be observed and used as high-risk indices.

The use of fetal acid–base assessment is invaluable where heart rate is abnormal in distinguishing the presence of true asphyxial changes. However, the practical difficulties of this method are substantially greater than those involved in the use of monitoring techniques. Most maternity units are familiar with the difficulties of providing a 24-h biochemical service for pH measurements, and the employment of medical staff in this capacity often leads to incorrect calibration of the pH electrode or damage to equipment from poor maintenance. Difficulties in obtaining blood samples may also lead to delay in management where urgent action is required or it may lead to unnecessary operative intervention because of uncertainty and insecurity about the actual readings when the results are obtained.

There is no doubt that excellent results can be obtained by devoting attention to detail and meticulous application of the present methods. It should be possible to guarantee survival for any child once labour has commenced, but too often incorrect usage of existing methodology still results in an unsatisfactory outcome to the pregnancy.

Perinatal mortality rates continue to fall. This is partly due to the reduction in the 'at risk' population, which has occurred over the last decade, but is also partly due to more sophisticated antepartum and intrapartum screening, and to the radical changes that have occurred in neonatal management. With increasingly sophisticated methodology, it should be possible to simplify application, and at the same time improve the precision of screening and monitoring methods applied to the fetus.

ACKNOWLEDGEMENTS

The assistance of Miss A. Williams, Sister P. C. Sharp, Miss J. M. Mawby and the Department of Audiovisual Services, Nottingham University Medical School, in the preparation of this chapter, is gratefully acknowledged.

REFERENCES

Althabe, I. Jr, Schwarcz, R. L., Pose, S. V., Escarcena, L. & Caldeyro-Barcia, R. (1967) Effects on fetal heart rate and fetal Po_2 of oxygen administration to the mother. *American Journal of Obstetrics and Gynecology*, **98**, 858–870.

Baillie, P. (1974) Non-hormonal methods of antenatal monitoring. In *Clinics in Obstetrics and Gynaecology*, ed. Beard, R. W., Ch. 6, pp. 103–122. London: W. B. Saunders Co. Ltd.

Beard, R. W. (1968) The effect of foetal blood sampling on Caesarean section for foetal distress. *Journal of Obstetrics and Gynaecology of the British Commonwealth*, **75**, 1291–1295.

Beard, R. W. & Morris, E. D. (1965) Foetal and maternal acid–base balance during normal labour. *Journal of Obstetrics and Gynaecology of the British Commonwealth*, **72**, 496–506.

Beard, R. W. & Roberts, G. M. (1970) A prospective approach to the diagnosis of intrauterine growth retardation. *Proceedings of the Royal Society of Medicine*, **63**, 501–502.

Beard, R. W., Morris, E. D. & Clayton, S. G. (1966) Foetal blood sampling in clinical obstetrics. *Journal of Obstetrics and Gynaecology of the British Commonwealth*, **73**, 562–570.

Beard, R. W., Morris, E. D. & Clayton, S. G. (1967) pH of foetal capillary blood as an indicator of the condition of the foetus. *Journal of Obstetrics and Gynaecology of the British Commonwealth*, **74**, 812–822.

Beard, R. W., Filshie, G. M., Knight, C. A. & Roberts, G. M. (1971) The significance of changes in the continuous fetal heart rate in the first stage of labour. *Journal of Obstetric and Gynaecology of the British Commonwealth*, **78**, 865–881.

Beischer, N. A., Holsman, M. & Kitchen, W. H. (1968) Relation of various forms of anaemia to placental weight. *American Journal of Obstetrics and Gynecology*, **101**, 801–809.

Beischer, N. A., Reid, S., Brown, J. B. & Macafee, C. A. J. (1970) Value of urinary oestriol estimation in patients with antepartum haemorrhage. *Australian and New Zealand Journal of Obstetrics and Gynaecology*, **10**, 191–204.

Bell, G. H. (1938) The human foetal electrocardiogram. *Journal of Obstetrics and Gynaecology of the British Empire*, **45**, 802–809.

Bergstrand, C. G., Karlsson, B. W., Lindberg, T. & Ekelund, H. (1972) Alpha-foetoprotein, albumin and total protein in serum from preterm and term infants and small-for-gestational-age infants. *Acta Paediatrica Scandinavica*, **61**, 128–132.

Blunt, A. (1971) Value of plasma oxytocinase in the assessment of feto-placental function. *Australian and New Zealand Journal of Obstetrics and Gynaecology*, **11**, 37–43.

Boddy, K. & Mantell, C. (1972) Observations of foetal breathing movements transmitted through maternal abdominal wall. *Lancet*, **2**, 1219–1220.

Boddy, K. & Robinson, J. S. (1971) External method for detection of fetal breathing in utero. *Lancet*, **2**, 1231–1233.

Boddy, K., Dawes, G. S. & Robinson, J. S. (1973) A 24-hour rhythm in the foetus. In *Foetal and Neonatal Physiology*, pp. 63–66. London: Cambridge University Press.

Bretscher, J. and Saling, E. (1967) pH values in the human fetus during labor. *American Journal of Obstetrics and Gynecology*, **97**, 906–911.

Brown, J. B. (1957) The relationship between urinary oestrogens and oestrogens produced in the body. *Journal of Endocrinology*, **16**, 202–212.

Brown, J. B., MacLeod, S. C., MacNaughton, C., Smith, M. A. & Smyth, B. (1968) A rapid method for estimating oestrogens in urine using a semi-automatic extractor. *Journal of Endocrinology*, **42**, 5–15.

Butler, N. R. & Alberman, E. D. (1969) Perinatal problems. In *The Second report of the 1958 British Perinatal Mortality Survey*. Edinburgh and London: Livingstone.

Campbell, S. (1968) An improved method of fetal cephalometry by ultrasound. *Journal of Obstetrics and Gynaecology of the British Commonwealth*, **75**, 568–576.

Campbell, S. (1974) Fetal growth. In *Clinics in Obstetrics and Gynaecology*, ed. Beard, R. W., Ch. 3. London: W. B. Saunders Co. Ltd.

Campbell, S. & Dewhurst, C. J. (1971) Diagnosis of the small-for-dates fetus by serial ultrasonic cephalometry. *Lancet*, **2**, 1002–1006.

Chard, T. & Klopper, A. (1974) The variability of plasma oestradiol concentration in late pregnancy. *Journal of Obstetrics and Gynaecology of the British Commonwealth*, **81**, 357–000.

Coltart, T. M., Trickey, N. R. & Beard, R. W. (1969) Foetal blood sampling. Practical approach to management of foetal distress. *British Medical Journal*, **1**, 342–246.

Crawford, J. S. (1972) The mother. *Principles and Practice of Obstetric Anaesthesia*, 3rd edn, p. 16. London: Blackwell Scientific Publications.

Crawford, J. W. (1975) Computer monitoring of fetal heart rate and uterine pressure. *American Journal of Obstetrics and Gynecology*, **121**, 342–350.

Cremer, M. (1906) Ueber die direkte Ableitung der Aktionsströme des menschlichen Herzens vom Oesophagus und über das Elektrokardiogramm des Fötus. *München Medizinische Wochenschrift*, **53**, 811–813.

Curzen, P. & Morris, I. (1965) Serum alkaline phosphatase in the hypertensive disorders of pregnancy. *Journal of Obstetrics and Gynaecology of the British Commonwealth*, **72**, 397–401.

Dobbing, J. & Smart, J. L. (1973) Vulnerable periods in brain development and behaviour. In *Ethology and Development*, ed. Barnett, S. A., Ch. 2. Spastics International Medical Publications. London: Heinemann Medical Books; Philadelphia: Leppincott.

Donald, I., MacVicar, J. & Brown, T. G. (1958) Investigation of abdominal masses by pulsed ultrasound. *Lancet*, **1**, 1188–1195.

Dweck, H. S., Huggins, W., Dorman, L. P., Saxon, S. A., Benton, J. W. & Cassady, G (1974) Developmental sequelae in infants having suffered severe perinatal asphyxia. *American Journal of Obstetrics and Gynecology*, **119**, 811–815.

Eastman, N. J. (1932) Foetal blood studies. The chemical nature of asphyxia neonatorum and its bearing on certain practical problems. *Bulletin of the Johns Hopkins Hospital*, **50**, 39–50.

Figueroa-Longo, J. G., Poseiro, J. J., Alvarez, L. O. & Caldeyro-Barcia, R. (1966) Fetal electrocardiogram at term labor obtained with subcutaneous fetal electrodes. *American Journal of Obstetrics and Gynecology*, **96**, 556–564.

Fliegner, J. H., Renou, P., Wood, C., Beischer, N. A. & Brown, J. B. (1969) Correlation between urinary estriol excretion and fetal acidosis in high-risk pregnancies. *American Journal of Obstetrics and Gynecology*, **105**, 252–256.

France, J. T. & Liggins, G. C. (1969) Placental sulfatase deficiency. *Journal of Clinical Endocrinology*, **29**, 138–141.

Fransden, V. A. & Stakemann, G. (1964) The site of production of oestrogenic hormones in human pregnancy. III. *Acta endocrinologica (Copenhagen)*, **47**, 265–276.

Goodlin, R. C. & Kaiser, I. H. (1957) The effect of ammonium chloride induced maternal acidosis on the human foetus at term. I. pH hemoglobin and blood gases. *American Journal of Medical Sciences*, **233**, 662–672.

Gruenwald, P. (1949) Necrosis in coronary arteries of newborn infants. *American Heart Journal*, **38**, 889–897.

Gruenwald, P. (1969) Stillbirth and early neonatal death. In *Perinatal Problems*, ed. Butler, N. R. & Alderman, E. D., Ch. 9. The second report of the 1958 British Perinatal Mortality Survey. Edinburgh and London: Livingstone.

Grumbach, M. M., Kaplan, S. L., Sciarra, J. J. & Burr, I. M. (1968) Chorionic growth hormone-prolactin (CGP): secretion, disposition, biologic activity in man and postulated function as the 'growth hormone' of the second half of pregnancy. *Annals of New York Academy of Science*, **148**, 501–531.

Hainsworth, I. R. & Hall, P. E. (1971) A simple automated method for the measurement of oestrogens in the urine of pregnant women. *Clinica Chemica Acta*, **35**, 201–208.

Halban, J. (1905) Die innere Secretion von Ovarium und Placenta und ihre Bedeutung für die Funktion der Milchdrüse. *Archiv für Gynaekologie (Berlin)*, **75**, 353–441.

Hellman, L. M., Johnston, H. L., Tolks, W. E. & Jones, E. H. (1961) Some factors affecting the fetal heart rate. *American Journal of Obstetrics and Gynecology*, **82**, 1055–1063.

Hon, E. H. (1963) The classification of fetal heart rate. I. A working classification. *Obstetrics and Gynecology*, **22**, 137–146.

Hon, E. H. & Huang, H. S. (1962) The electronic evaluation of fetal heart rate. VII. Premature and missed beats. *Obstetrics and Gynecology*, **20**, 81–90.

Hon, E. H. & Khazin, A. F. (1969) Biochemical studies of the fetus. I. The fetal pH-measuring system. *Obstetrics and Gynecology*, **33**, 219–236.

Hon, E. H. & Lee. S. T. (1963a) Electronic evaluation of the fetal heart rate. VIII. Patterns preceding fetal death, further observations. *American Journal of Obstetrics and Gynecology*, **87**, 814–826.

Hon, E. H. & Lee, S. T. (1963b) Noise reduction in fetal electrocardiography. II. Averaging techniques. *American Journal of Obstetrics and Gynecology*, **87**, 1086–1096.

Hon, E. H., Bradfield, A. H. & Hess, O. W. (1961) The electronic evaluation of the fetal heart rate. V. The vagal factor in fetal bradycardia. *American Journal of Obstetrics and Gynecology*, **82**, 291–300.

Hull, M. G. (1972) Perinatal coagulopathies complicating fetal blood sampling. *British Medical Journal*, **4**, 319–321.

Ito, Y. & Higashi, K. (1962) Studies on the prolactin-like substance in human placenta. *Japanese Journal of Endocrinology*, **8**, 279–287.

James, L. S. (1960) Acidosis of the newborn and its relation to birth asphyxia. *Acta paediatrica (Uppsala)*, **49**, Suppl. 122, 17–28.

Josimovich, J. B. & MacLaren, J. A. (1962) Presence in the human placenta and term serum of a highly lactogenic substance immunologically related to pituitary growth hormone. *Endrocinology*, **71**, 209–220.

Kantor, H. I., Bowman, A. & Abbott, P. D. (1966) Misdiagnosis of fetal life from an artifact in the electrocardiogram. *American Journal of Obstetrics and Gynecology*, **94**, 287–289.

Kaplan, S. & Toyama, S. (1958) Fetal electrocardiography. Utilising abdominal and intrauterine leads. *Obstetrics and Gynecology*, **11**, 391–397.

Kelly, A. M., England, P., Corimer, J. D., Ferguson, J. C. & Govan, A. D. T. (1975) An evaluation of human placental lactogen levels in hypertension of pregnancy. *British Journal of Obstetrics and Gynaecology*, **82**, 272–277.

Kendall, B. (1967) Abnormal fetal heart rates and rhythms prior to labor. *American Journal of Obstetrics and Gynecology*, **99**, 71–78.

Klebe, J. G., Winkel, P. & Lyngbye, J. (1974) Urinary oestriol excretion in diabetic pregnancy. The problem of reference intervalse. *Acta endocrinologica*, **75**, Suppl. 182, 52–56.

Klopper, A. & Billewicz, W. (1963) Urinary excretion of oestriol and pregnanediol during normal pregnancy. *Journal of Obstetrics and Gynaecology of the British Commonwealth*, **70**, 1024–1033.

Klopper, A. & Stephenson, R. (1966) The excretion of oestriol and of pregnanediol in pregnancy complicated by Rh isoimmunisation. *Journal of Obstetrics and Gynaecology of the British Commonwealth*, **73**, 282–289.

Komaromy, B., Gaal, J., Mihaly, G., Mocsary, P., Pohanka, P. & Suranyi, S. (1967) Data on the significance of fetal arrhythmia. *American Journal of Obstetrics and Gynecology*, **99**, 79–85.

Krumbhaar, E. B. (1916) Electrocardiographic studies in normal infants. *American Journal of Physiology*, **40**, 133.

Kubli, F. W., Kaeser, O. & Hinselmann, M. (1969) Diagnostic management of chronic placental insufficiency. In *The Feto-placental Unit*, ed. Pecile, A. & Finzi, C., pp. 323–339. Amsterdam: Excerpta Medica Foundation.

Larks, S. D. (1963) The abnormal fetal electrocardiogram: intrauterine fetal difficulty and fetal distress. *Obstetrics and Gynecology*, **22**, 427–432.

Larks, S. D. (1965) Estimation of the electrical axis of the fetal heart. *American Journal of Obstetrics and Gynecology*, **91**, 46–55.

Lee, S. T. & Hon, E. H. (1963) Fetal hemodynamic response to umbilical cord compression. *Obstetrics and Gynecology*, **22**, 553–562.

Letchworth, A. T. & Chard, T. (1972) Placental lactogen levels as a screening test for fetal distress and neonatal asphyxia. *Lancet*, **1**, 704–706.

Loeffler, F. E. (1967) Clinical foetal weight prediction. *Journal of Obstetrics and Gynaecology of the British Commonwealth*, **74**, 675–677.

Lovell, K. E. (1973) The effect of post-maturity on the developing child. *Medical Journal of Australia*, **1**, 13–17.

Low, J. A. (1963) Acid–base assessment of the fetus in the normal obstetric patient. *Obstetrics and Gynecology*, **22**, 15–18.

Lumley, J., McKinnon, L. & Wood, C. (1971) Lack of agreement on normal values for fetal scalp blood. *Journal of Obstetrics and Gynaecology of the British Commonwealth*, **78**, 13–21.

Macafee, C. A., Beischer, N. A. & Brown, J. B. (1972) Feto-placental function and antenatal complications when the fetus is malformed. *Australian and New Zealand Journal of Obstetrics and Gynaecology*, **12**, 71–85.

Macafee, J., Beischer, N. A., Fortune, D. W. & Brown, J. B. (1971) Obstetric complications when the fetus has congenital heart disease. I. Fetoplacental function when the fetal heat is malformed. *American Journal of Obstetrics and Gynecology*, **110**, 653–657.

MacDonald, R. R. & Kelman, G. R. (1967) Problems of foetal blood sampling. *Journal of Obstetrics and Gynaecology of the British Commonwealth*, **74**, 826–828.

MacLeod, S. C., Brown, J. B., Beischer, N. A. & Smith, N. A. (1967) Value of urinary oestriol measurements during pregnancy. *Australian and New Zealand Journal of Obstetrics and Gynaecology*, **109**, 375–377.

MacNaughton, M. C. (1969) The foeto-placental unit. In *Modern Trends in Obstetrics*, ed. Kellar, R. J., Vol. 4, pp. 110–134. London: Butterworths.

Macrae, D. J. & Palavradji, D. (1965) The effect of complications of pregnancy and labour on acid–base balance of the baby at birth. *Journal of Obstetrics and Gynaecology of the British Commonwealth*, **72**, 269–272.

Masson, G. M. (1973a) Plasma oestriol concentration during normal pregnancy. *Journal of Obstetrics and Gynaecology of the British Commonwealth*, **,80** 201–205.

Masson, G. M. (1973b) Plasma oestriol in pre-eclampsia. *Journal of Obstetrics and Gynaecology of the British Commonwealth*, **80**, 206–209.

Mendez-Bauer, C., Arnt, I. C., Gulin, L., Excarcena, L. & Caldeyro-Barcia, R. (1967) Relationship between blood pH and heart rate in the human fetus during labor. *American Journal of Obstetrics and Gynecology*, **97**, 530–545.

Morishima, H. O., Moya, F., Bossers, A. C. & Daniel, S. S. (1964) Adverse effects of maternal hypocapnea on the newborn guinea-pig. *American Journal of Obstetrics and Gynecology*, **88**, 524–529.

Morrison, G., Meigs, R. A. & Ryan, K. J. (1965) Biosynthesis of progesterone by the human placenta. *Steroids*, Suppl. II, 177–188.

Moya, F., Morishima, H. O., Shnider, S. M. & James, L. S. (1965) Influence of maternal hyperventilation on the newborn infant. *American Journal of Obstetrics and Gynecology*, **91**, 76–84.

Nesbitt, R. E. Jr & Aubry, R. H. (1969) High risk obstetrics. II. Value of semi-objective grading system in identifying the vulnerable group. *American Journal of Obstetrics and Gynecology*, **103**, 972–985.

Newman, W. (1963) Foetal distress. *Medical Journal of Australia*, **2**, 912–915.

Newman, W., McKinnon, L., Phillips, L., Paterson, P. and Wood, C. (1967) Oxygen transfer from mother to fetus during labor. *American Journal of Obstetrics and Gynecology*, **99**, 61–70.

Noguchi, M. (1937) On hydrogen ion concentration of umbilical blood of normal and asphyxiated newborns. *Japanese Journal of Obstetrics and Gynaecology*, **20**, 248–266.

Oakey, R. E. (1970) The interpretation of urinary oestrogen and pregnanediol excretion in pregnant women receiving corticosteroids. *Journal of Obstetrics and Gynaecology of the British Commonwealth*, **77**, 922–927.

Paul, W. M., Gare, D. J. & Whetham, J. C. (1967) Assessment of fetal scalp sampling in labor. *American Journal of Obstetrics and Gynecology*, **99**, 745–753.

Petrucco, O. M., Cellier, K. M. & Fishtall, A. (1973) Diagnosis of intrauterine fetal growth retardation by serial serum oxytocinase, urinary oestrogen and serum heat stable alkaline phosphatase (HSAP) estimations in uncomplicated and hypertensive pregnancies. *Journal of Obstetrics and Gynaecology of the British Commonwealth*, **80**, 499–507.

Prevention of Perinatal Mortality and Morbidity (1970) WHO Technical Report Series No. 457. Report of WHO Expert Committee.

Ratanasopa, V., Schindler, A. E., Lee, T. Y. & Hermann, W. L. (1967) Measurement of estriol in plasma by gas–liquid chromatography. Its significance in the treatment of high risk pregnancies. *American Journal of Obstetrics and Gynecology*, **99**, 295–302.

Reid, S., Beischer, N. A., Brown, J. B. & Smith, M. A. (1968) Urinary oestriol excretion in pregnancies complicated by proteinuria. *Australian and New Zealand Journal of Obstetrics and Gynaecology*, **8**, 189–196.

Saling, E. (1964) Technik der endoskopischen Mikroblutentnahme am Feten. *Geburtshilfe und Frauenheilkunde*, **24**, 464–469.

Saling, E. and Schneider, D. (1967) Biochemical supervision of the foetus during labour. *Journal of Obstetrics and Gynaecology of the British Commonwealth*, **74**, 799–811.

Schutt-Aine, J. C. & Drash, A. L. (1972) Human placental lactogen and human growth hormone for hypopituitarism. Absence of growth potentiation. *American Journal of Diseases of Childhood*, **123**, 475–479.

Sciarra, J. J., Kaplan, S. L. and Grumbach, M. M. (1963) Localisation of anti-human growth hormone serum within the human placenta: evidence for a human chorionic 'growth hormone-prolactin'. *Nature (London)*, **199**, 1005–1006.

Selinger, M. and Levitz, M. (1969) Diurnal variation of total plasma E3 levels in late pregnancy. *Journal of Clinical Endocrinology and Metabolism* **29** 995–996.

Seppala, M. & Ruoslahti, E. (1970) Serum concentration of human placental lactogenic hormone (HPL) in pregnancy complications. *Acta obstetricia et gynecologica scandinavica*, **49**, 143–147.

Seppala, M. & Ruoslahti, E. (1972) Alpha feto-protein in normal and pregnancy sera. *Lancet*, **1**, 375–376.

Shane, J. M. & Suzuki, K. (1974) Placental alkaline phosphatase a review and re-evaluation of its applicability in monitoring fetoplacental function. *Obstetrical and Gynecological Survey*, **29**, 97–105.

Shearman, R. P. (1959) Some aspects of the urinary excretion of pregnanediol in pregnancy. *Journal of Obstetrics and Gynaecology of the British Empire*, **66**, 1–11.

Shelley, T. & Tipton, R. H. (1971) Dip area. A quantitative measure of fetal heart rate patterns. *Journal of Obstetrics and Gynaecology of the British Commonwealth*, **78**, 694–701.

Short, R. V. & Eton, B. (1959) Progesterone in blood, III. Progesterone in the peripheral blood of pregnant women. *Journal of Endocrinology*, **18**, 418–425.

Siiteri, P. K. & MacDonald, P. C. (1966) Placental estrogen biosynthesis during human pregnancy. *Journal of Clinical Endocrinology*, **26**, 751–761.

Singer, W., Desjardins, P. & Friesen, H. G. (1970) Human placental lactogen. An index of placental function. *Obstetrics and Gynecology*, **36**, 222–232.

Singh, H. A. & Symonds, E. M. (1972) Red cell potassium in chronic fetal asphyxia. *Journal of Obstetrics and Gynaecology of the British Commonwealth*, **79**, 941–945.

Smyth, C. N. (1953) Experimental electrocardiography of the foetus. *Lancet*, **1**, 1124–1126.

Southern, E. M. (1957) Fetal anoxia and its possible relation to changes in the prenatal fetal electrocardiogram. *American Journal of Obstetrics and Gynecology*, **73**, 233–247.

Spackman, T., Fuchs, F. & Assali, N. S. (1963) Acid–base status of the fetus in human pregnancy. *Obstetrics and Gynecology*, **22**, 785–791.

Spellacy, W. N., Teoh, E. S., Buhi, W. C., Birk, S. A. & McCreary, S. A. (1971) Value of human chorionic somatomammotropin in managing high-risk pregnancies. *American Journal of Obstetrics and Gynecology*, **109**, 588–598.

Sureau, C. (1962) Technical difficulties and misinterpretations in foetal electrocardiography. *Journal of Obstetrics and Gynaecology of the British Commonwealth*, **69**, 1033–1035.

Suwa, S. & Friesen, H. (1969) Biosynthesis of human placental proteins and human placental lactogen (HPL) in vitro. I' Identification of 3H-labelled HPL. *Endocrinology*, **85**, 1028–1036.

Symonds, E. M. (1971) Configuration of the fetal ECG in relation to fetal acid–base balance and plasma electrolytes. *Journal of Obstetrics and Gynaecology of the British Commonwealth*, **78**, 957–970.

Symonds, E. M. (1972) Vectorcardiography and acid–base balance in the human fetus. *Journal of Obstetrics and Gynaecology of the British Commonwealth*, **79**, 416–423.

Symonds, E. M. (1972) Fetal cardiac arrhythmias and fetal acid–base status. *Australian and New Zealand Journal of Obstetrics and Gynaecology*, **12**, 170–175.

Touchstone, J. C., Stojkewycz, M. & Smith, K. (1965) The effect of methenamine mandelate (mandelamine) on determination of urinary estriol. *Clinical Chemistry*, **11**, 1019–1022.

Tovey, J. E. (1969) Serum oxytocinase. *Clinical Biochemistry*, **2**, 289–310.

Tulchinsky, D. & Korenman, S. G. (1971) The plasma estradiol as an index of fetoplacental function. *Journal of Clinical Investigation*, **50**, 1490–1497.

Tulchinsky, D. & Okada, D. M. (1975) Hormones in human pregnancy. IV. Plasma progesterone. *American Journal of Obstetrics and Gynecology*, **121**, 293–299.

Ursell, W., Brudenell, M. and Chard, T. (1973) Placental lactogen levels in diabetic pregnancy. *British Medical Journal*, **2**, 80–82.

Vara, P. & Halminen, E. (1952) Foetal electrocardiography. II. *Acta obstetricia et gynecologia scandinavica*, **31**, 179–185.

Venning, E. H. & Browne, J. S. L. (1936) Isolation of water-soluble and pregnanediol complex from human pregnancy urine. *Proceedings of the Society for Experimental Biology and Medicine*, **34**, 792–793.

Vermelin, H., Dellestable, B. & Muller, M. (1962) Interet de la mesure simultanee des gaz et du pH de sang de la reine ombilicale à la naissance particulierement en cas de souffrance foetale (etude de 160 cas). *Bullétin de la Fédération des sociétés de gynécologie et d'obstétrique de la langue française (Paris)*, **14**, 593–599.

Villee, C A. (1953) Regulation of blood glucose in human fetus. *Journal of Applied Physiology*, **5**, 437–444.

Walker, A., Phillips, L., Pose, L. & Wood, C. (1968) A new instrument for the measurement of tissue P_{O_2} of human fetal scalp. *American Journal of Obstetrics and Gynecology*, **100**, 63–71.

Ward, E. H. T., Letchworth, A. T., Niven, P. A. R. & Chard, T. (1974) Placental lactogen levels in rhesus isoimmunisation. *British Medical Journal*, **1**, 347–349.

Whitfield, C. R. (1966) A source of diagnostic error in fetal electrocardiography. *American Journal of Obstetrics and Gynecology*, **95**, 669–675.

Willman, K. & Pulkkinen, M. O. (1971) Reduced maternal plasma and urinary oestriol during ampicillin treatment. *American Journal of Obstetrics and Gynecology*, **109**, 893–896.

Willocks, J., Donald, I., Campbell, S. & Dunsmore, I. R. (1967) Intrauterine growth assessed by ultrasonic foetal cephalometry. *Journal of Obstetrics and Gynaecology of the British Commonwealth*, **74**, 639–647.

Wood, C., Lumley, J., Hammond, J. & Newman, W. (1968) The assessment of the foetus during labour in patients with hypertension. *Medical Journal of Australia*, 26th October, 707–710.

Wood, C., Ferguson, R., Leeton, J., Newman, W. & Walker, A. (1967) Fetal heart rate and acid–base status in the assessment of fetal hypoxia. *American Journal of Obstetrics and Gynecology*, **98**, 62–70.

Ylikorkala, O. (1973) Maternal serum HPL levels in normal and complicated pregnancy as an index of placental function. *Acta obstetricia et gynecologica scandinavica*, Suppl. 26, 25–52.

Zander, J. (1959) Gestogens in human pregnancy. In *Recent Progress in Endocrinology of Reproduction*, ed. Lloyd, C. W., pp. 255–282. New York: Academic Press Inc.

2
INFANTS DAMAGED DURING BIRTH
Pathology

J. K. Brown

Reflection on the nature of a delay of only a few moments in the substitution of pulmonary for the ceased placental respiration would lead to the apprehension that even the want of a few breathings, if not fatal to the economy, may imprint a lasting injury upon it. The observations I have recorded of the direct connection between suspended animation at birth and mental and physical impairment of the individual, prove that the proportion of entire recoveries from the effects of asphyxia neonatorum is smaller than has hitherto been supposed.

Little, 1861

The aim of the modern management of the handicapped child is early recognition with full multidisciplinary assessment followed by appropriate therapy. This has led to the idea of 'mass developmental screening' in order to detect handicap at an early stage. If this is accepted uncritically it will place an enormous load upon a financially insolvent health service and much energy will be spent detecting minor abnormalities for which there is no effective therapy. The services for those children with established handicap must be improved before they are overloaded by a search for 'deviant developmental' as well as 'abnormal developmental' problems.

Much more is now known about normal and abnormal neonatal behaviour, largely due to the work of Heinz Prechtl (1964, 1968). In the next two chapters the behavioural abnormalities and neurological findings of infants who have sustained possible cerebral birth injury will be considered in order to try to demonstrate that 'screening' of infants by good neonatal practice will identify the pathology which is treatable or preventable. 'At risk' registers yield a very poor return for the enormous amount of work involved (Rogers, 1971). We suggest that definite abnormalities of behaviour in the newborn period and not an 'at risk' score based on historical data should be the criteria for screening and for long-term follow-up.

Where figures are given without reference to their source they are derived from the annual report of the Simpson Memorial Maternity Pavilion (SMMP), or prospective data from follow-up studies on asphyxiated infants (Brown et al, 1973; Brown et al, 1974).

The article is confined to the effects of intrapartum asphyxia and birth trauma upon the brain of the child. The respiratory problems associated with perinatal asphyxia were comprehensively reviewed by Hull (1971) in the last edition in this series. The problems associated with low birth weight from the neurological point of view have recently been reviewed in depth by Davies and Stewart (1975). Congenital malformations affecting the central nervous system and primary biochemical abnormalities will not be considered.

INCIDENCE

Intrapartum asphyxia is the major cause of intrapartum fetal death at term (Towell, 1966; Lilien, 1970). If we look at the necropsy findings in fresh still-births we find that asphyxia plays some part in about 50 per cent of cases.

Table 2.1   Various disorders as a percentage of perinatal mortality (booked cases)

	1969	1970	1971	1972	1973
Birth trauma	0	4	3	1	0
Asphyxia (placenta and cord conditions)	12	14	22	20	22
Congenital malformations	28	34	43	35	39

Table 2.2 Incidence of 'asphyxia' at various stages of the infants' progress

Apgar score of 6 or less	200/1000 births
Umbilical arterial (pH < 7.2)	200/1000 births
Neonatal asphyxia (intubated)	50/1000 births
Perinatal mortality	4/1000 births
Abnormal behaviour	6/1000 births
Long-term neurological abnormality	1.5/1000 births
Minimal brain damage	1.5/1000 births

Most of the remaining stillbirths are congenitally malformed infants. In terms of neonatal death rate, if we accept that the idiopathic respiratory distress syndrome in the preterm infant is predisposed by asphyxia during birth then 33 per cent of neonatal deaths are primarily asphyxial. Over the years the incidence of asphyxial deaths due to placenta and cord conditions has not declined as much as death from mechanical trauma. Since the total perinatal mortality is falling, asphyxia, like congenital malformation, is rising as a percentage of total perinatal mortality (Table 2.1). The long-term morbidity from perinatal asphyxia is probably in the region of 1.5/1000 deliveries for severe handicap and similar for so-called minimal brain damage (Table 2.2). The importance of good obstetrics is seen if the total fetal wastage from placenta and cord conditions for mothers booked for hospital confinement (4/1000) is compared with those who are unbooked (21/1000).

Asphyxia is common but asphyxial brain damage is rare in the average maternity hospital population. Table 2.2 shows the approximate incidence at various stages of the infant's progress. Fetal distress as defined by a scalp pH of less than 7.2 is found in 14 per cent of monitored pregnancies (Saling and Schneider, 1967). Asphyxia at birth as defined by an Apgar score of less than three, or the need for endotracheal intubation occurs in 5 per cent of pregnancies. Only 0.6 per cent of all births will have abnormal behaviour suggesting cerebral asphyxia and 0.15 per cent will have lasting handicap of any severity. When fetal monitoring is considered it must be remembered that the morbidity is low and therefore the risks of the monitoring procedures must also be low.

Table 2.3 Association between perinatal abnormalities and cerebral palsy

A. Presumptive causes in 92 children referred with cerebral palsy under one year of age

Perinatal asphyxia	25%	Genetic	18%
Birth trauma	6%	Low birth weight	21%
Hyperbilirubinaemia	6%	Postnatal	9%
Intraventricular haem.	8%	?What	7%

B. Prospective study on early detection of handicap from perinatal abnormality (SMMP, three-year period 1968–70)

Aetiology	Number	Percentage	Incidence per 1000 live births
Asphyxia	23	51	1.6
Jaundice	3	7	0.2
Birth trauma	3	7	0.2
Prematurity			
(Drillien survey)	16	35	0.7
Total	45	100	2.7

Although cerebral palsy may be on the decline due to improved management of the traumatised, the jaundiced and the preterm infant, there does not appear to be any risk of the centres for handicapped children running out of work. Table 2.3A shows the percentage of cases of cerebral palsy seen under one year of age in the Scottish Council for the Care of Spastics, in which asphyxia was thought to have played a major aetiological role. Figures are also shown for a prospective survey of cerebral palsy performed five years ago (Table 2.3B). It can be seen that this is still an area where there is plenty of room for prevention. This is especially so since many of these children are amongst the group most severely handicapped (Hagberg, Hagberg and Olow, 1975).

CAUSES OF ASPHYXIA

The causes of perinatal asphyxia may be classified by the site of the abnormality, i.e. placental, cord, etc., or as acute and chronic, or as antepartum, intrapartum or postpartum (Table 2.4). Postpartum asphyxia is 'revealed', usually acute and can be terminated by artificial ventilation. It does not cause the same long-term morbidity as symptomatic intrapartum asphyxia. Infants with a Po_2 as low as 20 mmHg, with total apnoea, a severe metabolic acidosis and treated by intermittent positive ventilation for many days are at no great risk of brain damage if they survive (Brown, 1973). The infant with severe respiratory distress syndrome is usually immature and this may also enable him to withstand acute hypoxic stress provided he does not die of an intra-ventricular haemorrhage. There is more concern over intrauterine asphyxia which may be 'concealed', more chronic and is more difficult to treat even if its presence is recognised. The infant is also more likely to be full term and so possibly more vulnerable to the cerebral effects of asphyxia (Brown, 1974).

Table 2.4   Causes of perinatal asphyxia

	%
Maternal	
Shock (severe APH, epidural reaction, cardiac arrest)	4
Respiratory failure (chronic lung disease, pulmonaryembolus amniotic fluid embolus, eclampsia, Mendelsone syndrome)	1
Placental	
Placental insufficiency (PET, low oestriols, etc.)	22
Placental separation APH	13
Uterine	
Uterine tetanus, oxytocic overdose, impaired uterine blood flow	0
Cord disorder	
Prolapse	6
Tightly round neck (with fetal distress)	10
Compression head injury	
Malpresentation and disproportion	33
Miscellaneous	
Including postpartum causes and secondary to above	11

Hagberg et al (1975) in an analysis of 560 cases of cerebral palsy found 93 cases were due to or associated with placental insufficiency. The types of cerebral palsy included hemiplegia, diplegia, dyskinesia and teraplegia. Whilst most of these can be explained upon the basis of cerebral asphyxia as will be described later, the large number of hemiplegias (39) suggests that embolus from the placenta may play a part as described by Cocker, George and Yates (1965). There is a theoretical risk of thromboplastin released from damaged tissues causing thrombi to form in the umbilical veins and a risk of embolism (Perlman and Divilansky, 1975). This would be preferentially carried to the fetal brain due to the anatomy of the intra-uterine fetal circulation. In our own series of 94 infants with symptomatic perinatal asphyxia 50 per cent were due to placental or cord conditions and placental insufficiency was the major component in 35 per cent of all cases (Table 2.4). Abnormalities were also found on follow-up studies of infants selected because of placental insufficiency on the basis of a low maternal urinary oestriol excretion (Wallace and Michie, 1966).

CAUSES OF COMPRESSION HEAD INJURY

The head of the fetus may be injured during birth by compression and this is non-concussive, unlike the usual postnatal deceleration injury. As with all head injuries, the cervical spine is also at risk. Fracture dislocation is not uncommon after breech extraction (Towbin, 1969; Leventhal, 1960). This may be the cause of the infant's postnatal respiratory difficulties. Trauma to the vertebral arteries may also cause brain stem ischaemia and later respiratory problems (Yates, 1959).

Table 2.5   Mechanisms of damage in compression head injury in neonates

Compression
  Impaired cerebral circulation
  Cerebral oedema
  ?Intrauterine 'coning'
  Traumatic asphyxia
  Facial palsy

Moulding (distortion)
  Antero/posterior rupture of vein of Galen, traumatic thrombosis (infarction in
    deep white matter or subdural in middle fossa)
  Lateral—saggittal sinus entrapment
       —tears bridging veins
  Tentorial, sinus or dural tears

Traction (hyperextension or rotation)
  Cervical spinal damage
  Erb's, Klumpke's, or total plexus injury
  Vertebral or carotid traumatic thrombosis
  Sternomastoid tumour, ?postnatal squint baby syndrome

Secondary asphyxia
  Uteroplacental failure from uterine tetanus
  Fetal hypotension from intrauterine bradycardia
  Failure to establish breathing at birth

Compression of the head may damage in several ways (Table 2.5). Selective induction to avoid postmaturity and the policy of never to let the sun set twice on the same labour has abolished the grossly moulded 'Magoo head' with the dural structures being stretched beyond their elasticity with the resultant massive intracranial haemorrhage. The introduction of these measures has resulted in a drop in compression head injury from 4.8/1000 live births to 2/1000 over the last five years. However, lesser degrees of moulding in the lateral plane with marked overriding of one parietal bone may still sometimes damage the veins into sagittal sinus (sinus entrapment syndrome) and causes bleeding into the CSF and a temporary external hydrocephalus which may be unilateral. With lesser degrees of moulding infants may only show the signs of a headache, a cerebral cry, resentment at being handled and excess vomiting. Table 2.6 shows the presumed pathology and the associated lesions in 82 compression head injuries in the newborn studied five years ago; it illustrates a point that we shall return to when discussing the pathology of asphyxia, namely that the intermediary pathological mechanisms must be studied if treatment is to be rational and if we are to try to understand why so many long-term problems arise from one aetiology.

Table 2.6 Presumed pathological mechanisms in 82 cases of compression head injury in the newborn (15000 births, 1968–70)

Traumatic subarachnoid haemorrhage[a]	29
Subdural haematoma	7
Traumatic external hydrocephalus	5
Cerebral oedema (without haemorrhage)[b]	26
Cerebral contusion[c]	13
Presumed vertebral artery thrombosis	2
Associated lesions	
Cephalohaemotoma	12
Erb's palsy	9
Radial nerve palsy	5
Fractures[d]	4
Severe moulding or external trauma	48

[a] Proven by centrifugation and spectrophotometry
[b] Tense fontanelle, splayed sutures, fundal changes, with or without decerebrate rigidity
[c] Unilateral fits, persisting hemisyndrome, or asymmetrical EEG in the absence of haemorrhage or clinical evidence of brain swelling
[d] Two skull, one humerus, one cervical spine

The clinical problems posed by the infant with a compression head injury are very similar to those of intrauterine asphyxia. They often coexist. About 50 per cent will show fetal distress and 50 per cent will need intermittent positive pressure ventilation after birth. A third will continue to have apnoeic and cyanotic attacks and 50 per cent will have convulsions (Table 2.7). Homeostatic defects are less common than with simple asphyxia. As with a head injury at any age the two fundamentals of good management are to maintain the airway and treat raised intracranial pressure, both kill or may cause permanent secondary brain damage.

Obstetric manoeuvres are rarely a cause of significant trauma and the necessity to avoid asphyxial brain damage must come first. However, Keilland's rotation is not well tolerated by an infant who has had prolonged head compression or who is suffering from secondary asphyxia due to the failure of the utero-placental circulation. Long-term follow-up studies of infants

Table 2.7   Clinical problems and symptoms in 82 infants with compression head injuries

Fetal distress	47%	Irritable	15%
IPPR	49%	Jittery	36%
Apnoeic/attacks	35%	Abnormal tone	70%
Tube feeding	47%	Hemisyndrome	20%
Vomiting	14%	Absent Moro reflex	15%
Cerebral cry	26%	Raised intracranial pressure	35%
	Convulsions	47%	
	Hypothermia	14%	
	Hypocalcaemia	20%	
	Hypoglycaemia	11%	

In 32 cases (40%) asphyxia was thought to be a serious secondary complication

with trauma show that in the absence of asphyxia the prognosis is good (Purvis et al, 1975).

DIAGNOSIS OF PERINATAL ASPHYXIA

The infant may be born after a clinical event such as a prolapsed cord, antepartum haemorrhage or a pregnancy complicated by severe pre-eclamptic toxaemia with falling urinary oestriol concentrations and yet never have been subjected to any actual asphyxial episode. When the cord is tightly around the neck acidosis and hypoxia does occur, but only in a very few instances (Wood et al, 1967). Infusion acidosis from the mother may lower the fetal pH and drugs given to the mother may cause a low Apgar score (Beard, 1970). In other words, a clinical history known to be strongly associated with fetal asphyxia can occur without fetal hypoxia, and the criteria which is used to detect asphyxia may not always be measuring the correct parameter. Apnoea at birth is the end result of many pathological events and with modern management (i.e., intubation according to 1 min Apgar score) there should be no post-natal asphyxia; apnoea at birth represents what has gone before, drugs, head compression or asphyxia. Studies are hampered by the difficulty in defining asphyxia, the biochemical and physiological parameters may show that asphyxia is present, they do not demonstrate asphyxial brain damage has occurred. 'Cases of severe asphyxia pallida recover and exhibit no sequalae sufficiently common for this to be no freak occurrence' (Thomson, 1951). There is no absolute Po_2 at which brain damage will definitely occur; just as there is no absolute serum calcium concentration at which fits will occur; or bilirubin concentration at which kernicterus will develop or phenylalanine level at which severe mental defect will undoubtedly be produced. The currently available methods of diagnosing intrauterine asphyxia are reviewed in Chapter 1.

PATHOPHYSIOLOGY

Asphyxia is defined as a reduced Po_2 and a raised Pco_2 and is usually taken as a measure of respiratory failure. After birth hypoxaemia may occur without hypercarbia and vice versa. There is some evidence that the pattern of blood gases may affect the degree of brain damage (Bakay and Lee, 1968).

Oxygen is required in the cell so that the mitochondria can remove hydrogen ions and produce water, releasing energy. If there is a lack of oxygen then hydrogen ions build up and there is less energy available to the cell. The cell does not die providing that it can get rid of the hydrogen ions by some other means such as forming lactate, and lactate can then be discharged into the circulation. Thus a blood circulation is as important as a supply of oxygen. Ischaemia can devastate the tissues with a rapidly fatal intracellular acidosis. When the pH falls below 6.9 all the enzyme processes producing energy by anaerobic break down of glucose to lactate stop. The cell may die due to the acidosis whilst it still has a supply of energy-rich bonds such as ATP and creatine phosphate. There is a critical circulation even with oxygenated blood below which the lactate and pyruvate concentration will suddenly rise in the venous blood draining the tissue.

Hypoxaemia is said to cause respiratory failure at cellular level when there is a Po_2 less than 8 mmHg. This causes the mitochondrion to swell to several microns in diameter. This with the accumulation of glycogen in the astrocytes is the only histological finding in pure hypoxaemia (Bakay and Lee, 1968; Klatzo, 1967). Experimental evidence from isolated tissues suggest that they withstand hypoxia well. For example, slices of human fetal cerebral cortex resumed 80 per cent of normal oxygen consumption after 1 h of complete anoxia (Villee, 1967). Equally impressive is the observation that neurones survive 2 h perfusion with a red cell free fluid (Lindenberg, 1967).

For anaerobic metabolism a good supply of glucose or glycogen is needed. There are only two high energy rich bonds obtained from glycolysis of glucose to lactate compared with 38 when fully aerobically metabolised. However, it is not an inefficient process for when oxygen is available the liver or placenta can either break down the lactate fully or convert it back to glucose. The reason for the routine administration of glucose and bicarbonate to the asphyxiated infant is to buffer the lactate in the blood and to supply the cells with more glucose substrate to keep them going until aerobic metabolism becomes possible again. There would appear to be more glycogen in fetal than in the adult brain and the brain may also store glucose as glutamate (Jilek et al, 1967). Is is thought that the brain might get much of its energy anaerobically until the late stage in development.

If the cells energy supply fails then the membrane pumps fail so that substances in the cell such as amino acids, potassium, phosphate and magensium leave and other substances such as calcium and sodium enter with corresponding rises or falls in the serum concentrations. The finding that during asphyxia the cell is unable to synthesise protein and that some enzymes are lost may account for the apparent recovery of function after a time.

PATHOLOGY

The form of handicap of the injured child varies and the findings in the brain at autopsy many years after the event are so confusing that all the varieties of brain response must be considered in order to see why an apparent simple generalised insult produces such a miscellany of effects. It is also necessary in order to demonstrate the rationale of treatment during the acute phase. The pathology of the brains of children who have died after years of handicap have been reported to show a wide variety of lesions including ulegryia, status marmoratus, hydrocephalus, porencephaly, cerebral atrophy, Schilder's disease, Alper's disease, hemiatrophy, cystic leucomalacia or discrete changes in the number of neurones in the brain stem such as the cochlear nucleus (Malamud, 1963; Norman, 1963; Myers, 1972; Grunnet et al, 1974; Banker and Larroche, 1962; Courville, 1953). The clinical findings include diplegia, hemiplegia, tetraplegia, choreoathetosis, microcephaly, macrocephaly, mental handicap, epilepsy, speech retardation, clumsy children and hyperkinetic behaviour disorder. There is no simple relationship between asphyxia and brain damage, rather asphyxia sets off a cascade of intermediary pathogenetic mechanisms which may result in a whole range of brain damage.

Selective vulnerability of the brain to hypoxaemia

The developing fetal brain in the early stages is a mass of undifferentiated blast cells, there is no defined blood supply and there are no astrocytes to connect the neurone to its blood supply. The metabolism of the cells must depend upon diffusion and cells are anerobic as shown by the fact that cyanide has no effect at all on brain growth at this stage (Richter, 1967). Cytochrome oxidase only develops late in gestation in the cerebral hemispheres and the same is true for succinic dehydrogenase and ATPase (Himwich, 1958). Thus there is a critical period in development when cerebral hemispheres become sensitive to hypoxia. Dobbing (1974) has emphasised the idea of the brain growth spurt and critical periods of sensitivity to malnutrition. He has emphasised how data on animal experiments are meaningless unless one knows when the brain growth spurt occurs for that particular animal. The same is true for the sensitivity to asphyxia and one cannot extrapolate results from rats, fetal lambs or rhesus monkeys without this data. The guinea-pig at birth has gone through the critical period and is as sensitive to asphyxia as the adult but the rat and dog at birth are much more resistant to asphyxia than the corresponding adult animal (Himwich, 1958).

There is another reason why the newborn brain may be relatively resistant to hypoxia. In the adult brain it is the dendrites which appear to be very sensitive to oxygen lack. There are no dendritic connections in the cerebral hemispheres at birth, the neurones are nude, but in the brain stem they are well developed (Grossman and Williams, 1971).

The concept that in the newborn infant the brain stem is selectively more vulnerable than the relatively underdeveloped cortex is fundamental to our understanding of the symptomatology in the immediate postnatal period (Table 2.8). We are in great debt to workers such as Dr and Mrs Himwich (1958), Flexner, Belknap and Flexner (1953) and Windle (1969) who have provided most of the data in this area. Windle (1969) has shown that in the monkey the sensory brain stem nuclei are most affected.

Table 2.8   Metabolism of human fetal brain
(A) Fetus compared to adult brain

Free L-glutamic acid in mg/dl

Part of brain	20–40 weeks gestation	61–84 years
Cerebral cortex	142	293
Medulla oblongata	261	251
Cerebellum	220	295
Thalamus	215	284

(B) Brain stem compared to cortex (human fetus crown rump 13–16 cm)

	Brain stem	Cerebral cortex
Oxygen consumption	11.9	9.1
CO_2 produced	24.7	29.1
Lactate produced	4.4	4.1
Lactate under anaerobic conditions	9.5	6.2

After Himwich et al, 1955. Units μmol per gram tissue per hour

Damage to these structures is bilateral and symmetrical, the extent varies with the degree of asphyxia. In mild cases the thalamus and inferior colliculi only are affected. In severe cases basal ganglia and cerebellum are involved. Only in very severe cases are the depths of the sulci in the motor strip damaged but in this area there are vascular factors which may be important. The part of the temporal lobe, Ammon's horn, which is very sensitive to asphyxia in the adult is not affected in the infant but the part known as the h2 sector may be severely damaged (Norman, 1963). This was present in 14/17 cases studied by Malamud (1963). If one has the patience to count the neurones in a brain stem nucleus, then after asphyxia they may be shown to be remarkably reduced to less than 20 per cent of the normal number. The neuropathologist is used to looking for gliosis to indicate the area of damage, the infant brain does not always react in this way so changes may be missed on routine examination.

Under four years of age the brain takes about 50 per cent of the body's resting oxygen consumption. Oxygen consumption is not uniform throughout the brain, it is maximum in developing areas. The blood supply increases to an area about to myelinate (Kennedy et al, 1970). The oxygen consumption of grey matter is five times that of white matter (Grote, 1974). Autoradiographic techniques show that the areas most vulnerable to asphyxia have the highest oxygen uptake (Kety, 1963). The oligodendroglia are dividing in the last trimester prior to the phase of rapid myelination, although clinical

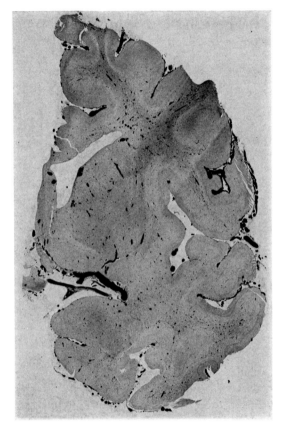

Figure 2.1 Loyez staining for myelin in a celloidin section of human infant's brain at term to show the leg area myelinating before that of the arm

development of the child is from head to leg, myelination occurs in the leg area first and again could be a reason for selective vulnerability of this area (Norman, 1963, Fig. 2.1).

Convulsions are responsible for a grossly increased local blood flow with increased oxygen uptake and lactate production, so again a convulsing part of the brain will be selectively more vulnerable to hypoxaemia. An adequate Po_2 is a prerequisite to convulse and one can start or stop a fit by varying the inspired oxygen (Richter, 1960). This mechanism may be responsible for transient dysfunction, a Todd's paresis, or a permanent hemiplegia.

Ischaemic and vascular lesions

  Systemic hypotension due to acute blood loss may result from an antepartum bleeding from a vasa praevia, a feto-maternal or twin-to-twin bleed, a placental transfusion at birth from holding the infant above the uterus, bleeding from the cord, or secondary bleeding into gut, lungs, intracranial or subgalael due to haemorrhagic disease. An infant may have a true oligaemic shock and this may cause severe brain infarction, with resultant cerebral atrophy. Aicardi, Gontières and Hodebourg De Verbois (1972) described hypotensive infarction in twin-to-twin transfusion as a cause of one type of hydranencephaly. Central circulatory failure due to myocardial depression or necrosis may be the result of asphyxia, the heart is as sensitive as the brain and is put under increased strain because it is called upon to increase its output and do more work due to sympathetic drive trying to increase tissue blood flow under anaerobic conditions. Bradycardia, hypotension and cardiac arrest may then result. The raised serum potassium, low calcium and effect of drugs may also depress myocardial contractility. A bradycardia in utero may represent periods of hypotension and one cannot reiterate strongly enough that ischemia is more dangerous than hypoxaemia—the fetal and infant brain do not have any increased ability to withstand a severe tissue acidosis. External cardiac massage should be commenced in asphyxia pallida even if there is a heart beat. Measurement of blood pressure is probably the most important and least measured parameter in the asphyxiated newborn infant.

  It might be expected that hypotension would have a generalised effect on the brain but here again there is selective vulnerability. Clearly the most metabolically active part of the brain will suffer most from the effects of hypotension. Certain areas are also more subject to ischaemia because of the vascular anatomy and this results in a different pattern of brain damage from that seen in pure asphyxia when the circulation is sustained. The circle of Willis allows an anastomosis between four arteries, these are damped by having a winding course, the vertebral arteries in the foramina of the cervical vertebrae and the carotid arteries in the siphon. There must be areas of no flow where the pressures balance out, otherwise retrograde flow would occur. The vertebral artery flow may change with the position of the neck and so the no-flow areas will change. The arterial territories of the anterior, middle and posterior cerebral arteries are separated and areas between them are called last field or watershed zones (Lindenberg, 1967; Brierley and Meldrum, 1971). In hypotension these areas are more likely to be infarcted. It is thought that these infarctions may occasionally liquidise to form porencephalic cysts (Courville, 1962).

  There is another set of arteries between the surface which penetrate into the brain and a further group from the ventricular surface which penetrate outwards, i.e. the ventriculofugal and the ventriculopetal arteries (Armstrong and Norman, 1974). The watershed zone between these two territories is in the deep white matter and infarction here causes a multicystic leucomalacia; some of the cysts may reach a centimetre or even more (Smith, 1974). This characteristic lesion of perinatal asphyxia is attributed to a failure of perfusion due to hypotension (Banker and Larroche, 1962; Aicardi et al, 1972; Armstrong and Norman, 1974). It may be associated with placental infarction. The presence of an astrocytosis with the presence of macrophages suggests that in some cases it may occur before birth (Armstrong and Norman, 1974). These penetrating vessels will vary in number and size with maturity. As myelination occurs the more central area of white matter becomes more vascular and this may explain why the characteristic lesion of the preterm infant is intraventricular haemorrhage and that in the full-term infant is periventricular leucomalacia. Massive haemorrhage can occur into the infarcted area. In very severe cases one large cavity may form in the white matter on each side so the brain appears to have four lateral ventricles. In mild cases only a reactive astrocytosis of the white matter is seen. It causes thinning of the white matter with compensatory dilatation of the ventricles and gliosis as well as cyst formation. It is postulated that microcephaly, mental handicap and quadriplegia might result.

If the brain is anoxic, the cerebral blood flow is increased, which may in turn increase sympathetic vasomotor tone and lead to a rise in blood pressure. If severe, and we have seen blood pressures in the order of 260/160 in infants only a few weeks old, it may cause a hypertensive encephalopathy with intense protective vasoconstriction and vasculitis as demonstrated by haemorrhages and exudates in the fundi and reduced cerebral blood flow. Blood vessels may also go into spasm due to blood in the CSF causing depletion of catecholamines in the vessel walls and prolonged vasospasm lasting several days. The substance which causes the spasm is not known but blood or xanthochromic CSF applied to the basilar artery in the experimental animal has the same effect. Oxygen toxicity in the fundus causes intense vasoconstriction with retinal ischaemia and then a fibrovascular proliferative phase. Brand and Bignami (1969) showed that there was a marked increase in vessels of up to 400 per cent in the brain stem of asphyxiated human infants, the neurones and glia appeared normal. The possibility arises that a high Po_2 in the cerebral circulation above the level of the ductus arteriosus could be responsible for 'oxygen brain' similar to its effect on lung and retina. We thus have three mechanisms of vasospasm which may shunt blood in different areas.

Cerebral vessels may be occluded by placental emboli (Cocker et al, 1965), emboli from umbilical catheters (Smith et al, 1974), disseminated intravascular coagulation (Hathaway, 1970) and trauma to the vertebral arteries (Yates, 1959), or carotid arteries (Courville, 1962). Polycythaemia from chronic intrauterine asphyxia may increase plasma viscosity to a point necessitating plasmapheresis in order to prevent vascular occlusion. Cerebral blood flow is regulated by the vasomotor tone in the cerebral blood vessels, carbon dioxide can override this and cause widespread cerebral vasodilatation and cerebral congestion which in turn causes a rise in intracranial pressure. Focal brain damage will paralyse the vasomotor tone in the blood vessels to that area so that it has no compensatory mechanism and is vulnerable to any further drop in systemic blood pressure. Blood flow may also be selectively influenced by drugs; general anaesthesia for example will reduce blood flow in grey more than white matter. Carbon dioxide has been held to offer some protection against very severe hypoxaemia by maintaining cerebral blood flow (Gibbs, Gibbs and Lennox, 1943). It should be apparent that hypotension will not only make the asphyxia worse but may focus the target for devastation. Maintenance of the circulation of the asphyxiated infant by the administration of glucose and buffer may be more important because of their effect upon the heart rather than the head.

Towbin (1969) has laid the blame for white matter infarction in the periventricular region and the basal ganglia lesions upon thrombosis of the vein of Galen. Although frequently torn with severe birth trauma, kinking or traumatic thrombosis appear to be rare. We prefer the explanation of Cammermeyer (1958) that the brain is rich in thromboplastin and so damaged areas will drain into the veins of the corresponding area which may then thrombose. Cortical venous thrombosis may be the external hallmark of underlying infarction reflecting effect and not cause.

Cerebral oedema

Raised intracranial pressure may occur in the asphyxiated neonate for a variety of reasons including a space occupying blood clot associated with birth trauma, secondary hydrocephalus, cerebral congestion due to a high P_{CO_2}, excess CSF production and oedema of the brain. Cerebral oedema may be due to albumin leaking out of the vessels into the extracellular space taking water with it, water intoxication or toxic substances such as hexachlorophene or raised metabolites in inborn errors of metabolism (Brown and Habel, 1975). Several of these factors may coexist in the same child. The syndrome of inappropriate antidiuretic hormone secretion with hyponatraemia, a low plasma osmolality and a high urine osmolality is seen in asphyxiated neonates (Feldman, Drummond and Klein, 1970). This may be due to hypothalamic damage to the osmoreceptors resulting in failure to correctly monitor tonicity of the plasma or due to a failure of membrane pumps so that extracellular sodium moves into the cells. Water intoxication readily occurs in the neonate and may be due to the mother or the infant being given excess of 5 per cent dextrose. It can occur also as a rebound phenomenon from hypernatraemia produced by sodium bicarbonate and used to defend the pH.

The brain of the preterm infant is 90 per cent water and at five years white matter is still 70 per cent and grey matter 84 per cent water. Only 2.5 per cent increase in brain water is needed to produce severe odema (Cammermayer,

1958). Autopsy recognition of a swollen brain is aided by estimation of brain water as well as sodium and potassium concentrations when potassium is found to be reduced and sodium increased (Anderson and Belton, 1974). The effect of cerebral oedema is to increase brain volume and this may or may not cause a rise in intracranial pressure. There are two results which are feared, firstly a brain shift with 'coning' and secondly interference with the cerebral circulation. At autopsy the gyri are flat, the dura tense and the ventricles compressed and the brain appears very pale due to squeezing out

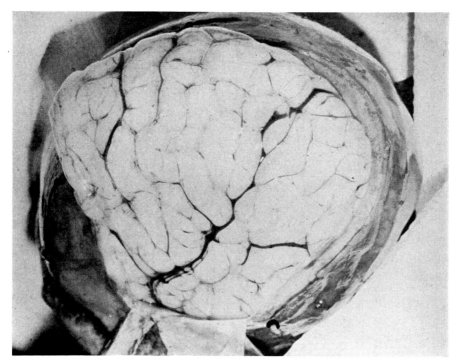

Figure 2.2   Cerebral oedema following perinatal asphyxia to show the brain under pressure and ischaemic with all the vessels compressed and empty

of blood. The blood pressure in the neonate may only be in the order of 50 mmHg and so the perfusion pressure is easily encroached upon. Studies using radioactive labelled antipyrene show that circulation can be arrested regionally in the brain by cerebral oedema (Adamsons and Myers, 1973). Infarction of the brain may cause the 'bag of mush' brain (Courville, 1962). Should the infant survive, severe cerebral atrophy with gross handicap can be expected. Figure 2.2 shows the brain of a neonate extruding under high pressure.

A cone at the level of the tentorium may be seen in the asphyxiated newborn infant with cerebral odema. There is also herniation of the medial portions of the temporal lobe alongside the midbrain. Clinically there may be decerebrate rigidity, sunsetting of the eyes, a change in alertness and changes in respiratory pattern. A cone at the level of the foramen magnum is rarely seen at postmortem examination. This may be because the brain is 90 per cent water and will not mould to show the compression at autopsy, or more likely the child dies from arrest of cerebral circulation before pressures are high enough to be transmitted to the medullary structures. It is difficult with open skull sutures to create high intracranial pressures. It takes only a 10 mmHg difference in pressure between the lateral ventricles and the cysterna magna to produce a cone (Kaufman and Clark, 1970). On the other hand a cone may occur without any rise in pressure simply due to the increase in brain volume (Brierley, 1971). The fontanelle tension cannot be used as a guide to the presence of brain swelling. Methods of monitoring intracranial pressures by non-invasive means such as applantion tonometry need further investigation.

Table 2.9   Types of intracranial haemorrhage seen at autopsy in the neonate (SMMP 1969–72)[a]

		No.	%
Total cases	59		
Mean/year	15		
Incidence	3/1000 births		
Intraventricular haemorrhage		38	65
Subarachnoid haemorrhage (not c̄ IVH)		14	23
Subdural haemorrhage		6	10
Intracerebral haemorrhage (all c̄ SAH)		3	5
Cerebellar haemorrhage		1	2

[a] By courtesy of Dr A. D. Bain and Dr J. A. Anderson

Intracranial haemorrhage

Birth trauma as already outlined may compress the baby's head causing compression of the brain and interference with the circulation so that one gets ischaemia or cerebral oedema. Excess compression causes distortion with traction on blood vessels and dural reflections causing bleeding into the subarachnoid or subdural space. Trauma may predispose to asphyxia and the two states may then be difficult to separate; an echoencephalogram and subdural space aspiration may still be necessary in doubtful cases. The causes of intracranial haemorrhage in a group of infants is shown in Table 2.9. There are two conditions which are associated with asphyxia and cause bleeding into the head, namely intraventricular haemorrhage and secondary haemorrhagic disease. Intracerebral haemorrhage is either due to a subependymal haemorrhage or bleeding into an infarct.

Intraventricular haemorrhage. This is now one of the most important causes of neonatal death. It is the usual cause of death in infants with low birth weight and often occurs after many hours of sweat and toil treating their idiopathic respiratory distress syndrome by artificial ventilation. Since on long-term follow-up the survivors have been found to do so well (Brown, 1973), prevention of intraventricular haemorrhage would reduce the mortality rate and as far as we can tell, it should not increase morbidity. Four out of five deaths from respiratory distress syndrome are due to intraventricular haemorrhage. Infants dying in units with intensive care facilities are more often found to have IVH at autopsy (Anderson, 1975; Grunnet et al, 1974). The incidence is given as 1.1/1000 births by Fedrick and Butler (1970), 2.2/1000 by Sřseň (1966) and the SMMP in 1973 was 2.8/1000 births. The figures will vary depending upon the autopsy rate and those given for the SMMP are for a 90+ per cent autopsy rate by paediatric pathologists.

IVH has no relation to mechanical trauma (Harcke et al, 1972) but is more common after pregnancies complicated by APH and pre-eclamptic toxaemia (Fedrick and Butler, 1970). The infants usually have been in poor condition at birth with variable evidence of intrapartum asphyxia. It is thought that the intrapartum asphyxia may damage the osmophil cells in the lung so that surfactant deficiency and idiopathic respiratory distress syndrome then occurs. Asphyxia in utero is rarely a direct cause of IVH, for only 25 per cent of deaths occur in the first 24 h, the remainder occurring between 24 and 72 h (Harcke et al, 1972). Most cases are associated with the respiratory distress syndrome (Harrison, Heese and Klein, 1968). Our infants were all under 37 weeks gestation (90 per cent are under 34 weeks gestation), 70 per cent are male. It is less common in Negro than Caucasian infants (Spears et al, 1969). An IVH appears to be a response of the immature nervous system to a protracted asphyxiating condition.

Towbin (1969) thought that venous thrombosis in the region of the vein of Galen caused infarction of the periventricular white matter and subsequent haemorrhage. This would not account for discrete unilateral lesions. Clotting defects are common but may antedate or postdate the bleed and prophylactic use of prothrombin complex does not appear to prevent IVH (Turner, 1975). Sodium bicarbonate could produce hypernatraemia and hyperosmolality with shrinkage of the brain and haemorrhage, but this should be subdural and subarachnoid and not be age-dependent and therefore is unlikely to play a part in IVH (Brown et al, 1973). The autopsy incidence of IVH has not changed over the last 10 years in the SMMP during which time the routine use of sodium bicarbonate has been introduced (Anderson et al, 1976). A high P_{CO_2} causing cerebral vasodilatation may be a possible cause but there is no difference between the P_{CO_2} of infants surviving normally, those dying with IVH, and those dying with no IVH, and IVH occurs in infants who have a normal P_{CO_2} (Harrison et al, 1968). A high central venous pressure especially due to intermittent positive pressure ventilation or constant positive airways pressure could cause back pressure and rupture of the delicate subependymal vessels. The subependymal region is very vascular at the age that IVH

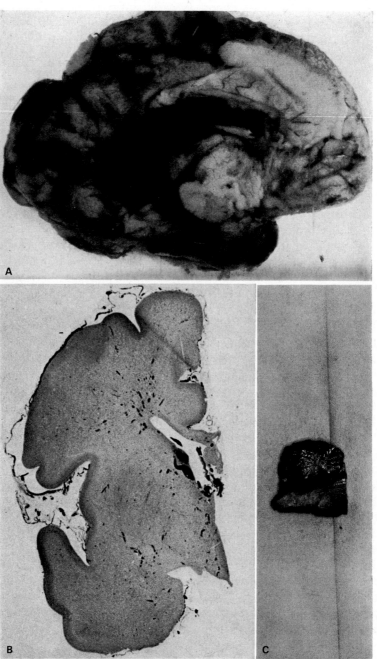

Figure 2.3   Intraventricular haemorrhage.   A, Cast of the lateral ventricle.   B, Vascularity of the subependymal region at 26 weeks gestation.   C, Blood clot in the fourth ventricle and encircling the brain stem

occurs (Fig. 2.3) and at this stage in development there is no myelin in this area to support the blood vessels. Subependymal vessels gradually involute and so the risk lessens with increasing maturity. The area is also a watershed zone and therefore very susceptible to ischaemic infarction. It is desirable therefore to avoid hypotension, a high P_{CO_2}, a high central venous pressure and clotting defects, for all may play a part in maintaining the bleed once it has occurred.

Most bleeds originate in the lateral half of the subependymal matrix in the anterior half of the lateral ventricle; 70 per cent are unilateral (Ross and Dimmette, 1965). They are only rarely seen in the temporal or occipital regions. They are venous in origin from the territory of the transverse caudate vein. Wigglesworth et al (1975) has recently challenged this and thinks the origin may be arterial. The area that they originate from is the last area to be active as germinal plate. The local bleed usually ruptures into the lateral ventricle then via the fourth ventricle into the subarachnoid space. A solid clot may encircle the brain stem, fill the fourth ventricle and give a cast of the lateral ventricles (Fig. 2.3). Occasionally, it dissects out the white matter as well as rupturing into the ventricle and gives a multicystic encephalopathy, (Fig. 2.4). The infant usually dies in the acute stage but if he survives then fibrinolysis occurs and the blood is broken down to chocolate coloured fluid and a secondary communicating hydrocephalus results (Ross and Dimmette, 1965). Occasionally the head of the caudate nucleus is infarcted. There may be an established reaction on histological examination at autopsy suggesting either the bleed occurred some time before death or there was a recent bleed into an area of previous infarction.

Clinically it is difficult to time when the bleed actually occurred. A drop in haemoglobin and haematocrit and evidence of shock from blood loss may help. If one taps the lateral ventricle either nothing may be obtained if the needle enters solid clot, or one may get clear CSF, the bleed being in the opposite ventricle. Echoencephalography will not detect the clot, carotid angiography via the umbilical arterial catheter may be developed in the future. Clinically sudden apnoea may be due to the cause or the effect of the IVH, sudden death is the usual arbiter in diagnosis. A tense fontanelle is unusual (4 out of 30 cases; Ross and Dimmette, 1965), fits are rare in the immature infant but tonic fits may be seen in up to one-third of infants at sometime during the course of the disease. Apathy, diminished moro and tendon reflexes or hypotonia are as likely to be due to the asphyxia which caused the bleed. The difficulty in diagnosing a mild non-fatal bleed means that it is impossible to disprove claims that the spastic diplegia of low birth weight is due to IVH (Churchill, Carleton and Berendes, 1970). One would have to perform diagnostic lumbar puncture with spectrophotometry of the CSF on every infant less than 37 weeks with an asphyxial episode.

Secondary haemorrhagic disease. Primary haemorrhagic disease of the newborn is due to vitamin K deficiency and is unusual now that prophylactic vitamin K is used routinely. We are not concerned here with the specific genetically determined clotting defects such as haemophilia or Christmas disease (factor VIII and IX deficiency). In infants who have been severely asphyxiated and especially those with a period of hypotension, a secondary disorder of clotting occurs. There is a deficiency in the prothrombin complex normally made in the liver with a prolonged prothrombin time, there is a reduction in platelets, a reduction in fibrinogen, a prolonged partial thromboplastin time and in many cases elevated fibrin degradation products (Hatha-

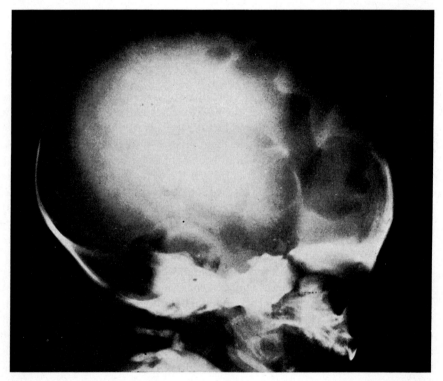

Figure 2.4 Subependymal haemorrhage dissecting white matter to produce a multicystic leucomalacia

way, 1970). This has given rise to the notion that the infant is suffering from disseminated intravascular coagulation (DIC). There is no doubt that DIC occurs in the newborn with severe rhesus isoimmunisation or septicaemia (Chessells and Wigglesworth, 1970). In true DIC there is clotting within the vascular compartment and so infarction of the tissue distal to the block will occur. This is especially likely in the kidney causing renal failure but may also occur in the head so that for example acute hemiplegia may develop in the haemolytic uraemic syndrome or septicaemia. The treatment for true DIC is to give heparin. In the asphyxiated neonate there is tissue infarction

Table 2.10   Intermediary pathogenetic mechanisms in the genesis of asphyxial brain damage and the theoretical clinical implications

Intermediary mechanism	Pathology	Clinical implications
Cerebral oedema		
Tentorial cone	Temporal lobe ischaemia	Temporal lobe epilepsy
	Midbrain and brainstem infarction or haemorrhage	Abnormal eye movements, ataxia, bulbar paresis
Cerebral circulation impaired	Cerebral atrophy	Mental handicap, microcephaly, epilepsy, tetraplegia
Subarachnoid haemorrhage	Block arachnoid granulations	Communicating hydrocephalus	Big head, ataxia, mild diplegia, clumsy child
Intraventricular haemorrhage	Hydrocephalus	Big head, ataxia, mild diplegia, clumsy child
	Subependymal cystic dissection	Hemiplegia, mental defect, tetraplegia
	Infarction in caudate and white matter leg area	Dystonia/diplegia choreoathetosis
Selective vulnerability	Ammon's horn	Temporal lobe epilepsy
	Cerebellar atrophy	Ataxia—truncal
	Status marmoratus of basal ganglia	Dystonia/choreoathetosis
	Brainstem nuclei	Squint, ataxia, bulbar palsy
	Thalamus	Lack attention, hyperkinetic behaviour
	Vertex myelination	Diplegia
	Convulsing brain	Hemiplegia
Ischaemia		
Severe generalised	Cerebral atrophy	Mental handicap, microcephaly, infantile spasms, epilepsy, spastic tetraplegia
Focal watershed	Anterior	Hemiplegia
	Posterior	Visuospatial problems, verbal performance discrepancies, schooling problems
Occlusion	Porencephaly, unilateral atrophy, ulegyria	Hemiplegia, epilepsy, schooling problems
Polycythaemia, trauma, DIC, embolus, compression, vasospasm		
Central watershed	Periventricular leucomalacia	Mental handicap, tetraplegia, diplegia, cerebral atrophy, microcephaly
	Schilder's sudanophilic dystrophy	Mental handicap, tetraplegia, diplegia, cerebral atrophy, microcephaly, progressive deterioration
	Alper's disease	Onset of fits about six months, with deterioration

3

in the brain, liver, kidney, adrenal and myocardium. There is also a true clinical haemorrhagic diathesis with bleeding into the head, gut, kidney and lung which one would feel should be treated. There is however no evidence at autopsy for disseminated arteriolar lesions, there are no glomerular lesions (Anderson, Brown and Cockburn, 1974). It would appear that the asphyxia and hypotension causes tissue death from infarction and that thromboplastin released from the damaged tissues causes local intravascular coagulation especially in the veins. There is therefore a consumption of coagulation factors, the asphyxial liver necrosis preventing them being replenished so that one has a consumption coagulopathy with localised intravascular coagulation secondary to tissue death. The presence of a coagulation defect especially one which returns after treatment is good evidence for widespread tissue damage and a bad prognosis (Turner, 1976). It should not be treated with heparin or fatal bleeding may occur into the brain, it should be corrected with fibrinogen, as cryoprecipitate, platelets and prothrombin factor complex. Secondary subarachnoid haemorrhage, a late subdural haematoma from a mild tentorial laceration or maintenance of intraventricular bleeding may all otherwise be seen (Visudhiphan et al, 1974). Adrenal haemorrhage due to haemorrhagic venous infarction of the adrenal gland causes a picture reminiscent of the Waterhouse–Friderichsen syndrome associated with meningococcal septicaemia. There is no way of diagnosing adrenal insufficiency during the acute stage as electrolyte estimations are affected by so many other factors in the asphyxiated infant that sodium and potassium concentrations may be high or low. This is another reason for considering the use of steroids in the severely asphyxiated neonate. Bleeding into the CSF may cause blocking of the arachnoid granulations and a secondary communicating hydrocephalus.

SUMMARY OF PATHOLOGY

The apparently random pathology attributed to perinatal asphyxia can all be explained depending upon which group of pathogenetic mechanisms occurs in that particular child. These are summarised in Table 2.10, and the theoretically possible clinical syndromes which may accompany the pathology is also shown. We shall see in the next section whether this concurs with the actual observed clinical state of the child. Although the obstetrician may not be able to prevent every antepartum haemorrhage or cord prolapse, a knowledge of the intermediary pathology does encourage the paediatrician to be more active in his management of the infant in the hope that further brain damage might be prevented.

REFERENCES

References are at the end of the next chapter (p.83).

3
INFANTS DAMAGED DURING BIRTH
Perinatal Asphyxia
J. K. Brown

In the previous chapter the difficulty in detecting intrauterine asphyxia with the methods currently available has been mentioned. Asphyxia may be present and not be recognised and, on the other hand, some of the investigations may give abnormal results without asphyxia being present. After birth, asphyxia can be recognised by the infant's breathing pattern and colour and the diagnosis is easily confirmed by blood analysis. For the present discussion we are concerned primarily with the recognition of the presence of cerebral asphyxia. Cerebral asphyxia may be suspected if there are abnormal symptoms or behaviour, abnormalities on neurological examination, abnormalities of the electroencephalogram, abnormalities of the cerebrospinal fluid or defects in body homeostasis.

THE SHORT-TERM EFFECTS OF PERINATAL ASPHYXIA

Abnormal symptoms or behaviour
There is evidence to suggest that at birth the brain stem is the part of the brain most sensitive to asphyxia. The neurological responses and the behaviour of the baby is mainly mediated by the brain stem. Significant cerebral asphyxia is unlikely to occur without it being easily detected clinically. It should be possible therefore to screen out infants at risk and identified infants could then be monitored intensely and actively treated in the hope of preventing at least to some degree any subsequent handicap. What abnormalities should we seek? The neonate has a relatively limited repertoire of symptoms and signs so very few will be specific indices of brain injury. Natelson and Sayers (1973) felt that apathy, pallor, absent Moro reflex, respiratory abnormality, poor sucking, a third nerve palsy and a bulging fontanelle constituted the clinical pattern with worst outlook. Craig (1950) reviewed the literature and again gives poor cry, tense fontanelle, hypertonicity, apathy, abnormal respiration, irritability, nystagmus, poor sucking, fits and an anxious scowling expression as the significant abnormalities.

De Souza and Milner (1974) found apnoeic attacks, absent Moro reflex and feeding difficulty were related to a poor prognosis. Amiel-Tison (1969) found in 41 babies studied intensely and followed up subsequently that fits, irritability, abnormal muscle tone, abnormal reflexes, abnormal eye signs, decreased consciousness level, abnormal respiration and signs of raised intra-cranial pressure were most significant. Schulte, Michaelis and Filipp (1965) felt that convulsions, coma and hemisyndromes represented true central nervous system syndromes whilst other abnormalities could be due to drugs or metabolic defects. Schulte summarises the abnormal behaviour patterns as hypertonia/hypotonia, hemisyndrome, coma, convulsions. Ewerbeck (1971) divides symptomatology from perinatal asphyxia into three grades. In slight hypoxic damage the infant is excitable, hyperreflexic, cries a lot, sleeps less and has nystagmus. With moderate hypoxia the infant is apathetic with hypotonia, poor sucking, diminished reflexes and unblinking eyes. In severe asphyxia, coma is accompanied by hypotonia, hemisyndromes, and an EEG which is flat or epileptic. Thorn (1969) in her excellent monograph says that symptoms are more frequent with asphyxia than trauma and there are more of them. Respiratory difficulties after birth with hypotonia and poor feeding together with fits, tremor and rigidity are noted to be common. She feels that fits with cyanotic attacks have a particularly bad prognosis. Donovan, Coves and Paine (1962) found that abnormalities such as tendon reflexes, presence of ankle clonus, blink to light, startle response, ATNR, grasp reflexes, etc., had no prognostic significance. Many of their observations were ones which are 'state' dependent such as stepping reflexes, feeding reflexes, spontaneous movements and these may be reduced or absent in the normal contented baby.

It can be seen that on the whole there is very good general agreement. Not every infant with abnormal behaviour or neurological findings will be abnormal in later childhood. Our own findings (Brown et al, 1972, 1974) are in agreement with most of these authors and especially the grading presented by Ewerbeck (1971).

With the present organisation of maternity services it is easier to separate those abnormalities which may be noted by nursing staff in order to select out the infant and those which are the result of a medical examination of the infant's nervous system. There are eight abnormalities which nursing staff may note: convulsions, apathy, hypothermia, apnoeic or cyanotic attacks, feeding difficulty, vomiting, cerebral cry, or jitteriness with irritability. The nurses will of course often bring an infant to medical attention because he is too floppy or too stiff but this is better discussed in relation to other neurological findings. One observation which is difficult to quantitate in routine clinical practice is the amount and type of sleep. It can be monitored over a 24-h period with a cerebral function monitor once the infant has been selected as being abnormal but clearly this is not practicable for all infants with a history of asphyxia. In most centres every infant with a history of fetal distress, a low Apgar score or the need for resuscitation will be admitted to a special care baby unit for 24 h. The nurses in these units are highly trained and will very soon recognise any infant with abnormal behaviour. It should be remembered that only a small percentage of infants with fetal distress will show abnormal behaviour after birth. Those infants with a history of intra-partum asphyxia and subsequently showing abnormal behaviour and neuro-logical signs we refer to as 'symptomatic neonatal asphyxia'.

Convulsions. Convulsions occur as a symptom in 50 per cent of cases, a fit is unusual under 37 weeks so that the asphyxiated preterm infant has a fit much less commonly than the infant at term. The fits may be focal clonic 'Jacksonian' type, generalised clonic or tonic in nature (Brown, 1973). They may be directly due to asphyxia or secondary to hypoglycaemia (12 per cent), hypocalcaemia (20 per cent), intracranial haemorrhage, water intoxication (5 per cent) or associated birth trauma. Treatment will depend upon whether any of these mechanisms are present. Status epilepticus may occur when further severe brain damage may arise not only from interference with ventilation but also by consumptive asphyxia; the 'fitting' part of the brain has a very high oxygen consumption. Post-convulsive brain swelling will further increase brain damage. Fits usually occur within 48 h of delivery, but because oxygen is necessary in order to maintain a fit they are rarely seen in the labour ward during resuscitation.

Apathy. It is difficult to know if a neonate is aware of 'self' and his surround-ings and therefore conscious in the way we understand it in older patients. We cannot test the infant's response to speech or painful stimulation nor assess the appropriateness of his response and so we speak of degrees of arousal or alertness rather than consciousness. The state of alertness of the infant may be graded according to Prechtl's five states (Prechtl and Beintema, 1964), alternatively into sleep (REM, and quiet), normoalert, hyperalert, hypoalert and apathetic states. The hyperalert infant is the ravenously hungry baby on the go all the time, the warm, dry, recently fed infant is usually hypoalert. Apathy or extreme lethargy is an abnormal state and is not seen in a normal infant (Fig. 3.1), there is no spontaneous movement and no response to touching the cheek with a teat, pinching the infant or giving him injections; Moro reflex and walking reflexes are usually absent as well. Fifty per cent of cases of cerebral asphyxia are apathetic but this is never the only clinical finding.

Hypothermia. We found a temperature of 95° or less to be present in 33 per cent of cases. Many mechanisms may be involved. Excess heat may be lost during resuscitation, the heat production tissues may not receive sufficient oxygen, asphyxia may directly damage the central nervous mechanisms controlling body temperature, or an intracranial haemorrhage or asphyxia may cause intense vasoconstriction and thus impair the response to cold (Bruck et al, 1962). In severe asphyxia loss of temperature control may be permanent, the infant remains poikilothermic and severely handicapped. Lagos and Siekert (1969) state that hyperthermia is a common accompani-ment of intracranial, especially intraventricular, haemorrhage in the newborn, but this has not been our experience.

Apnoeic or cyanotic attacks. Apnoeic and/or cyanotic attacks occurred in

66 per cent of our affected infants. Again apnoeic attacks may be due to many causes such as immaturity, respiratory distress, convulsions (Schulte and Jurgens, 1969), as well as intraventricular haemorrhage or hypoglycaemia. These must be borne in mind and respiratory abnormalities not dismissed as 'brain damage'. In the infants mentioned above immaturity and postnatal respiratory disorders were uncommon, most were full-term infants with intrauterine asphyxia.

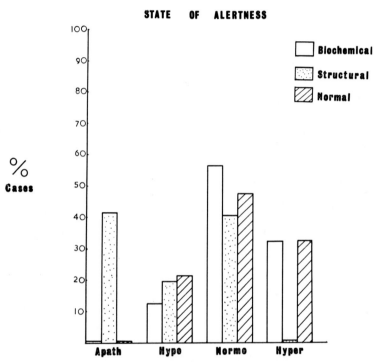

Figure 3.1   Comparison of the 'state of alertness' of three groups of infants, normal infants, those with biochemical fits (neonatal tetany) and those with structural brain damage from asphyxia or trauma

Other abnormal respiratory patterns may be seen in the neonate, e.g. the brain stem syndrome, central neurogenic hyperventilation, Cheyne Stokes breathing and gasping. In the brain stem syndrome with loss of CO_2 response, a high inspired oxygen concentration may cause apnoea, the environmental temperature may also induce apnoea if it is too high. Bradycardia may accompany 'physiological' apnoea of preterm infants and both are more likely to occur in non-eye movement sleep when they may appear at times to accompany the suppression bursts on the EEG of the tracé alternans (Deuel, 1973). Raised intracranial pressure may be signalled by a change in respiratory pattern (Moody, Ruamsuke and Mullan, 1969), and it may also cause pulmonary oedema (Balf, 1952).

Central neurogenic hyperventilation occurs in asphyxiated neonates especially if they have blood in the CSF, the respiratory rate gradually increases to 100/min with a true central drive so that the Pco_2 can be as low as 20 mmHg. There is an alkalosis and a normal Po_2; as the respiratory rate rises the tidal volume eventually approaches dead space volume and ventilatory failure, CO_2 retention then occurs (Brown and Habel, 1975).

Abnormal feeding. Feeding difficulties as indicated by the need to tube feed was the commonest abnormality in the mature asphyxiated infant. It was present in 76 out of 94 infants with cerebral asphyxia. It was associated with apnoeic and cyanotic attacks in 70 per cent, apathy in 60 per cent and convulsions in 45 per cent. There is a depression of the rhythmic bursts of sucking as well as suppression of the coordination of the individual reflexes, e.g. rooting, sucking, stripping, swallowing, arrest of respiration, closing glottis, initiation of oesophageal peristalsis which produce feeding behaviour as opposed to feeding reflexes. Aspiration occurs if respiration does not cease and the larynx does not close.

Vomiting. Although vomiting is often a major feature of neurological disease in older children it is surprising how rarely persistent vomiting is a major problem in the asphyxiated infant (8 per cent). It is more common in the infant with a mild compression head injury.

Cerebral cry. The irritable infant who resents handling, and lies curled up so that loud noise, bright light or rough movements cause a high pitched shrieking cry is again more characteristic of the infant with a headache from head compression or blood in the CSF. A severely asphyxiated infant does not cry at all.

Jitteriness. This is not the same as irritability but means tremor of the limbs upon movement which can be spontaneous or reflex, for example, associated with a Moro reflex. It is nearly always accompanied with brisk tendon jerks and ankle, knee and jaw clonus (Fig. 3.2). It is of no significance in isolation especially if muscle tone is normal. It may occur with excess hunger and hypoglycaemia (hunger drive), with thirst and hypernatraemia (thirst drive), due to peripheral hyperexcitability in hypocalcaemia or hypomagnesaemia, in the infant of the thyrotoxic mother or from drug withdrawal as in the mother taking barbiturates or narcotic drugs. The infant tends to be in the hyperalert state rather than apathetic. Monosynaptic reflexes recover before tonic reflex activity, so jitteriness may occur with hypotonia in the recovery period. It was found in 37 per cent of infants with perinatal asphyxia.

Neurological findings

It is easier in clinical practice to think in terms of 'patterns' of abnormality rather than a score system of abnormal signs. Since muscle tone is related to many of the other neurological abnormalities, the other neurological findings are considered in relationship to muscle tone. We recognise six patterns of muscle tone in the asphyxiated infants, hypotonia, transition from hypotonia to extensor hypertonus (decerebration), extensor hypertonus, normal flexor tone commensurate with gestational age, an asymmetry of muscle tone, i.e. a hypertonic or a hypotonic hemisyndrome and regression in muscle tone so that the infant behaves as if immature, for example the arms are more hypotonic than the legs. Very rarely a seventh pattern is seen in infants maintained on ventilation, when return to a very primitive spinal flexor muscle tone may be found.

Hypotonia. These infants are floppy and lie in posture in which they are placed. There is no recoil in arms or legs, no shoulder righting and no adduction in arms or legs. The infant either lies in the pithed frog position with

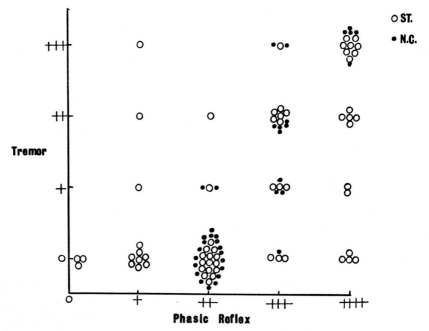

Figure 3.2 The relationship of tendon reflexes (phasic reflexes) with tremor in normal infants (NC) and those with asphyxial or traumatic births (ST)

arms abducted at the side of the head, or with the arms extended by the side (Fig. 3.3). There is marked head lag in the pull to sit movement, in the prone position the legs are not flexed and abducted under the abdomen as in a full-term infant but abducted sideways. The popliteal angle often approaches 180 degrees and the heels can be placed behind the ears with ease. There is no traction response in the arms with the grasp reflexes. The asymmetrical tonic neck reflex, trunk incurvation and Perez reflexes are usually difficult to elicit. The infant is usually apathetic (84 per cent) and shows little spontaneous movement. Moro is absent (43 per cent) or shows tonic abduction without a flexion and adductor phase. Progression reflexes such as walking, stepping and crawling are usually absent. Feeding reflexes are absent apart from spontaneous rhythmic sucking movements which appear in bursts. Ophthalmoplegia as shown by absent labyrinthine reflexes, conjugate spasm of the eyes, skew deviations or bilateral sixth nerve weakness are common (37 per cent). The pupils are usually pinpoint rather than dilated. Bulbar palsy as shown by absent gag and cough reflex and pooling of saliva may be present (40 per cent). This may persist later with long-term feeding difficulty and is not simply a function of conscious level. Asymmetry of tone, reflexes

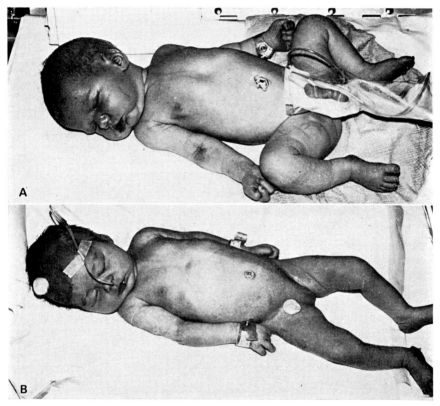

Figure 3.3 Hypotonia, (A) mild, arms extended by the sides, loss of adduction; (B) severe, no tone in arms or legs

or spontaneous movements may be present. The tendon reflexes at this stage may be very easily elicited with ankle clonus.

One of three things may then happen. The infant may remain hypotonic for several days and then gradually regain tone in the lower limbs and like an immature baby gradually return to neonatal flexion over a week or two. Secondly, it may go on to an extensor phase after about 12 h. Thirdly, it may go into a severe hypotonic phase which is often fatal.

Severe hypotonic phase. In the severe hypotonic phase tonic convulsions may occur, and there is often an associated loss of homeostasis with hypo-thermia, hypoglycaemia, hypocalcaemia, a consumption coagulopathy and an inappropriate secretion of antidiuretic hormone. Apnoeic attacks and tonic convulsions may be provoked by handling. The brain stem reflexes are 'cut off' from higher centres, rhythmic sucking movements may occur, and respiration becomes gasping in type. Stimulation of the mouth produces pouting with the orbicularis oris muscle kept in tonic contraction like an 'anal

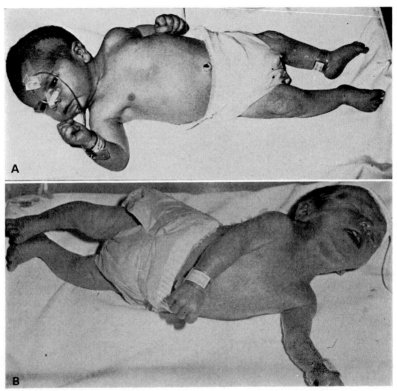

Figure 3.4   Extensor hypertonus: (A) moderate, legs extended with obligatory ATNR; (B) severe, opisthotonus with doggy paddling movements in the arms. (Reproduced by permission of the Editor of *Developmental Medicine and Child Neurology*)

sphincter'. The tendon reflexes disappear. Inspiration may cause tonic fits. Pressure on the nose may provoke inspiration and tonic extension of the limbs. Between these tonic episodes there is no muscle tone, the infant is profoundly hypotonic and arreflexic with little or no spontaneous movement other than convulsive or myotatic responses. Death is the rule in infants who enter this stage. If the infants are being supported by ventilation it may be difficult to decide when death has occurred.

Hypotonia to extension. After a varying period of 12 to 48 h, rarely longer, the infant who has been hypotonic shows changes. The asymmetrical tonic neck reflexes and the trunk incurvation reflexes appear (69 per cent). The tendon reflexes are usually brisk and the infant may be jittery (47 per cent). Extensor tone begins to appear and at first this may be asymmetrical so that one is not sure if one side is stiff or the other floppy (34 per cent). Both legs become rigidly extended with big toes extended (spontaneous Babinski) reaction (Fig. 3.4). Cycling movements may occur in the legs and 'doggy paddling' movements in the arms. Ophthalmoplegia (34 per cent) and bulbar palsy (43 per cent) with defects in homeostasis may still be a problem. Signs suggestive of raised intracranial pressure such as splaying of the sutures, distension of the scalp veins and a tense fontanelle appear in some infants (43 per cent) at this time and frank papilloedema may occasionally be seen. The infant may vary from lying with obligatory ATNR in the arms and extended legs to total opisthotonus. The infant may develop further central respiratory problems and die, or the hypertonus may gradually lessen over the next week to leave an infant showing signs of regression, that is, muscle tone pattern of a much more immature infant. This then improves until by about three weeks the infant may appear like a normal term infant. He may still need tube feeding.

Extensor hypertonus. These are infants who already show extensor hypertonus at the time of presentation with abnormal symptoms (Fig. 3.4). Extensor hypertonus is more evident in the legs than the arms, the extensor reflexes are brisk and the infants are more alert and show no evidence of bulbar palsy or ophthalmoplegia. The Moro response is usually present but may be held in tonic extension for 5 to 10 s. The infant is often jittery (56 per cent) with very brisk tendon reflexes (60 per cent) and ankle clonus. This stage may represent cerebral oedema or so-called postasphyxial rigidity.

Normal flexor tone. These infants have muscle tone appropriate to their gestational age as measured from the last menstrual period dates and from examination of cutaneous and general characteristics. The extensor reflexes are difficult to elicit and are never obligatory. Severe cranial nerve palsies are not present. Tendon reflexes tend to be neither exaggerated nor reduced. Moro is usually present and the infants are in the normally alert state. Hemi-syndromes either persisting more than 24 h or transient can occur in association with any of the patterns of muscle tone. The long-term prognosis in this group is very good.

Death on a ventilator

The infant will usually either have sustained a massive intraventricular haemorrhage or be in the severely hypotonic stage of intrapartum asphyxia. It is not ethical to leave junior medical staff, who are usually responsible for initial resuscitation, to decide whether or not to be 'active'. Our policy has always been that one treats all infants as intensively as possible not constantly worrying whether one was 'keeping alive a cabbage'. Half-hearted attempts to treat such as 'do everything but ventilate' may cause a child to survive with even more handicap. A decision is made, it must be to treat fully or not to treat at all, and if the latter then one has a moral duty to see that the child does not survive. We find that a diagnosis of 'failed resuscitation' can be more easily made after a period of intensive treatment rather than at of the moment after birth or of a catastrophe. Ventilation and support systems can be turned off when there appears to be cerebral death. Respiration may be absent or there may be terminal gasping, there will be an internal and an external ophthalmoplegia, that is no eye movements and no pupil reactions. Eye movements can be obtained by turning the babies head from side to side to get the doll's eye responses, rotating the whole baby for labyrinthine responses, and by caloric tests which are the easiest in infants on ventilators. Iced water is gently syringed in either ear to see if any eye movements occur (Plum and Posner, 1972). There should be no muscle tone, no spontaneous movement and no primitive reflexes (Moro, asymmetrical or tonic neck reflexes). Tendon reflexes will usually be absent. Muscles may contract on direct percussion, these myotatic responses may be confusing to the unwary. Lower cranial nerve function will be absent as shown by absent feeding reflexes, no sucking, no gag reflex, no cough and intubation is possible with the absence of tone in the floor of the mouth or tongue. There are certain neurological findings which may be retained in the profoundly brain-damaged infant. There may be a flexor withdrawal reflex in the leg after pinprick, the abdominal reflexes may be present together with myotatic responses described above, the foot may plantar flex on stimulation but must not show extension, the ankle jerk may be present (Ivan, 1973). Occasionally the small infant may not become profoundly hypotonic but shows a return of spinal flexion activity and this is confusing as one may think that it represents improvement. The EEG must be completely flat at high gain and with a lack of interference. Caloric testing must show absence of eye movements, atropine can sometimes be given to show that there is no vagotonia acting upon the heart and so there will be no acceleration. CSF lactic acid may be very high (Paulson, Wise and Conkle, 1972). Steiner and Neligan (1975) have recently provided us with some very useful practical data. They have shown that in the case of severely asphyxiated infants with a cardiac arrest at birth, if one restores the heart beat and then if spontaneous respiration is not restored within half an hour, the prognosis is very poor with gross handicap if the child survives. This would appear therefore to be a reasonable time to strive, in our own cases no infants in this group who were ventilated for a longer period did in fact survive.

Electroencephalography

The EEG is a sensitive indicator of acute cerebral hypoxia but is not a good guide to long-term prognosis. It is suggested that the reticular system is particularly susceptible to asphyxia (Golubeva, Elizarova and Farber, 1963); this is due to its multiple synapses and may account for the grouping together of the depressed EEG, feeding reflexes, breathing and reduced muscle tone as they are all mediated by the reticular formation. It is thought that the EEG flattens when the Po_2 falls to 20 to 40 mmHg (Fig. 3.5A) (Roberton, 1969); this is not invariable as can be seen from Figure 3.5B and 3.5C. The EEG may show asymmetry confirming that asphyxia can affect one hemisphere more than another and it may also show frank epileptic activity (Fig. 3.5D).

Defects in homeostasis

The brain monitors the milieu interieux by means of the carotid and aortic chemo and baroreceptors together with the receptors in hypothalamus and area postrema in the brain itself. By this means the blood pressure, heart rate, blood volume, plasma osmolality, temperature, blood pH, Pco_2, Po_2 and blood glucose are monitored and adjusted within fine limits via the autonomic nervous system and the hypothalamopituitary axis (Brown et al, 1972; Brown and Habel, 1975). In brain damage these systems may be disrupted leading to respiratory, temperature and cardiovascular abnormalities (Joseph, 1967), and also biochemical abnormalities like hypoglycaemia, hypoosmolality and hyponatraemia. Two other major defects in homeostasis are hypocalcaemia without hyperphosphatasia occurring in the first 48 h of life in 30 per cent of infants, and secondary haemorrhagic disease. All these parameters must be monitored and treated in the management of the asphyxiated neonate (Table 3.1).

Cerebrospinal fluid

Spectrophotometry of the cerebrospinal fluid for methaemoglobin, oxyhaemoglobin and bilirubin concentration should be performed if the fluid is bloodstained (Hellström and Kjellin, 1971). The enzyme creatine phosphokinase in the CSF is independent of blood concentration and can be a useful non-specific guide to brain damage (Belton, 1970). Thromboplastin may be released into the CSF and estimation of fibrin degradation products could also be useful as an indicator of brain damage (Anderson and Brown, 1972). The amino acids of brain are normally different from those in CSF and in the presence of brain damage the amino acid pattern of CSF changes to resemble more approximately that of the brain (Cockburn et al, 1975). The concentration of inorganic phosphate in CSF has also been considered to be of help and concentrations in the CSF of other enzymes such as lactic dehydrogenase and transaminases have also been used to indicate acute destruction of brain tissue (Lending, Slobody and Mestern, 1964).

Finally we must look at the acid base status of CSF. Carbon dioxide will diffuse easily from CSF to blood and vice versa, bicarbonate and lactate diffuse very slowly as does the hydrogen ion. The 'wonder' membrane within the head is the very vascular, very thin, arachnoid mater, this membrane can hold an osmotic gradient of 50 mosmol across it and also a sizeable hydrogen ion gradient. It is not known what mechanism controls arachnoid permeability, there must be some active transport system (Posner, Swanson and Plum,

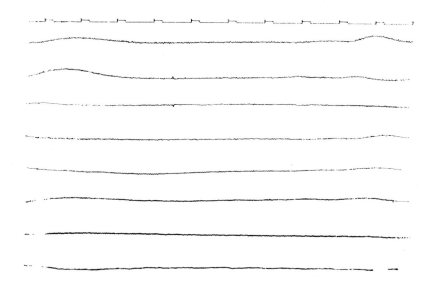

Y.R. I

Figure 3.5   (A) Flat EEG in severe neonatal asphyxia—eventful severe cerebral palsy

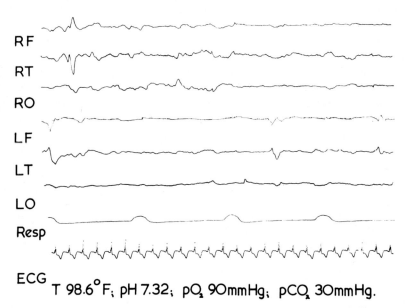

RF

RT

RO

LF

LT

LO

Resp

ECG   T 98.6°F; pH 7.32; pO_2 90mmHg; pCO_2 30mmHg.

Figure 3.5   (B) Activity with normal blood gases-respiration sustained by artificial ventilation

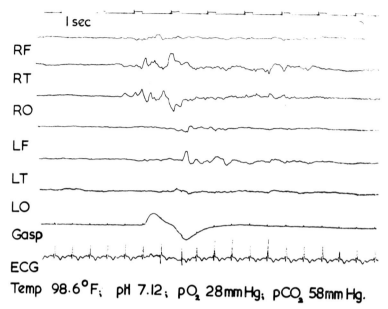

Figure 3.5 (C) Terminal gasping with hypoxia and acidosis and yet still EEG activity

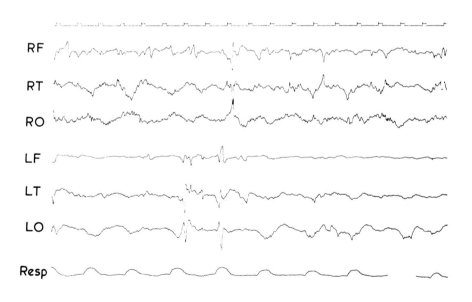

Figure 3.5 (D) Epileptic activity with asymmetrical brain damage from asphyxia

1965). The CSF Pco_2 is under normal conditions 9 mm more than that of arterial blood and the CSF pH is 0.10 unit less, with a mean of 7.31. Since there is no buffering power in CSF the pH will depend simply upon Pco_2 and HCO_3 concentrations or lactic acid production. If CO_2 diffuses into the CSF from a raised blood Pco_2 then the pH will change rapidly: if bicarbonate is then gradually produced to compensate for this and the child is subse-

Table 3.1   Management of the infant with established cerebral asphyxia

1. Nurse the infant in incubator, in neutral thermal environment; severe cases may be poikilothermic and require thermocouple with feedback.
2. Monitor apnoea with inspired oxygen 40 per cent if there are cyanotic attacks and adjust with blood gas tensions. Ventilate if (a) Po_2 not raised with raising F_{IO2}, (b) if high Pco_2 causing further cerebral vasodilation and congestion, (c) if pH cannot be controlled.
3. Fits and changes in colour are best seen if infant nursed naked. Phenobarbitone, 8 mg/kg/24 h, if no metabolic cause—theoretically also helps protect brain against hypoxia Phenytoin 5 mg/kg stat, then 8 mg/kg/24 h, no use i.m. must be given i.v., if fits continue after phenobarbitone. Status controlled by lignocaine or diazepam. Do not leave in status because of a theoretical risk of bilirubin binding.
4. Control raised intracranial pressure—if acute, give 20 per cent mannitol 7 ml/kg over 20 min, remember this is controlled dehydration and limit fluids to 75 ml/kg, only gradually increasing or will get rebound. Dexamethasone 2–4 mg stat and 1–2 mg 4 or 6 hourly dependent upon severity, tailed off after 48 h. Steroids also indicated as stabilise lysosomal membranes and there may be adrenal haemorrhage with insufficiency.
5. Monitor blood pressure and for cardiac arrhythmias—transfuse if hypotensive.
6. Check serum calcium as hypocalcaemia may occur in first 24 h usually with normal phosphorus, causing fits and cardiac arrythmias. Calcium given as electrolyte cocktail (Cockburn, 1976), i.v.
7. Test 4 hourly with Dextrostix and give glucose as bolus if hypoglycaemic. Give electrolyte cocktail which contains 10 per cent glucose if cyanotic or apnoeic attacks to provide adequate substrate for anaerobic glycolysis. Avoid water intoxication by not giving 5 per cent dextrose (avoid fructose because of possible severe metabolic acidosis).
8. Keep pH well buffered with sodium bicarbonate, monitor serum sodium, THAM theoretically better in treating cellular acidosis since HCO_3 is an extracellular ion. Beware of Posner effect.
9. Beware acute water intoxication with inappropriate ADH secretion, limit fluid in first 24 h to 75–100 ml/kg. If acute water intoxication treat with frusmide and mannitol.
10. Coagulation screen for consumption coagulopathy—no heparin, replace deficiencies by fibrinogen (as cryoprecipitate; fresh frozen plasma of little use due to large volume needed), platelet transfusion, prothrombin complex, vitamin K, whole blood.
11. Intracranial haemorrhage—echoencephalogram and exploration of subdural space. Cysternal puncture and release of CSF or ventricular puncture to lower intracranial pressure. Check coagulation screen, give prophylactic vitamin K and treat as above.
12. Beware development of hydrocephalus which may require twice daily ventricular aspiration or a Rickham reservoir until bood cleared prior to shunt procedure.
13. If in a 'metabolic mess' with hyperkalaemia, hypocalcaemia, acidosis difficult to control and large amounts of sodium bicarbonate already given, renal hypoxia with raised urea, perform exchange transfusion with fresh blood.

quently hyperventilated, the CO_2 will be removed from the CSF but not the bicarbonate so there will be an acute alkalotic change in pH. Equally if a large dose of bicarbonate is given intravenously to raise blood pH it will produce a marked hydrogen ion gap between blood and CSF so lowering CSF pH and raising that of blood. At a CSF pH of less than 7.15 coma results, and a Posner encephalopathy occurs (Posner et al, 1965; Posner and Plum, 1967). A respiratory acidosis will rapidly lower CSF pH whilst a metabolic acidosis may have no effect on it at all. Theoretically sodium bicarbonate has two possible hazards; firstly, the risk of producing an osmolar gap across the blood/CSF barrier and so intracranial haemorrhage (Simmons et al, 1974), secondly, of depressing the conscious level by lowering pH of CSF below 7.2. Asphyxia of the brain causes anaerobic metabolism with the production of lactate and pyruvic acid. The lactic acid can be measured in CSF if it is above 4 mmol; it can be used as an indicator of severe cerebral asphyxia (Simpson, 1974). The CSF lactate/pyruvate ratio was also found to be abnormal in neonatal asphyxia when it was accompanied by clinical symptoms in the series reported by Svenningsen and Siesjö (1972). Finally under normal steady state conditions the Po_2 of cerebrospinal fluid follows arterial Po_2 in a linear manner but if the cerebral blood flow increases then the CSF Po_2 rises as the brain extracts more oxygen. The difference between CSF and arterial Po_2 may be used as an index of oxidative metabolism in the brain (Rothman and Stern, 1973).

Summary

To summarise, the infant with asphyxia which is sufficiently severe to interfere with cerebral metabolism even if not severe enough to cause permanent damage will show a combination of the following features, apathy, hypothermia, the need to be tube fed, apnoeic episodes and tonic fits especially upon handling. On examination he is hypotonic with absent Moro, a bulbar palsy, ophthalmoplegia possibly progressing to decerebrate rigidity. There may be hypocalcaemia, hyponatraemia, hypoglycaemia and a consumption coagulopathy. The management of the asphyxiated infant is complex and depends upon anticipation of what may go wrong; the pathology must be borne in mind in order to lessen secondary brain damage. Treatment is summarised in Table 3.1. With the modern aggressive approach to treatment the strong clinical impression is that infants are now surviving with less handicap than similarly affected ones did five years ago.

LONG-TERM EFFECTS OF PERINATAL ASPHYXIA

Does perinatal asphyxia cause long-term morbidity? Even if the answer was no, the mortality rate is still sufficient to justify continued study of the problem. Keith, Norval and Hunt (1953) thought that it did not, Clark-Bailey (1958) found over 500 references to the relationship between asphyxia and long-term brain damage and found the evidence conflicting. Ingram (1964) thought there was a continuum of abnormality in pregnancy, delivery and the neonatal period rather than one isolated factor responsible for brain damage. Argument has raged since Little in 1861 claimed that cerebral palsy was caused by neonatal asphyxia. Fraser and Wilks (1959) in a study of 100 children in Aberdeen with asphyxia found only trivial abnormalities on long-term neurological and psychological follow-up study. Millar and Neligan (1968) found that delay in establishing respiration was not in itself predictive of long-term handicap. Berendes (1969) found no abnormality if infants were selected on the basis of bradycardia, and Schachter and Apgar (1959) none if they were selected upon the basis of oxygen saturation soon after birth. The Apgar score is equally unreliable as a screening test for cerebral damage (Drage et al, 1966).

Table 3.2   Long-term results in 93 cases of symptomatic neonatal asphyxia (mean age 20 months)

(A) Overall results

	Cases
Dead	20
Severely handicapped	11
Handicapped	13
Minimal brain damaged	15
Normal	34

(B) Types of handicap

No. cases	Mental handicap	Cerebral palsy	Epilepsy
11[a]	+	+	−
9[b]	+	+	+
3	+	−	−
2	−	+	−
2	−	+	+

(C) Types of cerebral palsy
23 cases (old enough to assess type)

Double hemiplegia	8
Diplegia	4
Hemiplegia	4
Ataxic diplegia	4
Diplegia with super imposed hemiplegia	2
Choreoathetosis with diplegia	1

[a] One late death
[b] Two late deaths, 10 microcephalic in whole group
Brown and Purvis, unpublished data

Figures given for the long-term effects of perinatal asphyxia are difficult to interpret as follow-up has often been on the basis of an Apgar score or some index which does not necessarily reflect the presence of cerebral asphyxia.

If we look at those infants selected upon the grounds of neurological abnormality in the newborn period following an asphyxial birth then a different picture emerges. Schulte et al (1965) found 32 per cent died or had cerebral palsy, 26 per cent minimal cerebral dysfunction and 40 per cent were normal. Our own long-term follow-up showed 44 per cent dead or handicapped, 15 per cent minimal cerebral dysfunction and 34 per cent normal (Brown et al, 1974). Amiel-Tison (1969) and De Souza and Milner (1974) also found abnormal neurological behaviour in the newborn period to be predictive as did Thorn (1969) who extensively reviews the literature. Possibly even more important is the reverse fact that an infant who is neurologically completely normal, no matter what the history has an excellent prognosis (Schulte et al, 1965; Brown et al, 1974).

Table 3.3 Long-term follow-up of infants with symptomatic neonatal asphyxia originally thought to be normal or to have suffered only minimal brain damage (age 4–6 years)

Handicap	Symptomatic asphyxia 32 cases	Normal controls 16 cases
Motor abnormality (clumsy children)	14	1 (choreoid)
Ataxia	5	0
Dyspraxia	3	0
Minimal hemiparesis	5	0
Minimal diplegia	3	0
Epilepsy (fits after neonatal period)	8	0
Speech retardation needing speech therapy	9	1
Behaviour disturbances	12	1 (Neurologically abnormal at birth)
Visual defects	3	0
Schooling problems (not all in school yet)	5	1
Intelligence quotient WPPSI		
Total	96	109
Verbal	99	112
Performance	93	104

After Burt et al, 1975
Normal controls matched for social class, all had normal behaviour in neonatal period but not necessarily normal births or pregnancies, no difference in 'mothering' scores assessed by health visitor. Normal accepted mean IQ on WPPSI is 110, a verbal performance discrepancy is usual

An association between cerebral asphyxia and handicap may be sought in two ways. Firstly by following infants selected on the grounds of symptomatic asphyxia (Tables 3.2 and 3.3) and secondly a retrospective enquiry for perinatal asphyxia may be made from handicapped children (Ingram, 1964; Hagberg et al, 1975). The numbers must inevitably be small in any longitudinal survey done from only one centre (Burt et al, 1975). Before we consider the diagnosis and nature of the individual types of handicap, the actual handicaps should be compared with those that were predicted upon theoretical grounds on the basis of the pathology (Table 2.10).

Early postnatal development

The duration of the abnormal signs in the neonatal period is of some significance and if they last more than five days the risk of handicap is increased (Balf, 1952). The infant gradually resumes flexor tone in the legs and then the arms and may enter a 'latent period' of about three months during which there may be no obvious neurological abnormality. In this period, however, the infant is often irritable and will not sleep at night so that parents are worn out by sleepless nights. There is a resistance to hypnotic drugs and this seems

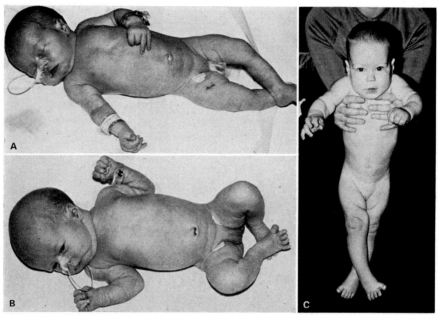

Figure 3.6 Sequential pictures of the same infant, brain-damaged from asphyxia. (A) At 72 h, in stage of extensor hypertonus. (B) At 14 days, now with flexor tonus but still with feeding difficulties. (C) Definite cerebral palsy at 10 months, developing choreoathetosis

to antedate the later hyperkinetic behaviour abnormality in which there is also an abnormal pharmacological response. Feeding is slow and they may take up to an hour per feed. In infants with a later ataxia they may remain floppy from birth and do not resume neonatal flexion. The other causes of the floppy baby syndrome will then need to be considered (Dubowitz, 1969).

By three months the brain damaged baby begins to show increasing extensor tone and this progresses to a marked 'dystonia' with retention of all the primitive reflexes (grasp, walking, stepping, symmetrical tonic neck reflexes and Moro), beyond the five months when they should normally all have been inhibited. The severe case progresses from a dystonia to a double hemiplegic (tetraplegic) type of cerebral palsy or a diplegia (spasticity restricted to the legs). Cerebral asphyxia illustrates well the fallacy of regarding cerebral palsy as a static disease entity (Fig. 3.6).

The grasp reflexes persist with no development of volition so that the normal hand regard and forced grasping at the clothes characteristic of the three-month infant is delayed; he may eventually develop an immature voluntary grasp with a spastic increase in muscle tone. In severe cases the hand remains permanently clenched in the 'mana obscena' posture with no learned hand skills. In mild cases full neurological maturation, with a well-coordinated pincer grip develops, but the child has difficulty learning skilled hand movements, he is dyspraxic. Because of the involvement of the basal ganglia the dyspraxia or spasticity is often mixed with an extrapyramidal dystonia and a choreoathetosis. The picture in the upper limbs is therefore often a complicated mixture of neurological disability.

Mental handicap

Cerebral atrophy and microcephaly may be associated with the most severe form of mental handicap so that the child has no learning at all above the four month level when recognition of the environment usually begins. Air encephalography will show cerebral atrophy which may be severe and asymmetrical. The head circumference is normal at birth but as a result of the brain damage there is gross slowing down of brain growth and so an apparently progressive microcephaly. The child may be dull for the family or there may be classical psychometric abnormalities of brain damage such as a verbal performance discrepancy on the WISC or poor function with spatial tests such as Frostig, Kohs' blocks, Raven's matrices and the Bender gestalt tests. In most children apparently recovered from symptomatic perinatal asphyxia the total IQ score will be normal and yet there may be enormous behaviour, educational, speech and coordination problems (Table 3.3).

Epilepsy

There is often neuronal loss and gliosis of the hippocampus after birth asphyxia (Gunnet et al, 1974). Ammon's horn is particularly affected by hypoxia (Norman, 1963), and there may be posterior temporal lobe infarction from posterior cerebral artery lesions in the newborn period leading to temporal lobe epilepsy later (Remillard, Ethier and Andermann, 1974). One-third of cases of temporal lobe epilepsy in children with a known aetiology other than pyrexial convulsions are ascribed to perinatal factors (Ounsted, Lindsay and Norman, 1966). Perinatal problems account for an incidence of later epilepsy of about 1/1000 population (Forfar, Brown and Cockburn, 1972). Fits tend to cease by the tenth day after birth and only recur at a later date. Infantile spasms may occur around six months in severely brain damaged infants, or pyrexial convulsions more correctly temperature precipitated epilepsy at the end of the first year. Pertussis immunisation must be avoided in these children for it may precipitate severe fits and an acute encephalopathy. Later epilepsy is more common following intrauterine asphyxia at term rather than postnatal asphyxia in the preterm infant. In very severely damaged infants any attempt at movement may cause sudden severe myoclonic jerks, or lying for any length of time in a particular position may initiate generalised myoclonus.

Cerebral palsy

All types of cerebral palsy, hemiplegia, diplegia, tetraplegia, dyskinesia or ataxia may result from perinatal asphyxia (Table 3.2C). This is not the place for a discussion of the multitude of clinical problems which are embraced by the 'cerebral palsies' (Ingram, 1964, 1974; Brown and Ingram, 1975). We have already delineated how a generalised insult such as asphyxia can result in different types of cerebral palsy. One form of cerebral palsy, cerebral diplegia, will be discussed in more detail later for the contribution of birth asphyxia is still a matter of controversy.

Speech disorder

Frank deafness is unusual in uncomplicated asphyxia, but with the selective involvement of cochlear nuclei and the inferior colliculli one would expect it to cause some degree of auditory 'inattention' and possible influence speech development. It is therefore of interest that 27 per cent of our cases with minimal brain involvement on follow-up needed speech therapy or had definitely delayed speech development. The motor involvement with mild ataxia or dyspraxia can result in a primary retardation of articulation. The mentally handicapped child will of course have delayed language and those with cerebral palsy, a true dysarthria from bulbar palsy. Psychometric testing shows statistically significant syntactical difficulties as shown by simple sentence repetition, and poorer performance on comprehension subtests of the WPPSI compared to matched control children. Care must be taken in dyskinetic children as asphyxia may cause a non-communicating child and a mistaken diagnosis of mental handicap.

Behaviour disorder

Symptomatic autistic behaviour may be seen in the children with severe mental handicap. In those with no obvious or trivial brain involvement it is of interest that 75 per cent were regarded by their mothers as difficult children to rear when compared to 10 per cent in normal controls matched for social class and 'mothering ability'. Thirty-seven per cent had a recognisable behaviour disorder. This is due to the feeding difficulty, irritability, reversed sleep rhythms, hyperkinesis, poor impulse control with rage reactions and occasionally panic attacks. Bad temper, back chat, rage, stubbornness and difficulty with discipline are more common complaints by parents than the typical hyperkinetic syndrome. Hyperkinesis is more like to occur with brain damage of a diffuse nature occurring before three years. One should not limit one's ideas as to the type of behaviour which may follow brain damage to the hyperkinetic syndrome. It has been shown that the full spectrum of neurotic behaviour and conduct disorders may follow brain damage (Shaffer, 1975).

Illness of the infant immediately after birth may affect the bonding of mother and her baby, and for this reason alone compromises the infant's progress (*see* Chapter 5).

Visual problems

Severe asphyxia in the toddler may result in a true cortical blindness. In the child surviving neonatal asphyxia there is a delay in the loss of forced visual pursuit (Gatev and Shikov, 1969), the optokinetic nystagmus which normally appears at about three weeks of age associated with visual fixation is often delayed. Blindness is only seen with severe mental retardation unless it is due to a complicating retrolental fibroplasia. Lesser degrees of retrolental fibroplasia may be associated with vascular tortuosity of the retina. Squints are common and may be paralytic or concomitant, loss of convergence and poor upward conjugate gaze are useful points to the 'minimally brain damaged'. Difficulties with cognitive function in the sense of concepts of space, shape and direction is common in the brain-damaged child. Nystagmus is unusually rare considering the brain stem involvement.

The clumsy child

We shall consider the neurological findings in the clumsy child in some detail as it offers more diagnostic difficulty than frank cerebral palsy. The clumsy child may have minor degrees of ataxia, dyskinesia or dyspraxia or can be suffering from a minimal type of cerebral palsy such as a hemiplegia or diplegia (Table 3.3).

Dyspraxia is the most difficult to diagnose as the child appears to have difficulty performing skilled movements, e.g. cutting with a knife and fork, fastening buttons, assembling a biro, using tools such as a screwdriver. He has nothing definite to find on neurological examination apart from possibly an excess of associated movements. He may write and spell without difficulty if language function is normal.

Ataxia may be divided into two types, postural ataxia and volitional ataxia. The cerebellum is postnatal in development as far as the control of volitional movement is concerned so nystagmus, dysarthria, intention tremor and dysmetria are less common than hypotonia, brisk reflexes, flat feet, genurecurvatum and clumsiness of a truncal ataxia. In these children there is a generalised hypotonia with exaggeration of joint angles so that the popliteal angle is 180 degrees, the tendo achilles is lax so that the dorsum of the foot can be approximated to the tibia, the hands can be hypersupinated to touch back to back. The arms are floppy, the tendon reflexes are very brisk. Postural development is delayed so that sitting and crawling are slow, the child may then appear to stop developing and spends many months walking around with furniture as a support before he has the balance to let go. He may swim, climb or ride a tricycle before he can walk independently. He cannot later stand on one leg, hop, crouch, walk a plank or walk backwards at normal ages, he falls easily and always has bruised legs.

Mild extrapyramidal syndromes might be expected in view of the selective vulnerability of the basal ganglia. The choreoid syndrome of jerky movements of the outstretched hands with shaky pencil control, and untidy penmanship is accompanied by mirror movements and associated movements as shown by getting the child to walk on the insides and outsides of his feet and on his heels (Fog test). Running causes the hands to assume athetoid postures. Forced movement of one hand may cause the mouth to open and the opposite arm to extend and show athetoid posturing.

The minimal hemiparesis shows as retention of the grasp reflex in the foot, a smaller foot with dwarfing of the nails, a temperature difference in the skin, slightly less dorsiflexion of the foot on the affected side, a spontaneous Babinski response on squeezing the leg, crossed adductor reflexes, brisker tendon reflex, inability to hop as well on one side, and stamping the foot (one hears the gait rather than sees it). The shoes wear unevenly, the toes scuffing and the heel showing no wear. The arm again may show dwarfing, an asymmetrical parachute response, some restriction of supination of the affected, side, left handedness without a family history, an asymmetrical Fog test, failure to swing the arm, assumption of the hemiplegic posture of the arm when running fast, poor fast tapping movements and the inability to touch each finger in turn with the thumb. Timed tests such as tapping with a pencil, insertion of pegs in a peg board or strength of grip or torque may also be used clinically to show clumsiness or asymmetry.

Minimal diplegia. There may be brisk reflexes and extensor plantar responses. Spasticity in the calves is best appreciated by rapidly flexing and extending the ankle when the range of dorsiflexion will suddenly lessen. The feet may be cold and blue with below knee wasting and chilblains, suspension of the child causes an active extension of the lower limbs which go into equinus with a bilateral spontaneous Babinski response to show that this is a true active extensor hypertonus. The child may waddle as if he had muscular dystrophy in those with mild proximal spasticity. He will run clumsily, fall readily and turns his toes inwards scuffing the toes of both shoes.

Educational problems

The child with frank mental handicap or cerebral palsy will need special schooling provision but the child who is placed in a normal school may have a large number of problems. If he has epilepsy then this readily allows him to be recognised and his potential learning difficulties evaluated (Holdsworth and Whitmore, 1974). His total intelligence quotient may not reflect his difficulties, but subtests scores usually indicate areas for further investigation. Hyperkinetic behaviour with a poor concentration span may not be impressive during a short interview by physician or psychologist due to the placebo effect of a change in environment. Speech retardation can be followed by reading retardation (Ingram, 1963). Clumsiness is easy to diagnose if the child shakes or grimaces but dyspraxia is less obvious and the child is often thought to be untidy, careless or lazy. Reading, writing and arithmetic are dominant hemisphere functions and so tend to develop at the expense of spatial concepts. Brain-damaged children often appear to underachieve in arithmetic. The child with a severe bulbar involvement which inhibits speech development may show a reversal of the usual pattern found on psychometric testing, and be very good with visuo-spatial concepts and poorer in language tests (Naughton, 1975). If the child fails to achieve in school due to specific learning problems yet is trying hard and if this is not recognised and he is constantly discouraged, he may withdraw and show secondary 'autistic' behaviour disturbance. Alternatively if schooling has no meaning he will cease to pay attention and may become disruptive in class or truant.

Diplegia and the contribution of asphyxia versus low birth weight
The leg area of the motor strip may be more susceptible to damage than the arm area because it is selectively myelinating at term, periventricalar leucomalacia or cysts may interrupt leg fibres, subependymal haemorrhages are more likely in this area and the head of the caudate nucleus and surrounding areas may be selectively infarcted; watershed lesions between anterior and middle cerebral artery may cause wedge-shaped infarcts maximum in this region, enlargement of the lateral ventricles with hydrocephalus will stretch the white matter in the leg area before the arm, a pure paraplegia may be caused by umbilical catheterisation (Aziz and Robertson, 1973).

The term asphyxiated infant may show a spastic diplegia in the legs but if he does the arms are usually involved to some degree often with additional dyskinetic movements, and epilepsy and mental handicap are common accompaniments. This must be contrasted with the pure paraplegic diplegia in the preterm infant when mental handicap and epilepsy are rare and dyskinesia in the upper limbs is never found even though an extrapyramidal type of dystonia always precedes the appearance of the spasticity in the legs and initially involves the arms (Ingram, 1964; Berenberg and Ong, 1964).

Dystonia
The preterm infant born at 28 to 30 weeks of gestation should go through the same pattern of maturation in his incubator as he would normally have passed through in utero, so that at the expected date of delivery, he should be behaving like a normal full-term infant (St Anne Dargassies, 1955). This does not happen, the infant develops flexor tone in the legs normally at first, but then the arms remain hypotonic with poor flexion. By 40 weeks gestation the legs begin to go into rigid extension so that at term instead of a nicely flexed adducted infant we have a stiff extended one. He shows arching of the back, ballet dances on tip toe, has brisk and often obligatory extensor reflexes

(Brown, 1971, Fig. 3.7). This can persist for several months and is associated with delay in postural development (allowing for prematurity) and a retention of primitive reflexes together with irritability, poor feeding, terrible sleeping and a resistance to conventional doses of hypnotic drugs (Drillien, 1972). When it persists beyond the fourth or fifth month of postnatal life cerebral palsy is suspected, it may persist till the end of the first year of life and several things may happen. It may suddenly disappear and the infant put on a developmental spurt and is then apparently normal, or it may persist as the dystonic phase of a diplegic cerebral palsy, eventually being replaced by a

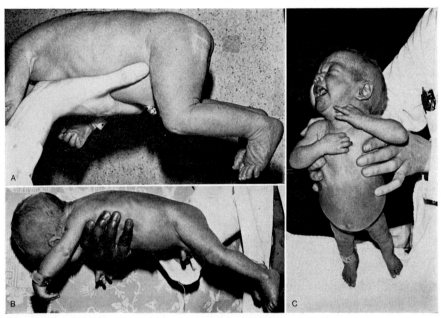

Figure 3.7 (A) Normal infant at term; (B) preterm infant on his expected date of delivery; (C) same showing gross extensor thrust

spastic stage, or it may be replaced by hypotonia and a truncal ataxia, or it may disappear and be replaced by hyperkinetic behaviour and schooling problems or it may be replaced by choreoathetosis if the infant also suffered from kernicterus in the neonatal period.

The spastic phase of diplegia

In severe cases the child may remain dystonic for many years but usually there is an increasing spasticity associated with brisk tendon reflexes which appears in the hip flexors, hip adductors, hamstring muscles and calf, i.e. in flexor muscles as opposed to the predominantly extensor pattern of dystonia. The child walks with his legs in the characteristic flexed and internally rotated posture with a waddle. He shows scissoring if suspended under the arms, due to the increased tone in the adductor muscles at the hip. This stage is marked by the appearance of severe fixed deformity from contractures and dislocation of the hips may occur extremely rapidly.

Aetiology of dystonia and diplegia

The idiopathic encephalopathy of low birth weight may cause a spectrum of abnormality ranging from transient dystonia or the clumsy child syndrome at one extreme to a severe spastic diplegia at the other extreme. The hypothesis was put forward by Drillien (1964, 1968), that the long-term handicap in low birth weight infants was due to some genetic predisposition in view of the high incidence of congenital malformations she found in her groups of infants. Stewart (1972) has contested this view since she could not find a high incidence of congenital malformations. Although the incidence of handicap in low birth weight infants has fallen dramatically (Davies and Tizard 1975), there has been no decline in the incidence of congenital malformations. The decrease in morbidity appears to be related to improvements in neonatal care of these infants.

McDonald (1967) felt that perinatal asphyxia played a part in the aetiology of the diplegia of low birth weight. Stewart and Reynolds (1974) found a high incidence of intrapartum asphyxia in the survivors with handicap during their study of very low birth weight infants. Churchill et al (1970) found a significant drop in haematocrit in children with diplegia and suggested that intraventricular haemorrhage was the cause.

This theory does not fit with all the clinical observations any better than the congenital malformations theory. The incidence of diplegia has dropped dramatically and yet there has been no change at all over the last 10 years in the incidence of IVH found at autopsy (Anderson et al, 1976). In fact Wigglesworth et al (1975) claims that IVH has increased among infants from the same population which Davies and Tizard say has shown a virtual disappearance of spastic diplegia. Preterm infants at high risk of IVH with severe postpartum asphyxia necessitating prolonged artificial respiration certainly die with IVH but the survivors do not show a high incidence of diplegia (Brown et al, 1973). The low birth weight infants with asphyxia described by Smith, Reynolds and Taghizadeh (1974) as suffering from periventricular leucomalacia with subependymal plate haemorrhage and hydrocephalus had nearly all suffered from neurological abnormalities such as fits or decerebrate rigidity. This is the type of history noticeable by its absence in cases of pure diplegia of low birth weight. In our experience, infants with intraventricular haemorrhage proven by ventricular puncture (aspirating large quantities of chocolate-coloured changed blood with positive spectrophotometry) go on to develop a hydrocephalus. They may be mentally retarded with ataxia or a hemiplegia. When a diplegia does develop it is usually in a floppy not a dystonic infant. Intraventricular or subependymal haemorrhage is more often unilateral and the paraplegic diplegia is remarkable for its symmetry in the two legs. It is possible that symmetrical white matter infarction occurs from asphyxia and in some cases there may be bleeding into one of the infarcted areas which causes the IVH.

If one accepts the spectrum of dystonia then the abnormal brain maturation pattern of the vast majority of low birth weight infants on their expected date of delivery makes it unlikely that they have all suffered from some degree of IVH or asphyxial brain damage (Thistlethwaite, 1975). In the past 40 per cent of infants less than 2000 g showed this maturation pattern beyond four months of age (Brown, 1971; Drillien, 1972), this is now very much reduced. unidentified improvement in neonatal care is responsible for the change but the evidence for congenital malformation, asphyxia, IVH, hypoglycaemia, hyperbilirubinaemia, hypertyrosinaemia, birth trauma or idiopathic respiratory distress syndrome is not at present convincing. Total nutrition or some more specific component in the improved nutrition of the low birth weight baby may play a part (Lubchenco et al, 1972). If the infant is born light for dates and does not show rapid catch-up growth then permanent stunting and dystonic maturation is more likely to be found (Drillien, 1972; Thistlethwaite, 1975). Nor is the evidence that asphyxia is responsible for the idiopathic encephalopathy of low birth weight convincing. On the other hand asphyxia certainly may cause a spasticity of the legs in mature infants but this is usually associated with other signs of brain damage. This group probably represents the second peak of the diphasic distribution of this type of cerebral palsy when related to maturity (Drillien, Ingram and Russell, 1962).

Summary

Asphyxia and its effects upon the brain forms one of the exciting areas in the neurology of childhood. It assumes a major role not only in the field of neonatal asphyxia but also in the effects of pyrexial convulsions, status epilepticus, poisonings, complications of cardiac bypass surgery and artificial ventilation therapy. It is still responsible for a significant mortality and morbidity. We have considered the effects of neonatal asphyxia in detail but the principles apply equally to the other areas of acute paediatric care.

The concept of cerebral palsy as a single disease entity has resulted in a neglect of pathology as the basis of disease. No excuse is offered therefore for trying to relate the immediate and long-term effects of perinatal asphyxia to the possible underlying pathological mechanisms.

Like society in general, 'medicine' has its fashions, we have recently seen the appearance of developmental paediatrics, educational medicine, community paediatrics and rehabilitation paediatrics. In most areas it still falls to the lot of the general paediatricians to manage the child's acute handicapping condition and subsequently the effect that this has upon the family. He can only perform this duty providing that he has the sapiential authority based upon an understanding of the total effects of the particular disease upon the child.

Prevention is the ideal, advances in obstetrics and neonatal paediatrics have gone a long way to making this a reality.

ACKNOWLEDGEMENTS

The work presented here is an overview of the last 10 years' discussions and research by my colleagues in Edinburgh. I am very grateful to Professor John Forfar and Forrester Cockburn with whom most of the work was done. Dr John Anderson, Consultant Paediatric Neuropathologist, Tom Turner, David Thistlethwaite and Richard Purvis have allowed me to draw upon their work, some of which is as yet unpublished.

REFERENCES

Adamsons, K. & Myers, R. E. (1973) Perinatal asphyxia—causes, detection and neurological sequalae. *Pediatric Clinics of North America*, **20** (2), 465–480.

Aicardi, J., Goutières, F. & Hodebourg De Verbois, A. (1972) Multicystic encephalomalacia of infants and its relation to abnormal gestation and hydranencephaly. *Journal of Neurological Sciences*, **15**, 357–373.

Amiel-Tison, C. (1969) Cerebral damage in full-term newborn. *Biologia neonatorum*, **14**, 234–250.

Anderson, J. M. & Brown, J. K. (1972) Brain ischaemia and D.I.C. *Lancet* (letter), **1**, 373.

Anderson, J. M. & Belton, N. R. (1974) Water and electrolyte abnormalities in the human brain after severe intrapartum asphyxia. *Journal of Neurology, Neurosurgery and Psychiatry*, **XXXVII** (5), 514–520.

Anderson, J. M., Brown, J. K. & Cockburn, F. (1974) On the role of disseminated intravascular coagulation in the pathology of birth asphyxia. *Developmental Medicine and Child Neurology*, **16**, 581–591.

Anderson, J. M., Bain, A. D., Brown, J. K., Cockburn, F., Forfar, J. D., Machin, G. A. & Turner, T. L. (1976) Hyaline membrane disease, alkaline buffer treatment and cerebral intraventricular haemorrhage, *Lancet*, **1**, 117.

Anderson, J. M. (1975) Personal communication.

Armstrong, D. & Norman, M. G. (1974) Periventricular leucomalacia in neonates. *Archives of Disease in Childhood*, **49**, 367–375.

Aziz, E. A. & Robertson, A. F. (1973) Paraplegia: a complication of umbilical artery catheterisation. *Journal of Paediatrics*, **82**, 1051–1052.

Bailey, C. J. (1958) Interrelationship of asphyxia neonatorum, cerebral palsy and mental retardation: present status of the problem. In *Neurological and Psychological Deficits of Asphyxia Neonatorum*, ed. Windle, W. F., Hinman, E. H. & Bailey, P., pp. 5–30. Illinois: Charles C. Thomas.

Bakay, L. & Lee, J. C. (1968) The effect of acute hypoxia and hypercapnia on the ultrastructure of the central nervous system. *Brain*, **91**, 697–706.

Balf, C. L. (1952) Birth injuries in relation to post-natal defects. II. The paediatric interpretation. *Transactions of the Edinburgh Obstetrical Society*, pp. 62–69.

Banker, B. Q. & Larroche, J. C. (1962) Periventricular leukomalacia in infancy. *Archives of Neurology*, **7**, 386–410.

Beard, R. W. (1970) Fetal blood sampling. *British Journal of Hospital Medicine*, **3**, 523–534.

Belton, N. R. (1970) Creatine phosphokinase—blood and CSF levels in newborn infants and children. (Proc. P.R.S.) *Archives of Disease in Childhood*, **45**, 600.

Berenberg, W. & Ong, B. H. (1964) Cerebral spastic paraplegia and prematurity. *Pediatrics*, April 1964, 496–499.

Berendes, H. W. (1969) Perinatal factors affecting human development. In *Scientific Publication 185*, p. 228. Washington: Pan American Health Organisation.

Brand, M. M. & Bignami, A. (1969) The effects of chronic hypoxia on the neonatal and infantile brain. *Brain*, **92**, 233–254.

Brierley, J. B. & Meldrum, B. S. (1971) Brain hypoxia. *Clinics in Developmental Medicine* 39/40. London: Heinemann.

Brierley, J. B. (1971) The neuropathological sequalae of profound hypoxia. In *Brain Hypoxia*, ed. Brierley, J. B. & Meldrum, B. S., pp. 147–151. London: Heinemann.

Brown, J. K. (1971) The dystonic syndrome of the low birth weight infant. *Proceedings XIII International Congress of Paediatrics, Vienna*, **8**, 13, 53–58.

Brown, J. K., Cockburn, F. & Forfar, J. O. (1972) Clinical and chemical correlates in convulsions in the newborn. *Lancet*, **1**, 135–139.

Brown, J. K. (1973) Convulsions in the newborn period. *Developmental Medicine and Child Neurology*, **15** (6), 823–846.

Brown, J. K., Cockburn, F., Forfar, J. O., Marshall, R. L. & Stephen, G. W. (1973) Problems in the management of assisted ventilation in the newborn and follow-up of treated cases. *British Journal of Anaesthesia*, **45**, Suppl., 808–817.

Brown, J. K., Ingram, T. T. S. & Seshia, S. S. (1973) Patterns of decerebration in infants and children: defects in homeostasis and sequalae. *Journal of Neurology, Neurosurgery, and Psychiatry*, **36** (3), 431–444.

Brown, J. K. (1974) Examination of the nervous system in the neonate. In *Neonatal Medicine*, ed. Cockburn, F. & Drillien, C. M. Edinburgh: Blackwell.

Brown, J. K., Purvis, R. J., Forfar, J. O. & Cockburn, F. (1974) Neurological aspects of perinatal asphyxia. *Developmental Medicine and Child Neurology*, **16**, 567–580.

Brown, J. K. & Ingram, T. T. S. (1975) The development of muscle tone in the infantile cerebral palsies. *Encyclopedia of Neurology, Neurosurgery, Psychology and Psychiatry* (in press).

Brown, J. K. & Habel, A. H. (1975) Toxic encephalopathy and acute brain swelling in children. *Developmental Medicine and Child Neurology*, **17**, 659–679.

Bruck, K., Adams, F. H. & Bruck, M. (1962) Temperature regulation in infants with chronic hypoxaemia. *Pediatrics*, **30**, 350.

Burt, A., Brown, J. K., Palmer, J. & Forfar, J. O. (1975) Long term follow-up of perinatal asphyxia (in preparation).

Cammermeyer, J. (1958) Neuropathology of asphyxia neonatorum In *Neurological and Psychological Deficits of Asphyxia Neonatorum*, ed. Windle, W. F., Hinman, E. H. & Bailey, P., pp. 156–172. Illinois: Charles C. Thomas.

Chessells, J. M. & Wigglesworth, J. S. (1970) Secondary haemorrhagic disease of the newborn. *Archives of Disease in Childhood*, **45**, 539.

Churchill, J. A., Carleton, J. H. & Berendes, H. W. (1970) Hematocrit of newborns of short gestation. *Developmental Medicine and Child Neurology*, **12**, 153–157.

Cockburn, F., Belton, N., Brown, J. K. & Forfar, J. O. (1975) A study of amino acids and enzymes in CSF as an index of brain damage in the newborn (in preparation).

Cockburn, F. (1976) Intravenous feeding of the newborn. *Clinics in Endocrinology and Metabolism*, **5**, 191.

Cocker, J., George, S. E. & Yates, P. O. (1965) Perinatal occlusion of the middle cerebral artery. *Developmental Medicine and Child Neurology*, **7**, 235–243.

Courville, C. B. (1953) *Cerebral Anoxia*. Los Angeles: San Lucas Press.

Courville, C. B. (1962) Antenatal and paranatal anoxia. *International Journal of Neurology*, **3**, 443–463.

Craig, W. S. (1950) Intracranial irritation in the newborn. *Archives of Disease in Childhood*, **25**, 325.

Davies, P. A. & Stewart, A. L. (1975) Low-birth-weight infants. *British Medical Bulletin*, **31**, (1), 85–91.

Davies, P. A. & Tizard, J. P. M. (1975) Very low birthweight and subsequent neurological defect. *Developmental Medicine and Child Neurology*, **17**, 3–17.

De Souza, S. W. & Milner, R. D. G. (1974) Clinical and CSF studies in newborn infants with neurological abnormalities. *Archives of Disease in Childhood*, **49**, 351–358.

De Reuck, J., Chattha, A. S. & Richardson, E. P. (1972) Pathogenensis and evolution of periventricular leukomalacia in infancy. *Archives of Neurology*, **27**, 229–236.

Deuel, R. K. (1973) Polygraphic monitoring of apnoeic spells. *Archives of Neurology*, **28**, 71–76.

Dobbing, J. (1974) Later development of the brain and its vulnerability. In *Scientific Foundations of Paediatrics*, ed. Davies, J. A. & Dobbing, John. London: Heinemann.

Donovan, D., Coves, A. B. & Paine, R. S. (1962) The prognostic implications of neurologic abnormalities in the neonatal period. *Neurology*, **12**, 910–914.

Drage, J. S., Kennedy, C., Berendes, H., Schwartz, B. K. & Weiss, W. (1966) The Apgar score as an index of infant morbidity. *Developmental Medicine and Child Neurology*, **8**, 141–148.

Drillien, C. M., Ingram, T. T. S. & Russell, E. M. (1962) Comparative aetiological studies of congenital diplegia in Scotland. *Archives of Disease in Childhood*, **37** (193), 282–288.

Drillien, C. M. (1964) The effect of obstetrical hazard on the later development of the child. *Recent Advances in Paediatrics*, 3rd edn, pp. 82–109.

Drillien, C. M. (1968) Causes of handicap in the low weight infant. *Proceedings of the 1967 Nutricia Symposium*. Leiden: H. E. Stenfert Kroese, N.V.

Drillien, C. M. (1972) Aetiology and outcome in low birth weight infants. *Developmental Medicine and Child Neurology*, **14**, 563–584.

Dubowitz, V. (1969) The floppy infant. *Clinics in Developmental Medicine*, 31. London: Heinemann.

Ewerbeck, H. (1971) Late cerebral damage after high risk birth. *Geburtshilfe und Frauenheilkunde*, **31**, 901–910.

Fedrick, J. & Butler, N. R. (1970) Certain causes of neonatal death—intraventricular haemorrhage. *Biologia Neonatorum*, **15**, 257–290.

Feldman, W., Drummond, K. N. & Klein, M. (1970) Hyponatraemia following asphyxia neonatorum. *Acta paediatrica scandinavica*, **59**, 52.

Flexner, L. B., Belknap, E. L. & Flexner, J. B. (1953) Biochemical and physiological differentiation during morphogenesis (to number XVI). *Journal of Cellular Physiology*, **42**, 151–161.

Forfar, J. O., Brown, J. K. & Cockburn, F. (1972) Early infantile convulsions and later epilepsy. In *Prevention of Epilepsy and its Consequences*, ed. Parsonage, M. J. London: International Bureau for Epilepsy.

Fraser, M. S. & Wilks, J. (1959) The residual effects of neonatal asphyxia. *Journal of Obstetrics and Gynaecology of the British Empire*, **66**, 748.

Gatev, V. & Shikov, N. (1969) Automatic visual pursuit in infants born normally and in asphyxia. *Developmental Medicine and Child Neurology*, **11**, 595–600.

Gibbs, F. A., Gibbs, E. L. & Lennox, W. G. (1943) The value of carbon dioxide in counteracting the effects of low oxygen. *Journal of Aviation Medicine*, October 1943, 1–12.

Golubeva, E. L., Elizarova, I. P. & Farber, D. A. (1963) The state of the CNS in newborn infants who have suffered from asphyxia during labour. *Akusherstova i Ginekologiya*, **6**, 25–29.

Grossman, R. G. & Williams, V. F. (1971) Electrical activity and ultrastructure of cortical neurones and synapses in ischaemia. In *Brain Hypoxia*, ed. Brierley, J. B. & Meldrum, B. S. *Clinics in Developmental Medicine*, **39/40**, 61–78. London: Heinemann.

Grote, J. (1974) Problems of cerebral oxygen supply. *Triangle*, **13** (4), 165–172.

Grunnet, M. L., Curless, R. G., Bray, P. F. & Hung, A. L. (1974) Brain changes in newborns from an intensive care unit. *Developmental Medicine and Child Neurology*, **16**, 320–328.

Hagberg, B., Hagberg, G. & Olow, I. (1975) The changing panorama of cerebral palsy in Sweden 1954–70. *Acta paediatrica scandinavica*, **64**, 187–192 (part 1), 193–200 (part 2).

Harcke, H. T., Jnr., Naeye, R. L., Storch, A. & Blanc, W. A. (1972) Perinatal cerebral intraventricular haemorrhage. *Journal of Pediatrics*, **80** (1), 37–42.

Harrison, V. C., Heese, H. de V. & Klein, M. (1968) Intracranial haemorrhage associated with HMD. *Archives of Disease in Childhood*, **43**, 116–120.

Hathaway, W. E. (1970) Coagulation problems in the newborn infant. *Pediatric Clinics of North America*, **17** (4), 929–942.

Hellström, B. & Kjellin, K. G. (1971) The diagnostic value of spectrophotometry of the CSF in the newborn period. *Developmental Medicine and Child Neurology*, **13**, 789–797.

Himwich, W. A., Sullivan, W. T., Kelley, B., Benaron, H. B. W. & Tucker, B. E. (1955) Chemical constituents of human brain. *Journal of Nervous and Mental Diseases*, **122**, 441,

Himwich, H. E. (1958) Introduction to round table discussion. In *Neurological and Psychological Deficits of Asphyxia Neonatorum*, ed. Windle, W. F., Hinman, E. H. & Bailey, P., pp. 141–151. Illinois: Charles C. Thomas.

Holdsworth, L. & Whitmore, K. (1974) A study of children with epilepsy attending ordinary schools. *Developmental Medicine and Child Neurology*, **16**, 746–758.

Hull, D. (1971) Asphyxia neonatorum. In *Recent Advances in Paediatrics*, ed. Gairdner, D. & Hull, D. London: J. & A. Churchill.

Ingram, T. T. S. (1963) Delayed development of speech with special reference to dyslexia. *Proceedings of the Royal Society of Medicine,* **56,** 199–203.

Ingram, T. T. S. (1964) *Paediatric Aspects of Cerebral Palsy.* Edinburgh: Livingstone.

Ingram, T. T. S. (1974) The long-term care of patients suffering from cerebral palsy. *Journal of the Irish Medical Association,* **67** (8), 205–212.

Ivan, L. P. (1973) Spinal reflexes in cerebral death. *Neurology,* **23,** 650–652.

Jilek, L. et al (1967) The metabolic adaptive reaction of the immature nervous tissue to stagnant hypoxia. *Development of the Nervous System—Proceedings of International Symposium, Prague,* 1967. Universitas Carolina Pragensis, 1968.

Joseph, M. (1967). Heart failure from brain damage. *Developmental Medicine and Child Neurology,* **9,** 772–773.

Kaufmann, G. E. & Clark, K. (1970) Continuous simulataneous monitoring of intraventricular and cervical subarachnoid cerebrospinal fluid pressure, to indicate development of cerebral or tonsillar herniation. *Journal of Neurosurgery,* **33** (2), 145–150.

Keith, H. M., Norval, M. A. & Hunt, A. B. (1953) Neurological lesions in relation of sequalae of birth injury. *Neurology,* **3,** 139.

Kennedy, C., Grave, G. D., Jehle, J. W. & Sokoloff, L. (1970) Blood flow to white matter during maturation of the brain. *Neurology,* **20,** 613–618.

Kety, S. S. (1963) Regional circulation of the brain under physiological conditions—possible relationship to selective vulnerability. In *Selective Vulnerability of the brain to Hypoxaemia,* Ed. Schodé, J. P. & McMenemy, W. H., pp. 21–26. Oxford: Blackwell.

Klatzo, I. (1967) Early effects of perinatal asphyxia on the brain. In *Brain Damage in the Fetus and Newborn from Hypoxia or Asphyxia,* pp. 31–34. 57th Ross Conference, Ross Laboratories, Ohio.

Kubli, F., Ruttgers, H. & Henner, H. (1972) Clinical aspects of fetal acid–base balance during labour, pp. 487–494. In *Respiratory Gas Exchange and Blood Flow in the Placenta,* Ed. Longon, L. & Bartels, H., pp. 73–361. Washington, DC: Department of Health, Education and Welfare.

Lagos, J. C. & Siekert, R. G. (1969) Intracranial haemorrhage in infancy and childhood. *Clinical Pediatrics,* **8** (2), 90.

Lending, M., Slobody, L. B. & Mestern, J. (1964) CSF glutamic oxaloacetic transaminase and lactic dehydrogenase activities in children with neurologic disorders. *Journal of Pediatrics,* **65,** 415–421.

Leventhal, H. R. (1960) Birth injuries of the spinal cord. *Journal of Pediatrics,* **56** (4), 447–453.

Lilien, A. A. (1970) Term intrapartum fetal death. *American Journal of Obstetrics and Gynecology,* **107,** 595–603.

Lindenberg, R. (1967) Patterns of damage in the human central nervous system. In *Brain Damage in the Fetus and Newborn from Hypoxia or Asphyxia,* pp. 12–16. 57th Ross Conference, Ross Laboratories, Ohio.

Little, W. J. (1861) On the influence of abnormal parturition, difficult labours, premature birth and asphyxia neonatorum on the mental and physical condition of the child, especially in relation to deformities. *Transactions of the Obstetrical Society of London,* **3,** 293.

Lubchenco, L. O., Papadopoulos, M. D., Butterfield, L. J., French, J. H., Metcalf, D., Hix, I. E., Jnr., Danick, J., Dodds, J., Downs, M. & Freeland, E. (1972) Long-term follow-up studies of prematurely born infants. Parts I and II. *Journal of Pediatrics,* **80** (3), 502–512.

Malamud, N. (1963) Patterns of CNS vulnerability in neonatal hypoxaemia. In *Selective Vulnerability of the Brain in Hypoxaemia,* ed. Schodé, J. P. & McMenemy, W. H., pp. 211–225. Oxford: Blackwell.

McDonald, A. (1967) Children of very low birth weight. *Spastics Research Monographs,* No. 1. London: Heinemann.

Millar, D. G. & Neligan, G. A. (1968) The Newcastle maternity survey and survey of child development. *Journal of Obstetrics and Gynaecology of the British Commonwealth,* **75,** 481–482.

Moody, R. A., Ruamsuke, S. & Mullan, S. (1969) Experimental effects of acutely increased intracranial pressure on respiration and blood gases. *Journal of Neurosurgery,* **30,** 482–493.

Myers, R. E. (1972) Two patterns of perinatal brain damage and their conditions of occurrence. *American Journal of Obstetrics and Gynecology,* **112,** 246–276.

Natelson, S. E. & Sayers, M. P. (1973) The fate of children sustaining severe head trauma during birth. *Pediatrics*, **51** (2), 169–174.

Naughton, J. (1975) The relationship of language to performance scores in cerebral palsied children with dysarthria. Course for Educational Psychologists, Stirling University. January 1975.

Norman, R. M. (1963) Patterns of symmetrical brain damage. In *Selective Vulnerability of the Brain in Hypoxaemia*, ed. Schodé, J. P. & McMenemy, W. H., pp. 243–250. Oxford: Blackwell.

Ounsted, C., Lindsay, J. & Norman, R. (1966) Biological factors in temporal lobe epilepsy. *Clinics in Developmental Medicine*, No. 22. London: Heinemann.

Paulson, G. W., Wise, G. & Conkle, R. (1972) Cerebrospinal fluid lactic acid in death and in brain death. *Neurology*, **22**, 505–509.

Perlman, M. & Divilansky, A. (1975) Blood coagulation status of small for dates and post-mature infants. *Archives of Disease in Childhood*, **50**, 424–429.

Plum, F. & Posner, J. B. (1972) *Diagnosis of Stupor and Coma*, 2nd edn, Contemporary Neurology Series. Philadelphia: F. A. Davis Co.

Posner, J. B., Swanson, A. G. & Plum, F. (1965) Acid–base balance in cerebrospinal fluid. *Archives of Neurology*, **12**, 479–495.

Posner, J. B. & Plum, F. (1967) Spinal fluid pH and neurologic symptoms in systemic acidosis. *New England Journal of Medicine*, **277**, 605–612.

Prechtl, H. & Beintema, D. J. (1964) The neurological examination of the full term newborn *Clinics in Developmental Medicine*, No. 12. London: Heinemann.

Prechtl, H. F. R. (1968) Neurological findings in newborn infants after pre- and paranatal complications. *Nutricia Symposium*, pp. 303–321. Leiden: H. E. Stenfert Kroese N.V.

Purvis, R. J., Brown, J. K., Cockburn, F. & Forfar, J. O. (1975) Compression head injury in the newborn (in preparation).

Remillard, G. M., Ethier, R. & Andermann, F. (1974) Temporal lobe epilepsy and perinatal occlusion of the posterior cerebral artery. *Neurology*, **24**, 1001–1009.

Richter, D. (1967) Biochemical changes in hypoxia. In *Brain Damage in the Fetus and Newborn from Hypoxia or Asphyxia*. Report of 57th Ross Conference on Paediatric Research, Ross Laboratories, Columbus.

Richter, D. (1960) Epilepsy and convulsive states. In *Modern Scientific Aspects of Neurology*, ed. Cumings, J. N., p. 314. London: Arnold Ltd.

Roberton, N. R. C. (1969) Effect of acute hypoxia on blood pressure and electroencephalo-gram of newborn babies. *Archives of Disease in Childhood*, **44**, 719–725.

Rogers, M. G. H. (1971) The early recognition of handicapping disorders in childhood. *Developmental Medicine and Child Neurology*, **13**, 88–101.

Ross, J. J. & Dimmette, R. M. (1965) Subependymal cerebral haemorrhage in infancy. *American Journal Diseases of Children*, **110**, 531–542.

Rothman, S. J. & Stern, L. (1973) Cerebrospinal fluid oxygen tension in newborn infants. *Neurology*, **23**, 1292–1296.

Saint Anne Dargassies (1955) Maturation neurologique du prématuré. *Etudes Neonatales*, **4**, 71.

Saling, E. & Schneider, D. (1967) Biochemical supervision of fetus during labour. *Journal of Obstetrics and Gynaecology of the British Commonwealth*, **74**, 799–811.

Schachter, F. F. & Apgar, V. (1959) Perinatal asphyxia and psychologic signs of brain damage in childhood. *Pediatrics*, **24**, 1016–1025.

Schulte, F. J., Michaelis, R. & Filipp, E. (1965) Neurology of the newborn, Parts I and II. *Zeitschrift für Kinderheilkunde*, **93**, 242–276.

Schulte, F. & Jurgens, U. (1969) Apnoen bei reifen und unreifen Neugeborenen. *Monats-schrift für Kinderheilkunde*, **117**, 595–601.

Schulte, F. J., Hinze, G. & Schrempf, G. (1971) Maternal toxemia, fetal malnutrition and bioelectric brain activity of the newborn. *Neuropädiatrie*, **2** (4), 439–460.

Shaffer, D. (1975) Behavioural and cognitive aftereffects of localised head injury in children. Paper presented to UK group of Paediatric Neurologists. Bristol.

Simmons, M. A., Adcock, E. W., Bard, H. & Battaglia, F. (1974) Hypernatraemia, intracranial haemorrhage and $NaHCO_3$ administration in neonates. *New England Journal of Medicine*, **291**, 6–9.

Simpson, H. (1974) Personal communication and paper presented to British Paediatric Research Society.

Smith, J. F. (1974) *Pediatric Neuropathology*. New York: McGraw-Hill.

Smith, J. F., Reynolds, E. O. R. & Taghizadeh, A. (1974) Brain maturation and damage in infants dying from chronic pulmonary insufficiency in the postneonatal period. *Archives of Disease in Childhood*, **49**, 359–365.

Spears, R. L., Hodgman, J. E., Cleland, R., Tatter, D. & Hanes, B. (1969) Relationship between HMD and IVH as cause of death in low birth weight infants. *American Journal of Obstetrics and Gynecology*, **105**, 1028–1031.

Sršeǔ, Š. (1966) Intraventricular haemorrhage in the newborn and 'low birth-weight'. *Developmental Medicine and Child Neurology*, **9**, 474–480.

Steiner, H. & Neligan, G. (1975) Perinatal cardiac arrest. *Archives of Disease in Childhood*, **50**, 696–702.

Stewart, A. (1972) The risk of handicap due to birth defect in infants of very low birth weight. *Developmental Medicine and Child Neurology*, **14**, 585–591.

Stewart, A. L. & Reynolds, E. O. R. (1974) Improved prognosis for infants of very low birth weight. *Pediatrics*, **54**, 724–735.

Svenningsen, N. W. & Siesjö, B. K. (1972) Cerebrospinal fluid lactate/pyruvate ratios in normal and asphyxiated neonates. *Acta paediatrica scandinavica*, **61**, 117–124.

Thistlethwaite, D. (1975) Personal communication on results of research project studying growth, nutrition and neurological maturation of low birth weight babies.

Thomson, J. (1951) Birth injuries in relation to post-natal defects. *Transactions Edinburgh Obstetrical Society*, Session CIV, 45–61.

Thorn, I. (1969) Cerebral symptoms in the newborn. *Acta paediatrica scandinavica*, Suppl. 195. Copenhagen: Munksgaard.

Towbin, A. (1969) Latent spinal cord and brain stem injury in newborn infants. *Developmental Medicine and Child Neurology*, **11**, 54–68.

Towbin, A. (1968) Cerebral intraventricular haemorrhage and subependymal matrix infarction in the foetus and premature newborn. *American Journal of Pathology*, **52**, 121–139.

Towbin, A. (1969) Cerebral hypoxic damage in fetus and newborn. Basic patterns and their clinical significance. *Archives of Neurology (Chicago)*, **20**, 35.

Towell, M. E. (1966) The influence of labor on the fetus and the newborn. *Pediatric Clinics of North America*, **13** (3), 575–598.

Turner, T. L. (1976) Neonatal coagulation defects. *Clinics in Endocrinology and Metabolism* **5**, 89.

Villee, C. A. (1967) Bioenergetic considerations in fetal and mature tissues, pp. 47–56. In 57th Ross Conference, Ross Laboratories, Ohio.

Visudhiphan, P., Bhanchet, P., Lakanapichanchat, C. & Chiemchanya, S. (1974) Intracranial haemorrhage in infants due to acquired prothrombin complex deficiency. *Journal of Neurosurgery*, **41**, 14.

Wallace, S. J. & Michie, E. A. (1966) A follow-up study of infants born to mothers with low ostriol excretion during pregnancy. *Lancet*, **2**, 560–563.

Wigglesworth, J. S., Keith, I. H., Girling, D. J. & Slade, S. (1975) Relation between intraventricular haemorrhage and hyaline membrane disease in the newborn infant. Paper presented to 46th Annual Meeting BPA, York.

Windle, W. F. (1969) Brain damage by asphyxia at birth. *Scientific American*, **221** (4), 77–84.

Wood, C., Ferguson, R., Leeton, J., Newman, W. & Walker, A. (1967) Fetal heart rate and and acid base status in the assessment of fetal hypoxia. *American Journal of Obstetrics and Gynecology*, **98**, 62–70.

Yates, P. O. (1959) Birth trauma to the vertebral arteries. *Archives of Disease in Childhood*, **34**, (177), 436–441.

4
INFANTS OF VERY LOW BIRTH WEIGHT

An appraisal of some aspects of their present neonatal
care and of their later prognosis

Pamela A. Davies

Infants of very low birth weight, those of 1500 g and less, account for just
over 1 per cent of total births, but rather less than 1 per cent of live births.
Early neonatal mortality is also near to 1 per cent, and most of these deaths
are in babies of very low birth weight. Those of them who are liveborn,
also have the highest neonatal complication rate, and the highest tally of
handicap at later follow-up. They are in essence the raison d'être of today's
neonatal intensive care service, which perpetually requires more staff and
more highly specialised and expensive equipment in order to function to its
satisfaction. As our understanding of the biology and pathology of the newborn has increased, so has the scope and complexity of the care offered. There
are however important questions to be asked. To what extent are present
practices soundly based and safe both in the short and long term? And to
what extent can the recently reported improvement in the quality of survivors
offset increased survival rates, and so justify the very large expenditure of
resources?

There are inherent difficulties in trying to provide answers to these and
related questions. First, the factors affecting neonatal mortality and morbidity
are varied and complex, and few units look after large enough numbers of
very low birth weight infants to be able to carry out satisfactory controlled
trials. Multicentre trials are not necessarily the solution, for populations
differ, and so many subtle features of treatment have to be held constant over
the period involved. Second, follow-up studies cannot give immediate help,
and thus are of limited value, for a number of years must elapse before the
children are old enough to be tested for less obvious defects such as learning
disorders. Third, all students of neonatal medicine know that today's 'advance'
may become tomorrow's iatrogenic disaster. With these reservations in mind
I will seek to review the evidence available. Mortality trends of very low
birth weight infants will be considered. The nature of their present neonatal
care will be discussed with particular emphasis on its main preoccupations—
respiratory support, nutrition, temperature control, biochemical homeostasis,
and the prevention and control of infection. The recent follow-up studies will
be reviewed, and finally the extent of later handicap will be judged in the
context of present survival rates.

MORTALITY

It has been possible to obtain the numbers and mortality of very low birth weight live births ($\leqslant 1500$ g) in England and Wales since 1953, and of numbers of still births since 1955. Alberman (1974) has standardised these data from the Annual Reports of the Chief Medical Officer to the Department of Health and Society Security. During the 20-year period from 1953 to 1973, when neonatal mortality for all registered births fell from 18 to 11/1000 live

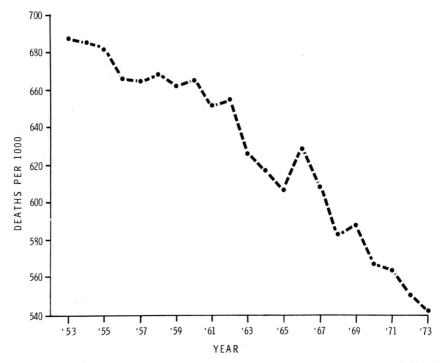

Figure 4.1   Neonatal mortality rate for infants weighing up to 1500 g, 1953 to 1973 (England and Wales). Reproduced from data of Alberman (1974). (I am grateful to Dr Alberman for supplying the additional figures for 1973)

births, that for infants 1500 g and less at birth fell from 687 to 542/1000. The pattern of this 20-year decline for the very low birth weight infants is shown in Figure 4.1, and deaths in the first 24 h of life (day 0), in the remainder of the first four weeks (days 1–28) and stillbirths are shown in Figure 4.2. As in the other birth weight groups below 2500 g (1500–2000, 2001–2250, 2251–2500 g), but to a greater extent than in them, deaths on the first day of life are those which show least improvement. It can be seen too that there is considerable fluctuation in day 0 deaths which actually rose during the latter years of the 1950s, and again quite sharply in 1966.

It seems almost certain that aspects of clinical care must be associated at least in some measure with these fluctuations, though it is almost impossible to assign them with any accuracy retrospectively. For instance it has been suggested (Cross, 1973; Bolton and Cross, 1974) that the failure of the 1950s first-day death rate to fall in the low birth weight group was due to restrictive oxygen practices introduced then to prevent retrolental fibroplasia (RLF). This decade saw the first tentative entry of paediatricians to labour wards

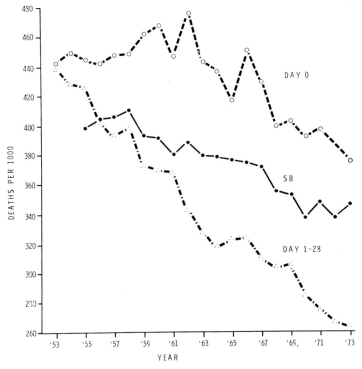

Figure 4.2 Perinatal mortality for infants weighing up to 1500 g; stillbirths, and deaths on first and subsequent days, 1953 to 1973 (England and Wales). Reproduced from Alberman (1974). (I am grateful to Dr Alberman for supplying the additional figures for 1973)

and newborn nurseries on a wider scale than hitherto. It must be said that theirs was not an instant success story, and they may also have been respon-sible for the failure of the death rate to fall in the first half hour of life (Lewis, 1974). Faced suddenly with the resuscitation at birth of very small infants, often done efficiently previously by anaesthetists or obstetricians, they did not cut dashing figures. Intubation was positively avoided as a last and desperate measure; infant laryngoscope design was poor, and the endotracheal tubes available were rubber and all too often miserable flaccid things which deflected off at a tangent as they approached the target area. A number of practices grew up to aid this subterfuge, such as 'rocking', intragastric oxygen, phrenic nerve stimulation, and the use of analeptic drugs, most of them without any sound physiological basis. The writer remembers the vivid impact of a lecture on neonatal resuscitation given by the late Virginia Apgar to the junior house staff of a New York City hospital engaged in somewhat similar practices in 1957, for here for the first time was someone actually teaching them the technique of intubation. Other harmful features of neonatal care over this period which could have been responsible for failure of first day deaths to fall must include the increasing use of incubators in which naked infants were nursed at insufficiently high ambient temperatures, and a much more liberal prescription of drugs at inappropriate dosages, some of which were to prove lethal. We do not know too whether births of infants < 1000 g fluctuated as a proportion of the total ≤ 1500 g. Since their mortality approached 100 per cent in those years, a higher proportion born at any one period would influence first-day deaths very considerably. This certainly was the experience at Hammersmith Hospital for instance between the years 1964 to 1968.

Alberman (1974) points out that there is no support for the hypothesis that in recent years there has been a tendency to postpone death, thus shifting stillbirths into neonatal deaths, or first-day deaths into 1–28 day deaths. It is quite possible of course that in individual centres pioneering new methods of perinatal treatment such a shift may have occurred in the 1970s though the numbers concerned would be too small to be reflected nationally. Certain of these well-staffed units too have a much higher survival rate of very low birth weight infants than the national average, despite receiving the illest infants from elsewhere. For instance at University College Hospital, London, 54 per cent of inborn infants and 55 per cent of outborn infants ≤ 1500 g survived between 1966 and 1970 inclusively (Stewart and Reynolds, 1974). If these figures are broken down for the outborn and presumably illest group, we find 5 per cent survival at birthweights 501–750 g, 32 per cent at 751–1000 g, 62 per cent at 1001–1250 g, and 75 per cent at 1251–1500 g. Further improvements have occurred since 1970 in various parts of the world, and the later status of these children as potential citizens will clearly be a crucial question. It is most unfortunate though that comparison of mortality statistics of very low birth weight infants between various perinatal centres continues to be beset by various pitfalls. The most important of these, relating largely to infants < 1000 g, are the widely differing interpretations of the terms viability, livebirth and stillbirth. Thus some calculated mortality rates still exclude deaths less than 28 weeks gestation, though any such babies who lived would undoubtedly be included to swell the survival rate! Since gestational age is so often uncertain the WHO recommendation of a particular weight for viability, 500 g, is convenient for this purpose for fresh stillbirth or livebirth. The former should continue to be defined as one in which there is no sign of life—that is neither detectable heart beat nor respiratory gasp at birth, whereas any infant of 500 g or above who displays these signs for however short a time would be liveborn. Differences in social class continue to be one of the most important factors in mortality differences, however, and these are rarely specified.

PRESENT NEONATAL PRACTICES

Respiratory support

The adaptation of mechanical techniques for ventilatory support for the smallest newborn infant has been one of the technical advances of the past 10 years, and some further progress has been made since Scopes (1971) reviewed this subject in the last edition of this book. Apart from initial resuscitation at birth, the conditions most likely to require intervention of this nature in those of very low birth weight are hyaline membrane disease (HMD) and severe recurrent apnoea.

Hyaline membrane disease. It was logical that attempts to treat the established disease after birth, now accepted as due to a deficiency of pulmonary surfactant causing alveolar collapse, should have been either medicinal or mechanical. However, medicine in the form of attempted cortisol acceleration of lung maturity and hence of pulmonary surfactant, known to be valid when delivered to the preterm fetus via the mother for a certain period before birth (see review by Avery, 1975), has been unsuccessful after birth (Baden et al, 1972), as has the attempted replacement of pulmonary surfactant as an aerosol (Robillard et al, 1964).

Mechanical measures to keep the air sacs open on the other hand have been more fruitful (see review by Reynolds, 1975), though it has to be said that there is as yet no wholly satisfactory evidence to prove that they have influenced survival in infants of 1500 g and less. Mortality from HMD in general however has almost certainly fallen—Roberton and Tizard (1975) report one of under 10 per cent for those over 1000 g—but there may be contributory causes other than later respiratory support by mechanical means. For instance there is some retrospective evidence from Newcastle (Omer, Robson and Neligan, 1974) suggesting that improved resuscitation in the delivery room and careful supervision of the environmental conditions during transfer to the nursery might contribute to a fall in mortality. These authors investigated the records of infants weighing 1000 to 2000 g who were born between 1960 and 1967. The mortality from HMD of those that were 'blue' on arrival in the nursery was four times that of those that were 'pink'. During the years 1971 to 1972, the number of such infants given intermittent positive pressure ventilation (IPPV) immediately after birth nearly doubled, the numbers arriving 'blue' in the nursery were cut by two-thirds, and the mortality fell, though the fall did not achieve statistical significance. Roberton and Tizard (1975) have shown that the mortality from HMD for all babies weighing over 1000 g who are breathing spontaneously by 15 min after birth is about a tenth of that seen in those who have not established adequate breathing by this time.

At present respiratory support is given either as mechanical ventilation using positive pressure respirators or negative pressure tanks, or, to the spontaneously breathing infant, as some form of continuous distending pressure (CDP), either continuous positive airway pressure (CPAP) (Gregory et al, 1971), or continuous negative pressure (CNP) (Vidyasagar and Chernick, 1971). Ventilation in the course of HMD is generally reserved for two eventualities: apnoea which cannot be terminated by other means and/or an inability to maintain P_aO_2 above 30 mmHg in high concentrations of oxygen (Davies et al, 1972). Intermittent positive pressure ventilation is usually delivered by an endotracheal tube passed either through the nose or the mouth, or by a tightly fitting face mask, using a pressure limited ventilator. The survival rate of infants artificially ventilated for HMD increased by nearly 50 per cent in one centre when positive end expiratory pressure was applied during ventilation and CPAP was maintained during the weaning period (Cumarasamy et al, 1973). Others also found that the survival rate for severe HMD increased suddenly in intubated IPPV treated infants after they started using a square pressure wave form, a slow respiratory frequency (30 cycles/min), a high inspiration:expiration ratio (up to 2:1), and a positive end expiratory pressure of 5 cm H_2O. By this means they were able to achieve adequate oxygenation at much lower peak airway pressures (25 cm H_2O) with a reduced inspired oxygen concentration as well, and believed the fall in mortality was due to a corresponding fall in the incidence of bronchopulmonary dysplasia (Reynolds and Taghizadeh, 1974). This term has been used to describe either lung necropsy findings involving mucosal, alveolar and vascular tissues, or a characteristic radiological appearance of the lungs during life (Northway, Rosan and Porter, 1967). It has variously been ascribed to oxygen toxicity, mechanical ventilation or a combination of both, and it is generally agreed that the two are difficult to separate (Banerjee, Girling and Wigglesworth, 1972; Reynolds, 1975; Philip, 1975). Some support for Reynolds' view that it is the high peak pressures of IPPV rather than high inspired oxygen concentrations that are primarily responsible, has been provided by Berg et al (1975) who never saw the condition following CNP, and by Stocks and Godfrey (1976) who showed that a raised airways resistance was present later in the first year of life in ventilator survivors, but not in those HMD infants who had been treated with CPAP and/or high inspired oxygen concentrations only. Controlled data to show that mechanical ventilation, however delivered, favourably affects survival in those $\leqslant 1500$ g is not available. Reid, Tunstall and Mitchell (1967), the first to publish results in this country showed a significantly lower mortality among a very small number of infants weighing 1000 to 2000 g treated with IPPV via tracheal intubation compared with non-ventilated controls. Others have shown such significance only in infants of over 2000 g (Murdock et al, 1970). This may well be because of the hazards of tracheal intubation in the smallest babies (see below). A recent survival rate of 87.5 per cent in infants with HMD or recurrent apnoea whose median birth weight was 1096 g and median gestation 29 weeks ventilated or given CPAP by face mask must command respect (Allen et al, 1975).

Continuous distending pressure has been applied in various ways. Gregory et al (1971), the pioneers of CPAP, delivered a pressure of up to 12 mmHg to the spontaneously breathing infant with HMD either via a head box or via an endotracheal tube. Others have used a plastic hood (Barrie, 1973), a face mask (Rhodes and Hall, 1973) or nasal cannulae (Caliumi-Pellegrini, 1974) in an effort to avoid intubation. Alternatively CNP, applied round the chest, has been advocated by some (Vidyasagar and Chernick, 1971; Bancalari, Garcia and Jesse, 1973). Controlled trials have been relatively few, sometimes contradictory, and almost without exception relate to small numbers of infants only. One of the first, delivering CPAP by face mask, demonstrated a significant increase in survival, though again only for infants over 1500 g (Rhodes and Hall, 1973); and a sequential trial of CNP using a body chamber in infants greater than 1000 g showed that CNP improved oxygenation in HMD and significantly reduced both the duration of exposure to higher concentrations of oxygen, and the need for later IPPV (Fanaroff et al, 1973). Continuous distending pressure had also been used to wean infants from IPPV, but the primary indications for it in HMD are still being sought. For instance Dunn (1974), using a head box, has advocated that CPAP should be given soon after birth in most infants to prevent further deterioration. Krouskop, Brown and Sweet (1975) were able to use lower concentrations of ambient oxygen in infants treated early with nasal CPAP, and found they ran a less severe clinical course than late treated controls. They could demonstrate no difference in mortality, duration of CPAP therapy, total time of oxygen administration or complications however, and found that the very few infants < 1500 g in their trial did badly regardless of when CPAP was applied. Similarly others using endotracheal and nasal CPAP, have been able to report an increase in survival only in infants above 1500 g when they compared mortality in HMD with the pre-CDP era (Kamper et al, 1974; Boros and Reynolds, 1975). Two other controlled trials of early versus late CNP (Gerard et al, 1975; Mockrin and Bancalari, 1975) found the course of HMD modified by its early application. Thus although in general there is little clear-cut evidence of advantage relating to the infant of very low birth weight alone, it would seem that in a few cases the need for mechanical ventilation might be averted by early intervention with some form of CDP. Every effort however should be made to avoid endotracheal intubation for the smallest babies, and some other form of delivery, face mask, nasal cannulae or a simple negative pressure device, is desirable. It should go without saying that this form of treatment should be embarked upon only when constant supervision of the infant is available, and frequent blood gas measurements possible.

Recurrent apnoea. Low birth weight infants may develop periods of apnoea after birth, usually defined as a cessation of respiratory movement for 20 s or longer, as a warning symptom of some underlying illness. However in many no associated condition is found; they are merely of extremely immature birth weight and gestation. Their management has always posed a considerable problem, for the episodes of recurrent apnoea may continue for several weeks after birth in the smallest infants. Those who have studied such babies in detail have suggested various explanations. Thus the infants are considered to be hypoxic because of hypoventilation primarily due to mechanical abnormalities of the lungs, and unresponsiveness to this hypoxia, a feature of gestational and postnatal age, is thought to be mainly at the respiratory centre or central receptors (Rigatto and Brady, 1972a, b; Rigatto, Brady and Verduzco, 1975a, b). A loss of surfactant leading to a gradual loss in lung volume has been postulated (Krauss, Klain and Auld, 1975). The heart rate usually falls during an apnoeic attack and Girling (1972) found this occurred after the onset of apnoea in most babies he studied, the pulse pressure commonly rising at the same time. Major resuscitative measures were usually required if the pulse pressure did not rise as the heart rate fell.

It was inevitable that many such infants should have been attached to ventilators if serious apnoeic episodes persisted with any frequency. However, clinical experience over the last decade suggests, as already stated, that intubation as a means of applying IPPV or CPAP, known to be effective in reducing attacks (Kattwinkel et al, 1975), should be avoided, particularly in those less than 1000 g, and in most less than 1500 g. If respiratory support seems necessary, the face mask, fixed so as to avoid distortion of the head, seems to be the best method for these tiny infants, and it can be quickly adapted for mechanical ventilation should this become necessary (Allen et al, 1975). There is also sequential or controlled trial evidence to suggest that frequent peripheral stimulation (Kattwinkel et al, 1975), nursing on a gently oscillating waterbed (Korner et al, 1975) or the administration of theophylline (Kuzemko and Paala, 1973; Shannon et al, 1975; Uauy et al, 1975) to produce serum levels in the range 6 to 11 μg/ml, will significantly reduce the frequency and severity of apnoeic episodes.

With the help of cardiac and respiratory monitors though, an ever-vigilant nurse can gently and successfully prod these babies back to life at the first warning sign, and so often prevent major episodes. Even the most skilful and constant attendant however is defeated sometimes, and if very frequent or severe attacks are recurring, this writer prefers the use of the face mask to deliver CPAP with just a few centimetres of water pressure at ambient oxygen concentration, or if necessary IPPV, to drug therapy. There should be someone at or very near the baby's side throughout the 24 h whatever form of treatment is being given.

Hazards of mechanical ventilation and CDP. The presence of an endotracheal tube for only a few hours in the very low birth weight infant will lead to mucosal swelling and superficial epithelial damage in the very small airway. Ulceration and necrosis, focal in the larynx, extensive in the trachea, are seen as the duration of intubation increases (Rasche and Kuhns, 1972)

Serious scarring in survivors however seems rare, though subglottic stenosis has been known to occur. The upper respiratory tract is usually sterile at birth, but the rate of bacterial colonisation steadily increases over the first few days of life. Thus positive cultures from endotracheal tube secretions do not necessarily indicate infection, though very heavy growths and profuse or viscid secretions almost certainly do, and varying degrees of pneumonia are not uncommon at autopsy. Efficient removal of these secretions without further damaging the mucosa or disturbing the baby unduly presents a prob- lem, and the use of the indwelling oxygen electrode (Goddard et al, 1974) reveals how quickly arterial oxygen tensions fall during any nursing or medical procedure.

The question of whether nasotracheal or orotracheal tubes are to be used must largely rest on the personal preference and skill of the individuals who pass them. Nasotracheal tubes are easier to fix, but slower to pass in an emergency, and there are at least theoretical objections to this route in that infected nasal secretions could be carried down into the larynx. Bacteraemia has been reported to occur just significantly more often following nasotracheal intubation than following orotracheal intubation for surgical operations in older patients (Berry, Blankenbaker and Ball, 1973), but whether this would apply to the situation in the neonatal period is not known. As the newborn infant breathes entirely through the nose, the mucosal swelling and increased secretions which may be present following extubation could compromise easy weaning from the ventilator. Prolonged nasal intubation may also lead to some nostril deformity later, but in the writer's experience this is minimal when care is taken in the neonatal period. The slight difference in size which is sometimes present may not be obvious on casual inspection, but has to be consciously sought. More serious deformities such as stenosis of a nostril, or ulceration of nasal cartilage have been reported elsewhere (Baxter et al, 1975).

There are more immediately life-threatening hazards of IPPV and CDP therapy in the form of pneumothorax, and pneumomediastinum. While these complications can occur spontaneously in the course of HMD, there seems little doubt that the introduction of both IPPV with positive end expiratory pressure and CPAP has been associated with a significant increase in their occurrence. In one study the prevalence of pneumothorax, pneumo- mediastinum and interstitial emphysema nearly doubled from 20.7 to 39.7 per cent when a positive and expiratory pressure was added to IPPV, whereas they occurred in only 4.9 per cent of cases treated with CNP, similar to that occurring spontaneously. Even more alarming was the fact that once lung rupture occurred, 73 per cent of the infants died (Berg et al, 1975). Others have reported a 17 per cent incidence of pneumothorax in CPAP treated infants (Baum and Roberton, 1974). On the other hand no increase, but rather a slight decrease in incidence was noted by Reynolds and Taghizadeh (1974) when they added positive and expiratory pressure, but this was presumably because they had been able to drop peak airway pressures significantly at the same time. Pneumoperitoneum and pneumopericardium have also been reported (Leonidas et al, 1974). Continuous distending pressure has undoubtedly been of benefit in the treatment of HMD, particularly in infants over 1500 g. Stahlman and Cotton (1975) point out however that its use when the alveolar volume is not low to begin with can lead to CO_2 retention, an increasing functional residual volume and decrease in tidal volume, with consequent increased ratio of dead space to tidal volume. They emphasise that using CDP either when alveoli have a normal volume or with higher pressures than necessary to achieve such a normal volume may decrease or obstruct completely the alveolar wall capillary blood flow in areas of normal compliance. Thus very abnormal rather than improved ratios of ventilation to perfusion may occur, especially when the disease process is not uniformly distributed throughout the lung fields. Reduction of venous return can also lead to low output failure. It is clear that indiscriminate application of CDP, especially without very careful and frequent blood gas monitoring, may be actively harmful.

So far only complications associated with the upper and lower respiratory tract have been discussed. Intracranial haemorrhage is common in very low birth weight infants, with or without HMD and is probably now the most important single cause of death. It is usually found in the lateral ventricles and/or the subarachnoid space; hydrocephalus may develop as a result in survivors. However intracerebellar haemorrhage, not previously described, has recently been reported at necropsy from Toronto (Pape, Armstrong and Fitzhardinge, 1975) in about one-fifth of infants who also had the more usual intraventricular and/or subarachnoid bleeding. They weighed 1500 g and less at birth, all had HMD, and most were receiving CPAP or IPPV by face mask fixed in position by a band across the acciput; this was noted to cause severe compression in the occipital area and a tower skull deformity. Infants with intracerebellar haemorrhage had received IPPV by mask for a just significantly longer period of time than those without such haemorrhage. Others have been able to avoid this complication by fixing the mask with elastic netting applied uniformly over the whole head (Allen et al, 1975). Although considerable facial oedema occurs with the face mask, ophthalmologists have not found its use hazardous to the eyes (Pape et al, 1975). Concern has also been felt about the possibility of an increased incidence of intracranial haemorrhage with the use of CPAP delivered by head box, or of CNP using a negative pressure ventilator, for both require a tightly fitting neck seal to function effectively. A group of French workers (Vert, Andre and Sibout, 1973) reported an increased incidence of hydrocephalus after adopting the head box method of CPAP but this does not seem to have been reported from elsewhere. Certainly dangerous ulceration of skin and deeper tissues has been reported with the seal (Krauss and Marshall, 1975) and meticulous nursing supervision with careful padding of the neck is needed to prevent this happening. Erb's palsy has also occurred during the course of head box treatment (Turner, Evans and Brown, 1975). Care has to be taken to see that temperature drops do not occur when the head box or plastic bag are used, and the torrential flow of oxygen which may be delivered must be effectively warmed and humidified. Follow-up studies have not yet been published on hearing in children nursed in this way in the neonatal period. Noise levels of 80 dB may be reached at the higher pressures, which could theoretically be damaging to the VIIIth nerve (Svenningsen and Blennow, 1973).

It is relatively easy to put a very low birth weight infant on a ventilator; it is often much more difficult to get him off. Much activity has been directed recently at assessing the contribution made by patent ductus arteriosus to heart failure in association with HMD. For it is felt that the effects of a significant ductal shunt could be masked while artificial ventilation improves oxygenation, increases intrathoracic pressure, decreases pulmonary venous return and so reduces exudation into the alveoli. Once this support is withdrawn, the cardiovascular status may quickly deteriorate, and further ventilation be necessary. Thus ligation of the ductus in such infants—no mean surgical feat at birth weights less than a 1000 g—is now being undertaken in some cases (Baylen et al, 1975).

Nutrition

The fountain pen filler of 50 years ago filled with breast milk to be dripped into the mouth, and the central venous or arterial catheter of today filled with carefully calculated amounts of amino acids, carbohydrate, electrolytes, and sometimes fat for the circulation, illustrate the evolution of feeding of very low birth weight infants. The inadequacy of sucking and swallowing reflexes which have resulted in the past in the early death of these babies from aspiration pneumonia, was countered by a demand for early starvation (Clifford, 1947; Smith et al, 1949; Gaisford, 1950; Corner, 1962), a practice in direct contrast to that of early pioneers such as Hess (Hess, Mohr and Bartelme, 1934), and one stoutly opposed by the few (Yllpo, 1954; Gleiss, 1955).

Improving nursing techniques for gavage feeding, followed by the introduction of the indwelling nasogastric polyvinyl feeding catheter, and the increasing skill of young doctors at entering small veins probably led to a gradual relaxation of this policy of fluid and calorie restriction. As a consequence bilirubin levels were lowered (Laurance and Smith, 1962; Wu et al, 1967), protein catabolism reduced (Auld, Bhangananda and Mehta, 1966) and hypoglycaemia and ketonuria decreased (Beard et al, 1963). In the early 1960s too it was suggested that very early and much more liberal feeding of breast milk might reduce the time taken to regain birth weight, and thus allow an earlier resumption of growth; for growth would have proceeded fast but for untimely expulsion from the uterus (Smallpeice and Davies, 1964). Early and liberal feeding was gradually adopted and was given much impetus by the experimental work of Dobbing (1968) and Winick (Winick and Noble, 1966). The questions to be answered are whether this is justifiable, and to what extent the various methods of feeding larger amounts of food are safe and effective.

The basis of the relevant experimental work in the fetal and newborn animal is that undernutrition at a period of very rapid growth results in permanent stunting of final mature size. This is true of body growth (e.g. Widdowson and Kennedy, 1962; Winick and Noble, 1966, 1967), and of brain growth (Dobbing, 1968). Providing the nutritional stress occurs through-out the period of the brain growth spurt, later liberal feeding cannot reverse the final stunting of brain or body (Dobbing, 1974). Enthusiastic extrapolation to the human has caused Dobbing to point out that although the sequence of events described holds true in different kinds of animals, there are important species differences in the timing of the brain growth spurt in relation to birth. In the human brain there are two important spurts (Dobbing and Sands, 1970). The first occurs between 15 and 20 weeks of gestation, and is a neuronal cell multiplication; and the second, starting at 25 weeks gestation and extend-ing into the second year of life is predominantly a glial cell multiplication with myelination continuing into the third or fourth year.

Intrauterine growth in the human fetus can be restricted by a variety of maternal factors, but usually does not begin to fall off until the third trimester is reached, and any deficiency in brain growth must then be one of glial cells. Clearly glial cell deficiency and intellectual deficiency should not be equated, but Dobbing also points out that in addition to glial cell multiplication and myelination which alone have been investigated in the past, there are other extremely important events occurring in the second brain growth spurt whose measurement is only just becoming technically possible. These include a large increase in dendritic complexity and the development of synaptic connections, as well as various metabolic and hormonal changes and may be important for intelligence, although this is by no means certain. The velocity of brain growth reaches a peak at term. The velocity of cerebellar growth may be greater than that of the rest of the brain for it starts its spurt a little later at about 30 weeks gestation and finishes much earlier at the end of the first year (Dobbing and Sands, 1973).

Thus the very immature infant leaves the uterus near to the start of the second brain growth spurt, while the very low birth weight infant destined to be small for dates stays in the uterus longer receiving less than enough food. If there is an analogy to be drawn between the experimental animal work and the human, undernutrition in the latter would probably have to continue well into the second year of life and not for just a few weeks after birth or in the uterus to have any permanent stunting effects. This is very unlikely to happen in the majority to children in this country today. On the other hand, malnutrition at a time of growth acceleration may be more important.

Head circumference is said to be an accurate reflection of cellular growth of the brain in the first year (Winick and Rosso, 1969), and of intracranial volume (Bray et al, 1969). It also bears some direct relationship to intelligence in children (Nelson and Deutschberger, 1970; Weinberg et al, 1974; Babson and Henderson, 1974), and before changes in bony growth and muscle bulk occur at puberty, seems to be a valuable measurement. It was however rarely measured in the follow-up studies of infants born in the 1950s, when delayed feeding of preterm infants was widely practised, but in those few in which it was, there are an unusually large number of children or young adults with small head circumferences (Baum and Searls, 1971; Wright, 1972). An abnormal distribution of head circumference percentiles at later follow-up was also evident in both small for dates (SFD) and appropriately grown (AFD) very low birth weight infants born in 1961 to 1964 who had relatively small feeds in the first week of life and body temperatures below the ideal for four weeks. In the years 1965 to 1968 however, when these two factors were to a large extent corrected, the distribution of head circumference percentiles of the infants of normal weight for gestation at birth was more normal though that of the SFD infants remained abnormal (Davies and Davis, 1970). A somewhat similar state of affairs appeared to exist for monozygous twins of very discrepant weight born 1950 to 1958, where one member of the pair was very severely growth-retarded by comparison. The undersized twin continued inferior in both growth (height, weight and head circumference) and intelligence into adult life (Babson et al, 1964; Babson and Phillips, 1973). Similar findings have been reported by Hohenauer (1971), and as regards intelligence, by Churchill (1965). However in discrepant weight twins born in recent years no significant differences in intelligence have been reported (Fujikura and Froehlich, 1974; Buckler and Robinson, 1974) and it may be that greater attention to nutrition after birth has resulted in this change. The weight of evidence suggests then that the immature or SFD very low birth weight infants' food requirements should be met as soon as possible after birth. Since there is nothing physiological about being born very immaturely, it follows that attempts to meet these requirements by whatever means are in themselves to some extent unphysiological by comparison with the intrauterine supply.

Parenteral feeding. The application of parenteral feeding to the smallest sick infants needs technical skill and a meticulous and continuing attention to detail on the part of all concerned. It has been used successfully for the most immature ill infants either alone, or to supplement oral intake. If the expertise is not present throughout the 24 h and seven days a week, it is best not attempted. The hyperosmolar solutions are usually fed into central veins or the right atrium, but if the infusion site is changed every 24 h, peripheral veins can be used first, thus lessening the risks of infection (Harries, 1971). Few controlled trials have demonstrated its unequivocal superiority where early mortality is concerned, and it is too early yet for differences in late morbidity to be assessed among the young survivors. A 3.5 per cent fibrin hydrolysate and 10 per cent dextrose solution has been compared with 10 per cent dextrose alone in infants 1300 g and less at birth (Bryan et al, 1973), and a 3.4 per cent amino acid and 10 per cent dextrose solution with 5 per cent dextrose in 0.2 per cent saline in infants 1500 g and less (Pildes et al, 1973). There were no significant differences in mortality but birth weight was regained sooner in the protein supplemented group in both studies, and discharge weight reached more quickly in the latter study. Others have found that similar parenteral supplementation of oral feeding in preterm infants weighing 1500 g and less and SFD infants reduced the time taken to regain birth weight compared with orally fed controls but did not influence the time of discharge; and length, head circumference and skin fold measurements were no different in the supplemental group suggesting that increased initial weight gains were due to water retention rather than tissue accretion (Brans et al, 1974). Although no significant difference in mortality could be shown in one study comparing parenteral supplements with conventional oral feeding in infants < 1200 g, it was stated that the non-survivors died at a mean time of 30 days in the supplemented group compared with a mean time of five days in the other (Abitbol et al, 1975). Fat emulsions have not been widely used, but small for dates infants have been shown to have a reduced capacity for dealing with them compared with preterm low birth weight babies (Gustafson et al, 1974; Olegard et al, 1975).

The complications reported are many, with infection, either bacterial or monilial being the most immediately dangerous. Possible long-term hazards of hyperaminoacidaemia such as those described by Menkes et al (1972) in another context are not yet known. Other metabolic abnormalities, acidosis, hyperammonaemia, hyperglycaemia, hypophosphataemia, hypocalcaemia, make careful monitoring and adjustments of the infused fluids important. Essential fatty acid supplements will be necessary when fat emulsions are not being used, and multiple vitamin supplements are vital if intravenous feeding continues for more than a few days. At present parenteral nutrition, surgical conditions apart, is likely to find most application in infants of exceptionally low weight (< 1000 g), in those with continuing and severe recurrent apnoea, and in those with severe respiratory distress syndrome. It will continue to be life saving in some such infants in whom oral feeding cannot be safely and adequately established. The obsessional attention to detail needed for its complete success should not be underestimated, and it cannot be undertaken without the additional support of laboratory and pharmacy.

Oral feeding. It is fair to say there has always been controversy about the amount and nature of milk suitable for the very low birth weight infant. Basal metabolic rate has been calculated as 45 to 60 cal/kg/day in the resting, non-distressed infant (Krauss and Auld, 1969) and calorie requirements of growth as 120 cal/kg/day (Sinclair et al, 1970), and somewhat higher for SFD infants. The protein content of human milk has been considered by many insufficient to allow adequate nitrogen retention and weight gain in very low birth weight infants since the report of Gordon, Levine and McNamara (1947). Recent studies on protein intake have been reviewed by Cox and Filer (1969) who conclude that daily protein intakes in the range of 2.25 to 5.0 g/kg are optimum. Stevens (1969) has pointed out that very low birth weight infants given pooled *early* human milk containing 1.85 ± 0.24 g/dl of protein will get a protein allowance of 3 to 5 g/kg/day, so that past strictures on this valuable but alas rare commodity may not have been valid. The anti-infective properties of breast milk could be of considerable importance to the LBW infant. The very high numbers of *Escherichia coli* in the bowel of such infants fed cow's milk (Graham, 1975) and possibly those of other bacteria such as *Klebsiella* species might be markedly decreased. There might also be less risk of such conditions as necrotising enterocolitis if early breast milk could be collected safely and used without sterilising, for sterilisation destroys heat labile fractions such as the immunoglobulins, macrophages and lysozymes.

The most important complication of oral feeding in the sick very low birth weight infants has always been the risk of aspiration into the lungs. Recent developments in feeding techniques have been concerned with reducing this while at the same time increasing the amounts offered. Stomach emptying time is known to be quicker after gastric tube feeding than bottle feeding, and there is less gaseous distension but this does not stop aspiration in very sick infants, and nasojejunal feeding has recently been suggested as an alternative to nasogastric, with the main aim of reducing the risk of regurgitation (Rhea, Ghazzawi and Weidman, 1973). Perforation of the gut has followed the use of polyvinyl tubes instead of the silastic ones originally recommended, presumably due to the rigidity of polyvinyl when it has been in situ some time (Boros and Reynolds, 1974; Sun et al, 1975). Care also has to be taken to see that the feed given is not excessively hyperosmolar (Rhea, Ahmad and Mange, 1975). However, taking these precautions, and given a rapid passage of the tube past the pylorus, nasojejunal feeding solves many of the problems associated with oral intake and it is quite feasible to give before the end of the first week of life in very sick and small infants as much as 200 ml/kg/day of expressed breast milk. Although the weighted end to the tube seems essential, it is not always necessary to use the introducer described by Rhea and colleagues, and it can safely be left in place for several weeks. This method is likely to find more widespread application than intravenous feeding because of its simplicity.

A feeding tube passed through the nose to stomach or jejunum is easier to keep in place than one through the mouth, but its presence must compromise the airway to some extent, however small the tube, and gavage feeding should be substituted as soon as possible. Continuous infusion of feed, now made easier for very small babies by the use of infusion pumps, has been preferred by some (Valman, Heath and Brown, 1972) to interval feeding, and may have some advantage in view of the finding of a fall in arterial oxygen tension and a rise in heart rate and blood pressure, shortly after a milk feed in ill newborns (Wilkinson and Yu, 1974). Food is likely to leave the stomach more quickly if the infant is lying prone or in the right lateral position rather than supine or in the left lateral position (Yu, 1975).

Temperature control

Although 10 to 20 years have elapsed since controlled trials demonstrated that even small changes of environmental temperature could significantly influence neonatal mortality (see reviews by Scopes, 1970; Hey, 1971), the importance of this aspect of care for the very low birth weight infant is still insufficiently appreciated. As Hey (1971) reminded us in the last edition of this book, deaths in infants under 1500 g can be reduced by a quarter or more if their body temperature is maintained above 36°C, and great care taken to reduce heat loss to a minimum. Clinical experience suggests that the battle for heat conservation is not waged ardently enough in labour wards. It has been shown that the use of an overhead infrared servo-controlled radiant heater with power set at 400 W, fixed 70 cm above the infant can maintain body temperature in asphyxiated and immature newborns, while allowing access to them (Dahm and James, 1972). While many infant resuscitation areas in delivery rooms are now fitted with heaters of some sort this is not invariably the case, and wattage of existing devices is often inadequate. The simple measure of drying the infant to reduce evaporative loss should of course always be carried out. If sick and immature babies have to be transported from their place of birth to a neonatal intensive care unit it is possible to conserve or even raise temperature on the journey by transporting them in an incubator, wrapped in a plastic swaddling device which reduces evaporative radiant and convective heat loss (Storrs and Taylor, 1970).

Nearly all very low birth weight infants are nursed in some form of incubator initially. Many stay there, unclothed, far too long. Although it was shown some years ago that radiant heat loss from naked infants in incubators could be effectively reduced by the use of an open-ended plastic shield placed over the infant (Hey and Mount, 1967), this simple device is not in universal use. The shield will reduce by 25 per cent the insensible water loss from infants of very low birth weight which represents an important source of heat loss (Fanaroff et al, 1972). These authors determined insensible water loss from measurements of insensible weight loss and found it to be greater than 2.5 g/kg/h, some three times higher than that of full-term infants, a fact not always appreciated when apportioning fluid requirements. Hey (1975) has calculated from his observations the mean temperature needed to provide thermal neutrality for healthy naked babies of differing weights and postnatal ages nursed in draught-free surroundings of uniform temperature and moderate humidity, and these are shown in Table 4.1. These temperatures are arrived at by allowing that evaporative heat loss is usually proportional to resting metabolic rate, while insulation increases with size. Thus the estimates may not be valid where resting metabolic rate is abnormal; it is for instance higher than normal in small for dates babies (Bhakoo and Scopes, 1974) and lower than normal in those with severe respiratory distress (Hey, 1972).

There is a growing tendency to nurse infants of very low birth weight, particularly those who because of illness need frequent nursing and medical attention, in open cradles under radiant heaters with servo-control mechanisms, the humidity obviously the low one of room air. Thermal regulation of infants nursed in this way has not as yet been fully investigated. It is known however that infants in servo-mechanised closed incubators have apnoea significantly more often during periods of rising air temperature (Perlstein, Edwards and Sutherland, 1970). Furthermore when humidity is low in such incubators, the rectal temperature of infants nursed in them drops signifi-

Table 4.1 The mean temperature needed to provide thermal neutrality for a healthy baby nursed naked in draught-free surroundings of uniform temperature and moderate humidity after birth[a]

Birth weight (kg)	Operative environmental temperature[b]			
	35°C	34°C	33°C	32°C
1.0	For 10 days	After 10 days	After 3 weeks	After 5 weeks
1.5	–	For 10 days	After 10 days	After 4 weeks

[a] From Hey, E. (1975)

[b] To estimate operative temperature in a single-walled incubator subtract 1°C from incubator air temperature for every 7°C by which this temperature exceeds room temperature

cantly below that of the abdominal skin temperature. The temperature is lower on naked skin than on skin covered by adhesive tape, such as that under the temperature probe, since skin is the predominant site of evaporative skin loss. Servo-control with low humidity thus increases evaporative skin loss and sets in train a lowering of body temperature as the incubator temperature rises (Belgaumkar and Scott, 1975a). A significantly greater proportion of severe apnoea was found by these authors in infants in low rather than high humidity, presumably due to the increased and widely fluctuating ambient temperature (Belgaumkar and Scott, 1975b).

One final aspect of temperature control which might conveniently be re-emphasised here is its association with growth. If infants are nursed at temperatures below the thermoneutral range some calories derived from food have to be diverted to heat production and are not available for growth. It has been suggested that a combination of a relatively low calorie intake and a lower than optimal body temperature in the first week and month of life respectively may have curtailed later head growth in very low birth weight infants who were AFD (Davies and Davis, 1970). Glass et al (1975) have now shown that the head growth of infants nursed at temperatures below the thermoneutral range and given a relatively low calorie intake’ was significantly retarded over the period of study in the early weeks of life.

Management of jaundice of immaturity

Some degree of non-haemolytic jaundice is common in the very immature, but the incidence of hyperbilirubinaemia (> 15 mg/dl) has fallen since the introduction of earlier and more liberal feeding. During the years 1961 to 1970 inclusive, two-thirds of the infants weighing ≤ 1500 g cared for at Hammersmith Hospital had serial estimations of bilirubin because of clinically recognisable jaundice. The mean maximum total bilirubin in the years 1961 to 1964 was 15.0 mg/dl (S.D. ± 4.4; $n = 40$), whereas in the years 1965 to 1970 following a significant increase in milk intake in the first week of life, there was a highly significant fall to a mean of 11.7 mg/dl (S.D. ± 4.3; $n = 78$). Exchange transfusion apart, two other methods of lowering serum bilirubin which have found most application in the very low birth weight infant are the use of phenobarbitone and phototherapy, and the separate mechanisms by which they act are well known, and will not be enlarged upon here (see respective reviews by Behrman and Fisher, 1970, and Lucey, 1972). The protagonists can rightly claim that there is good controlled evidence to show that both are effective in lowering bilirubin levels. A combination does not appear to be more effective than the one alone (Valdes et al, 1971).

The detractors of phenobarbitone tread largely theoretical ground, the relevance of which for those of very low birth weight is as yet uncertain. A dosage of 8 mg/kg/day for the first seven days of life given to babies of less than 36 weeks gestation was stated to be unassociated with any noticeable side effects (Carswell, Kerr and Dunsmore, 1972). It seems likely that were standardised examinations made of treated infants and compared with controls, subtle differences in behaviour would be found. Studies on experimental animals suggest that phenobarbitone therapy might have long-term effects on the smooth endoplasmic reticulum of the liver, on the metabolism of other drugs, an influence on steroid metabolism in turn affecting behaviour mechanisms and interfering with normal imprinting, on growth and sexual maturation, and on coagulation (Wilson, 1969).

Phototherapy has some well-documented side effects including a raised respiratory rate and increased stool water loss and insensible water loss for which allowance must be made in deciding fluid intake and which is greatest at lowest gestation (Oh and Karecki, 1972; Wu and Hodgman, 1974). The latter is probably due to evaporative water loss from the skin and the respiratory tract (Oh et al, 1973). Skin temperature and skin blood flow increase during phototherapy, and in the very immature sick infant the metabolic demands of this may be too great (Wu et al, 1974). A polygraphic study of healthy mature infants without jaundice has shown differences in behaviour under light treatment, which are reversible within a short time of stopping it. These include a slight increase in ‘physiologic apnoea’ (lasting longer than 3 s), a non-significant increase in heart rate, a slight decrease in the number of spontaneous startles, a significantly higher number of rapid eye movements, a relative increase of active sleep states with an unchanged total length of sleep cycles, and a more immature EEG pattern (von Bernuth and Janssen, 1974). The stools are often darker brown or green, presumably because they contain photodegradation products, but their number and frequency is probably not greater than those of controls (Washington, Brown and Starrett, 1972), though gut transit time is said to be increased (Rubaltelli and Largajolli, 1973). Increased tanning of the skin has been noted in some Negro infants exposed to phototherapy and is thought to be due to reoxidation of preformed melanin causing pigment darkening (Woody and Brodkey, 1973). Rapid bronzing of the skin of a very low birth weight Caucasian infant after only 48 h exposure to phototherapy has occurred and here pre-existing hepatic disease, resulting in a failure of biliary excretion of the photodegradation products of bilirubin was thought to be the cause (Kopelman, Brown and Odell, 1972).

There is a significant decrease in the affinity of fetal red cells for oxygen when they are exposed to blue light in the presence of bilirubin, suggesting photodynamic membrane injury (Ostrea and Odell, 1974). Phototherapy significantly alters the biliary bilirubin excretion pattern, for more bilirubin is excreted as the unconjugated variety, and the colour of the bile changes from yellow to dark brown (Lund and Jacobsen, 1974). Although the exact nature of all the photodegradation products of bilirubin is not known, they would appear to be non-toxic (Ostrow, 1972). Visible light is known to be an important controlling factor in various neuroendocrine functions, maturation of the gonads, and circadian rhythms (Behrman, 1974) and concern has been expressed at possible alterations of these by phototherapy. Other experimental or in vitro hazards do not seem to have materialised in vivo; thus there does not seem to be damage to the eyes provided they are shielded (Dobson, Riggs and Siqueland, 1974), or to red blood cells (Blackburn, Orzalesi and Pigram, 1972).

There has been a good deal of confusion about the units of measurement of the light in phototherapy. Thus the US committee on phototherapy in the newborn infant (Behrman, 1974) states that light meters have been inappropriately used since they measure illuminance: 'the density of electromagnetic radiation specially weighted to the response of the human eye'. What is needed apparently is a measure of spectral irradiance: 'the radiative power density of the incident light, expressed in watts per square centimetre per unit wavelength over the entire spectral range incident on the patient'. The average paediatrician may well feel bewildered by these statements especially when he learns that only a spectroradiometer—'complex, expensive and probably unsuited for use in a nursery'—can measure this spectral irradiance. The committee believes practical alternatives can be developed, and recommend at present that the phototherapeutic dosage be defined as the product of irradiance and time, with irradiance expressed in watt-seconds per square centimetre, and time in hours of phototherapy. It seems very doubtful that all the large variety of lamps in use will measure up to the committee's criteria. Acute observation led Cremer, Perryman and Richards (1958) to embark on phototherapy. After initial reluctance paediatricians have rushed to follow them, and have found themselves in a field of great complexity, which they only partly understand.

In the writer's experience the introduction of earlier and more liberal feeding meant that the need for exchange transfusion, to keep bilirubin levels below the conventional 20 mg/dl, virtually disappeared. However the realisation that some very low birth weight infants, all seriously hypoxic and acidotic during life, were found to have bile staining of the basal ganglia at autopsy when bilirubin levels had been below 20 mg/dl and sometimes below 10 mg/dl (Stern and Denton, 1965; Gartner et al, 1970; Ackerman, Dyer and Leydorf, 1970), gave impetus to the view that bilirubin levels in those of very low birth weight should be kept as low as possible. Neither phenobarbitone treatment nor phototherapy however have prevented kernicterus in such infants; a maximum total bilirubin level of 9 mg/dl was reported in association with yellow staining of the basal ganglia by Carswell et al (1972) in a phenobarbitone treated infant, and levels of unconjugated bilirubin between 8 and 18 mg/dl in four infants receiving phototherapy with similar autopsy findings by Keenan et al (1972).

Although Boggs, Hardy and Frazier (1967) have suggested there is a positive relationship between increasing bilirubin levels and the incidence of low motor scores attained at eight months, their evidence is not entirely satisfactory because of small numbers in the low birth weight groups, and because a comparison is made of developmental status of term and pre-term infants at eight months of age without making allowance for gestational age. In an era when the incidence of neurological and intellectual deficit following low birth weight was higher than at present, others have been unable to find such a correlation with bilirubin levels between 18 and 24 mg/dl (Koch, 1964; Vuchovich et al, 1965; Wishingard et al, 1965; Culley et al, 1970) A further breakdown of Hammersmith data (Francis-Williams and Davies, 1974), does not show any correlation between the level of maximum total bilirubin and either full-scale IQ or the presence of a significant (>15 points) discrepancy between performance and verbal IQ. Such a 'pure' correlation would be difficult to find in those of very low weight, since marked jaundice usually accompanies other neonatal problems. Another difficult state of affairs which persists despite a great deal of work is the absence of an entirely satisfactory laboratory test for the presence of free, diffusible and hence potentially brain damaging bilirubin, as opposed to the readily measureable total or unconjugated bilirubin. An indirect method, the saturation index has been used, and Odell, Storey and Rosenberg (1970) have shown a significant association between 'brain damage' and a high index, but not one with maximum bilirubin concentrations. However the index showed no association with IQ scores, or neurological abnormality on examination, and it was on tests of cognitive function that the children were pronounced damaged. More than half of these children had had a maximum bilirubin of greater than 20 mg/dl, and a third one above 24 mg/dl, in the neonatal period.

In the writer's view, the evidence at present justifies the use of photo-therapy to keep levels of total bilirubin below 20 mg/dl only, and with attention to an adequate calorie intake it should be very rarely needed. Since phenobarbitone has to be given from birth to be effective, its use is not justified for the very low birth weight, at least when there is no racial predisposition to excessive jaundice. But as exchange transfusion has a mortality of 1 per cent or more depending on the experience of the operator, and a varying morbidity, phototherapy is undoubtedly helpful in the few cases which would otherwise need this procedure. Its use must not preclude the investigation of other causes of jaundice than the immaturity and care must be taken to supervise fluid balance and temperature carefully.

Hypocalcaemia of immaturity

About one-third of preterm infants have serum calcium levels below 7 mg/dl between 12 and 72 h of age and the values are significantly correlated with gestational age (Tsang et al, 1973). This early hypocalcaemia is not to be confused with that occurring mainly in large, mature and artificially fed infants towards the end of the first week of life associated with convulsions, for there are no really clear-cut symptoms or signs which are pathognomonic for the former. Infants who have birth asphyxia are also found to have lower serum calcium and higher serum phosphorus levels than controls matched for gestational age (Tsang et al, 1974). Much calcium is deposited in the fetal skeleton during the last eight weeks of pregnancy, and is therefore lacking in preterm infants of very low birth weight. So are many other substances, but there seems little published evidence as yet to confirm that wholesale efforts to replace them with intravenous supplements is desirable or necessary.

Late metabolic acidosis

A number of otherwise well infants of very low birth weight are found to have a late metabolic acidosis persisting between the first and third weeks of life (Kildeberg, 1974). It is more common in those with a high dietary protein intake (Svenningsen and Lindquist, 1974) and these babies appear to have a lowered renal bicarbonate threshold level, a lowered capacity to compensate for the resulting bicarbonate leak, and an inadequate renal tubular hydrogen ion excretion with a decreased ability to lower urinary pH (Svenningsen, 1974). Nevertheless these functions mature rapidly, the protein intake perhaps even playing some role in the maturation, and most infants are in normal acid–base equilibrium by six weeks.

Prevention and control of infection

It cannot be said that there have been major advances in this very important sphere of neonatal care in recent years, yet the problems increase in parallel with the complexity of the apparatus surrounding the ill, very low birth weight infant. It is now well established that, in the past decade at least, these babies whether ill or well, are colonised soon after birth predominantly with Gram-negative aerobic bacteria (Farmer, 1968; Davies et al, 1970), which may be resistant to multiple antibiotics (Dailey, Sturtevant and Feary, 1972; Graham, 1975). The increased permeability of the skin of the most immature infants allowing absorption of hexachlorophane, which may then be concentrated in brain tissue, has made it unwise to continue the use of this antibacterial phenolic derivative in such infants. Its withdrawal (from low birth weight infants only), has made no difference to their pattern of colonisation in the writer's experience. The different influence of human and breast milk on the nature of the aerobic and anaerobic bowel flora has been known for three-quarters of a century. In a recent study of bacterial colonisation in ill low birth weight and normal infants, Graham (1975) has shown, with careful calculation of viable counts, that the numbers of *Escherichia coli* in the rectum of ill low birth weight infants fed on a cow's milk derivative are significantly greater than those of normal babies fed the same milk, both of course easily outnumbering those found in the entirely breast-fed baby. The geometric mean counts of *Escherichia coli* in these three groups of infants on the seventh day of life were $10^{8.2}$, $10^{5.9}$ and $10^{2.5}$, with colonisation with *Escherichia coli* being 85, 65 and 29 per cent respectively. The patterns of bowel colonisation in infants solely on parenteral nutrition have not yet been reported, but it would seem that for those infants who can be fed orally, and they should be the majority, greater efforts should be made to obtain early pooled human breast milk under sterile conditions so that it could be fed to them without prior heating. In addition to limiting the number of *Escherichia coli* in the bowel, breast milk influences the serotypes found there, and strains with K1 antigen are much more commonly isolated in the artificially fed (Ørskov and Sorensen, 1975). This capsular polysaccharide antigen is now known to be of importance in the causation and outcome of neonatal *Escherichia coli* meningitis (McCracken et al, 1974; Sarff et al, 1975). It seems very likely that the nature of the bowel flora is an important contributory factor in necrotising enterocolitis, the incidence of which has appeared to increase in many neonatal intensive care units in recent years. Functional stasis of bowel segments may have several underlying causes, but when it occurs it will be accompanied by bacterial multiplication. If numbers of bacteria are high to begin with, as in the artificially fed ill low birth weight baby, it is easy to see how invasion of the bowel wall occurs. Serotyping of *Escherichia coli* and pyocine typing of *Pseudomonas aeruginosa* in a neonatal intensive care unit revealed that individual types tended to occur in clusters at certain periods suggesting cross colonisation (Graham, 1975), and this is doubtless true of other bowel organisms. Cases of necrotising enterocolitis, relatively rare in this same unit, have also seemed to occur with a certain periodicity; production of enterotoxin by certain strains (Rudoy and Nelson, 1975) may also be of importance in this condition. A surgically conservative approach substituting intravenous for oral feeding, and the use of antibiotic therapy may avert the complete clinical picture; but where it is established, surgical mortality is lessening in recent years (Stevenson et al, 1971). Once again the use of fresh breast milk might do much to prevent this condition.

There seems as yet no wholly satisfactory evidence to suggest that anti-biotic prophylaxis is worthwhile. Thus recent studies have not shown any benefit of prophylactic use of antibiotics following umbilical vessel catheteri-sation (van Vliet and Gupta, 1973), respiratory distress syndrome with umbili-cal vessel catheterisation (Bard et al, 1973) or with naso- or orotracheal intubation (Harris, Wirtschafter and Cassady, 1975) or the prevention of necrotising enterocolitis (McCaffree, Fletcher and Avery, 1975). In all low birth weight infants given antibiotics from birth, Graham (1975) found that both the numbers of organisms recovered and the precentage of infants colonised remained lower than in untreated infants to begin with. *Klebsiella, Enterobacter, Serratia* species and *Pseudomonas aeruginosa* were then the dominant organisms to emerge and their numbers and incidence, compared with non-treated infants, became significantly higher towards the end of the first week. This seems an unpleasant price to pay for the early suppression. Since there is good evidence that very low birth weight infants acquire their bacterial flora largely from their environment, prevention of infection in intensive care units must continue to rest on obsessional attention to effective handwashing, and the efficient and regular sterilisation of apparatus, rather than the wholesale use of antibiotics.

Possible hazards of present day practice

Most practitioners of neonatal medicine, particularly those of them who are old enough to remember the 1950s, are acutely aware that their well-intentioned therapy may one day prove harmful. One of the striking differences between then and now which strikes the writer is the much greater use now of 'diagnostic' radiography. When the only treatment available for HMD was raising the ambient oxygen concentration as cyanosis increased, chest radio-graphs to affirm the diagnosis were often not taken. Now they are a routine, with abdomen frequently included, so that the position of umbilical catheters and sometimes feeding tubes can be checked. Continuous distending pressure has increased the risk of pneumothorax and pneumomediastinum, and as this diagnosis is not always made easily on clinical grounds, further x-rays may be called for, sometimes at frequent intervals as the clinical course fluctuates. It is very doubtful if the benefit to the patient is directly proportional to the numbers of films taken, and in some units these have increased enormously for certain sick infants. The testes are abdominal organs in the very immature male, so that gonadal radiation in the two sexes may be equal, and the cumulative dose to the reproductive organs of some very low birth weight survivors long before they have reached the expected date of delivery should not be dismissed as insignificant. Although radiographic techniques have improved greatly since the work on the effects of fetal radiation (Stewart, Webb and Hewitt, 1958; Stewart and Kneale, 1970; Newcombe and McGregor, 1971) we must surely be mindful of this aspect of neonatal care.

Intraventricular haemorrhage (IVH) is one of the most important causes of death in the very low birth weight. Attention has been drawn recently to the possibility of an association between hypernatraemia due to high sodium bicarbonate administration and non-traumatic intracranial haemorrhage (Simmons et al, 1974). Wigglesworth et al (1976) found a significant difference in the total quantity of alkali and in the total quantity of sodium bicarbonate given to infants subsequently dying of IVH, compared with infants of similar gestation dying of other causes. Although the incidence of metabolic acidosis was no different, the IVH infants received considerably more bicarbonate. Babies who died with HMD and germinal layer haemorrhage without IVH had also received significantly more alkali than those who died with HMD alone. They point out that it is not possible to say whether or not the alkali was given before or after the onset of IVH. Baum and Robertson (1975) have found that both bicarbonate and THAM cause a significant rise in blood volume especially if injected rapidly. Machin (1975), in a new survey of perinatal deaths, has noted a threefold increase of IVH, from 0.7 to 2.2/1000 births, when comparing his figures with those of the National Birthday Trust's Perinatal Mortality Survey of 1958. The newer methods of respiratory support should enable many infants with HMD to correct their acid–base status without recourse to frequent and rapid injection of hypertonic alkali solutions.

Since the widespread introduction of polyvinyl tubes and catheters, plasticiser has been identified and measured in the tissues of infants who have died and who had undergone umbilical vessel catheterisation. Higher levels were associated with blood transfusion, more extensive use of catheters and early death. Levels in gastrointestinal tissue were significantly higher in infants with necrotising enterocolitis than in those without the disease. The significance of these observations to the individual infant is unknown, though of importance to patients in general (Hillman, Goodwin and Sherman, 1975).

LATER PROGNOSIS

Follow-up studies of low birth weight infants have been in progress for a number of years, but it is only in the past two decades or so, as survival rates have improved, that the very low birth weight have been included in any numbers. Essential though such surveys are, their role in guiding neonatal care is a limited one. Major handicap can usually be ascertained by the age of six months, or at least one year, but more subtle damage may not be detected until the early school years. By then the nature of the treatment given in the intensive care nursery may have changed in some major as well as many minor ways so that it can be extraordinarily difficult to pinpoint cause and effect. The independent variables of socio-economic status, maternal pregnancy details, birth weight, gestation and intrauterine growth all have to be taken into account too when assessing final outcome, and completeness of follow-up becomes of first importance because of the relatively small numbers involved.

The well-known and comprehensive reports of infants born in the late 1940s and early 1950s (Lubchenco et al, 1963; Drillien, 1964; McDonald, 1967) drew rather depressing conclusions regarding the future potential of the smallest babies, for they described results in an era when iatrogenic handicap was much in evidence; and mental retardation, cerebral palsy, blindness and deafness could affect up to a third or more of the survivors. The application of a veritable explosion of recent knowledge of the fetus and newborn does appear to have resulted in a significant lessening of handicap among infants born in the 1960s (see review by Davies and Stewart, 1975). A selection of these reports will be considered under three main headings: physical growth, neurological handicap, and intelligence.

Physical growth

It is difficult to make anything more than general statements about the later physical growth of very low birth weight infants, for the numbers reported by individual authors are so limited. Thus one cannot assess the individual effects of social class, sex, birth order and number of younger siblings, maternal age, genetic factors, smoking in pregnancy and intrauterine growth rates, all of which have been shown to have some bearing on later size in a large national cohort of births (Davie, Butler and Goldstein, 1972), without separating the children into impossibly small groups from which nothing of statistical validity could emerge. In addition available growth standards may have been collected several decades ago, and it seems likely that in all but exceptionally and uniformly prosperous countries secular trends in children's growth continue, so that plotting measurements of very low birth weight children against these standards may give a false impression.

Possibly one of the largest groups of very low birth weight children to have their growth followed in recent years is that cared for at Hammersmith Hospital, London, between 1961 and 1970. Approximately one-third of the 165 children weighing $\leqslant 1500$ g at birth were small for dates, that is their birth weight lay below the tenth percentile for gestational age. At later follow-up the distribution of growth percentiles in this group was significantly different for height, weight and head circumference, in that in general they were shorter, lighter and had smaller heads when compared with those whose birth weight had been appropriate for gestation (Davies, 1975). These differences between SFD and AFD babies were not seen throughout the 10⁻ year period however, and mention has already been made of the possible growth restricting effects of low temperature and limited food intake in the early weeks of life in the years 1961 to 1964. During this period there were *no* significant differences in the distribution of height, weight and head circumference percentiles at later follow-up suggesting that the AFD infants had been artificially converted into SFD infants after birth. When food intake was increased, and body temperature maintained at a higher level, the significant differences noted for the entire group were again apparent for the SFD and AFD infants born 1965 to 1970, at least where head circumference and height were concerned. Other surveys of LBW infants which have included small numbers of infants ≤ 1500 g have shown similar growth trends for AFD and SFD (Fitzhardinge and Ramsay, 1973; Brandt and Schroder, 1974; Fitzhardinge, 1975).

Although it is difficult to compare the results directly with the older surveys of children born in the 1940s and 1950s, few of which recognised differences in intrauterine growth rates, an overall impression is gained of some stunting of growth potential among many children who must have been AFD at birth. It seems possible that food and temperature deficits in the first weeks and after could have had a restricting effect. Although SFD infants are very heterogeneous, only a tiny minority of the Hammersmith group might have had impaired growth associated with congenital anomaly; most appeared to have been malnourished in the uterus and the effects of this and preterm birth imposed a definite handicap where later growth was concerned.

Neurological handicap

Spastic diplegia. This has always been regarded as the commonest form of cerebral palsy seen in those of very low birth weight. Spasticity involves the legs more than the arms, which occasionally appear quite normal; spasticity can be asymmetrical, and the intelligence is near to normal. Lubchenco and colleagues reported its presence in 33 per cent of infants born 1949 to 1953 weighing 1500 g and less at birth (Lubchenco et al, 1963). While this was an exceptionally high figure compared with other surveys even from the same era, there is recent evidence that it is becoming very much less common from regional and individual surveys. In an area of Sweden particularly well controlled from the point of view of case finding, there has been a continuing fall in the total incidence of all forms of cerebral palsy from 1954 to 1970. Further analysis of the types of cerebral palsy has shown that this reduction in incidence—nearly 50 per cent—is largely due to a highly significant drop in cases of spastic/ataxic diplegia in very low birth weight children (Hagberg, Hagberg and Olow, 1975a, b). These authors equated this with the provision of neonatal intensive care for the region. A somewhat similar state of affairs has been seen at Hammersmith Hospital between 1961 and 1970 (Davies and

Tizard, 1975). The division of their 165 cases into two unequal time periods has been previously explained. Six cases of spastic diplegia occurred among the 58 infants born 1961 to 1964, while none occurred among the 107 born 1965 to 1970, a highly significant difference.

Apart from its very clear association with immature gestation and very low birth weight, the exact cause of spastic diplegia has never been defined. In discussing aetiology in relation to their case material Davies and Tizard found that the mean lowest temperature of the diplegics (usually on the first day of life) was just significantly lower ($P=0.05$) than that of the non-diplegics. Others have reported a lower haematocrit reading on the second day of life in diplegics compared with non-diplegics of similar birth weight and gestation (Churchill et al, 1974). The possibility of intraventricular haemorrhage as a cause was considered by both groups as low body temperature may be a factor contributing to haemorrhage in the neonatal period (Chadd and Gray, 1972). Other reported incidences of the condition which are available

Table 4.2   Recent incidence of spastic diplegia in infants of very low birth weight

Author	Year of birth	No. in study	% Spastic diplegia	Birth weight
Fitzhardinge and Ramsay, 1973	1960–66	32	3%	≤1250
Davies and Tizard, 1975	1961–70	165	4%	≤1500
Stewart and Reynolds, 1974	1966–70	95	3%	≤1500
Drillien, 1972	1966–71	87	16%	≤1500
Fitzhardinge, 1975	1970–72	44	2%	≤1500

from recent reports are shown in Table 4.2. With one surprising exception (Drillien, 1972) the incidence is considerably lower than one of the lowest estimates in this weigh group—9 per cent—of earlier years (Wright et al, 1972).

Other forms of cerebral palsy. These have always been very much less common among those of lowest weight and gestation. For instance spastic quadriplegia occurred in 0.6 per cent of the recent Hammersmith series (Davies and Tizard, 1975) and hemiplegia in 1 per cent of the University College Hospital series (Stewart and Reynolds, 1974). However a disquieting report of infants born 1970 to 1973 has appeared from Canada (Fitzhardinge et al, 1976) concerning 73 infants of 1500 g and less, all of whom survived varying periods of mechanical ventilation after birth. Nineteen (26 per cent) of these very ill infants later developed cerebral palsy: no fewer than 15 of the 19 had either spastic quadriplegia or hemiplegia, and only four had spastic diplegia. Thus it is possible that some who would previously have died before mechanical ventilation was available (from the mid-1960s onwards in many units) will now survive and show different patterns of neurological handicap. Somewhat similar findings in a group of 77 ventilator survivors with a median birth weight of 1760 g have been reported by Marriage and Davies (1976); though the incidence of neurological abnormality (15 per cent) was less. In both these series recurrent fits before or during ventilation carried a particularly poor prognosis where later neurological handicap was concerned.

Visual and hearing defects

Retrolental fibroplasia was and still is the most important cause of visual impairment in very low birth weight babies. Its incidence has almost certainly increased in the past few years. For instance in Sweden, where as elsewhere a dramatic fall in the condition occurred in the early 1950s, 46 cases were reported between 1960 and 1966, of whom 23 had irreversible changes (Svedbergh and Linstedt, 1973). A 23 per cent incidence was found among infants weighing less than 1000 g and born 1965 to 1970 in Seattle (Alden et al, 1972). Three of the 165 children of ≤ 1500 g cared for at Hammersmith Hospital between 1961 and 1970 developed it and were partially sighted as a result. The increase may be associated with an increase of survival of infants with recurrent apnoea, for they are the group most at risk (Mushin, 1974). Accurate and frequent monitoring of oxygen tension by repeated arterial puncture may become very difficult in these tiny infants whose episodes of apnoea and cynosis can continue for weeks. The factors which may modify the effects of oxygen on the retinal vessels of the very immature are not perfectly understood. For instance the disease may be asymmetrical; it has occurred in a preterm infant with severe cyanotic congenital heart disease; and a sustained high arterial oxygen tension (in very immature eyes) has not produced it (Aranda and Sweet, 1974).

There would appear to have been a genuine reduction in the incidence of deafness in recent years. Lubchenco et al (1963) found a 10.5 per cent incidence among very low birth weight infants born 20 to 25 years ago. Recent studies have reported an incidence of moderate to severe deafness of under 2 per cent (Stewart and Reynolds, 1974; Davies and Tizard, 1975). Safer dosage schemes of ototoxic drugs seem to be the most likely explanation for this.

Intelligence

As the incidence of cerebral palsy, blindness and deafness in children of very low birth weight has fallen in recent years so has the incidence of mental retardation. Francis-Williams and Davies (1974) recorded a mean full scale IQ of 97 among 105 children born 1961 to 1968 inclusive weighing ≤ 1500 g at birth, using the Wechsler tests. There was a significant difference between that of SFD children and that of AFD children (92 vs. 99). Neonatal illnesses such as respiratory distress tended to lower the mean IQ a few points, but not significantly. Several previous studies of children born in the 1950s had shown mean IQs in the 80 to 85 range; they had also reported boys to be at a disadvantage, as were those of lowest weight and gestation. However this was no longer found to be true, and the only highly significant correlation, as might be expected, was with social class. The AFD children born 1965 to 1968 whose head circumference percentiles at follow-up had been more normally distributed than those of AFD children born 1961 to 1964 did not have a higher mean IQ, though more of them had values over 100. A significantly higher IQ was found in those whose head circumference was above the fiftieth percentile rather than below it. Learning difficulties were present in one-fifth of these Hammersmith children, many of whom had a normal full scale IQ. Results for 32 AFD Montreal children weighing $\leqslant 1250$ g at birth were somewhat similar, with a mean IQ of 88 for males and 92 for females (Fitzhardinge and Ramsay, 1973). The IQ of 65 University College Hospital children born 1966 to 1969 was tested at a mean age of $3\frac{1}{2}$ years, and the distribution of IQ found to be no different from that of one of their parents (Stewart and Reynolds, 1974).

Total handicap

Isolated figures for neurological handicap, for sensory defects and for low intelligence or learning disorders do not give us an overall picture of the numbers of handicapped children from which we may judge the results of neonatal intensive care units. Three main studies of children born in the 1960s will be considered for this purpose: from Montreal (Fitzhardinge and Ramsay, 1973*); from University College Hospital, London (Stewart and Reynolds, 1974); and from Hammersmith Hospital, London (Francis-Williams and Davies, 1974; Davies and Tizard, 1975). At the outset it should be said that the great majority of children in all three studies were attending normal school, or were expected to be able to go there. The Montreal study involved 32/39 survivors, all AFD, weighing $\leqslant 1250$ g, and all born 1960 to 1966 in the Royal Victoria Hospital, Montreal. One child had died at three months, and six had been lost to follow-up. The University College Hospital study involved 95/109 children, 21 per cent of them SFD, either born in or admitted to the hospital between 1966 and 1970, weighing $\leqslant 1500$ g. Eleven children had died between 29 days and 25 months; three had been lost to follow-up. The Hammersmith Hospital study involved 120/123 children, 33 per cent SFD, born in or admitted from elsewhere between 1961 and 1968, weighing $\leqslant 1500$ g. Three children died between 28 days and six months. One of the 120 had been lost to follow-up after one year, when she was developing normally. If handicap is defined as an IQ < 70, neurological abnormality, whether major or minor, and moderate to severe hearing or visual handicap, then 13.7, 10.5 and 18.3 per cent respectively of the children are involved. This is a rather narrow view. Children with IQs between 70 and 85 are likely

* I am grateful to Dr Fitzhardinge for further details of the infants under her care.

to be at considerable disadvantage, particularly if they are of poor socio-economic status. A sizeable proportion of children in the Montreal study were adjudged as having percepto-motor difficulties though IQ in many was normal; a fifth of the Hammersmith sample had more than a 15-point discrepancy between performance and verbal IQ, again many having normal full scale IQs; the University College Hospital children are too young as yet for this data to be available. Thus if the concept of handicap were broadened to include children with learning difficulties and an IQ < 85, then 59.4 per cent of the Montreal children were handicapped, and 46.7 per cent of the Hammersmith group. Of the University College Hospital group, 21.5 per cent had IQs less than 85 (65/95 tested); these figures for Montreal and Hammersmith are 18.7 per cent (all tested) and 25.7 per cent (105/120 tested). In giving these figures together in this way it must be stressed that there may be very little comparability of population between the three groups, particularly since the Canadian study involved infants of lower birth weight (≤ 1250 g vs. ≤ 1500 g) who were all AFD. The social class distribution of the two London hospitals was different too; thus 38.8 per cent of the University College Hospital sample of 98 children came from social classes I and II, compared with 17.5 per cent of the Hammersmith Hospital group. Their 28-day survival rates (collected in a comparable way) also differ. That for inborn babies at the two hospitals for the periods of study involved being 54 and 38 per cent, and for outborn babies 57 and 41 per cent respectively. Handicapping congenital anomaly was a rarity in the Hammersmith Series, and this has been the experience of Stewart (1972). Drillien (1972) believes a proportion of very low birth weight handicapped infants are thus because of developmental anomaly. Intrauterine infection could be one cause of this, but may not always be identified as such.

It is possible to give a little more detail about the Hammersmith children with regard to outcome and their intrauterine growth rates. Thus taking the first and narrow view of handicap defined above 15.8 per cent of AFD and 23.7 per cent of SFD children are involved; taking the broader view and including children with IQs 70 to 85 and with learning difficulties as handicapped, then these figures become 42.7 and 55.3 per cent respectively. The figures for outborn infants are marginally worse than for inborn. The handicap rate for AFD dropped quite significantly in 1965 to 1968 compared with 1961 to 1964 (taking a 'narrow', but not a 'broad' view). Using Alberman's (1974) figures, it can be calculated that 18500 children ≤ 1500 g survived in England and Wales during the period of the Hammersmith study (1961 to 1968). Thus since mortality is not uncomparable, and assuming for the moment that the results in a generously staffed unit are applicable to the rest of the country, one could imagine that just over 3000 children have been launched from neonatal intensive care during this period with an IQ < 70, neurological abnormality, and moderate to severe visual or auditory handicap. If again the wider view of handicap is adopted, then nearly 8000 children, approximately 1000 per year, will be involved. Assumptions are dangerous however. Generously staffed regional neonatal intensive care units tend to imagine they produce better results than others less fortunate. On the other hand some 'advances' pursued in such institutions may be responsible ultimately for a higher incidence of iatrogenic disease. Continuing information on this subject is badly needed. Also it is short-sighted to abandon the very low birth weight child once he has been followed to school and help has been arranged for his learning difficulties should he have them. Behavioural problems in children, sometimes severe, may stem from their school learning difficulties and failures, even in the absence of impaired IQ or such perceptual problems. Birch and Gussow (1970) have reported an excess of behavioural and personality disorders in the low birth weight, which are worst among those of lowest socio-economic status, again whether or not associated with overt handicap (Wortis and Freedman, 1965). This may not augur well for their future as adults, and ideally a record linkage system should follow them to adult life, and preferably their offspring too. We know too little of their adult potential.

CONCLUSIONS

Very low birth weight infants have been surviving in slowly but steadily increasing numbers in the past 20 years. During that time the nature of their care has greatly increased in technical complexity, and the quality of their survival has improved. The main causes of handicap of 20 years ago, cerebral palsy, blindness and deafness, were largely though not entirely responsible for the mental retardation which was present in a third or more of the survivors. As all these three conditions have become less frequent, there are now many fewer retarded children, and the general level of intelligence may also have improved. This suggests that a majority of the previous handicap was preventable; indeed much of it may have been iatrogenic. There is evidence to suggest, improved obstetric care apart, that relatively simple measures such as the prompt treatment of birth asphyxia, the conservation of body temperature and more attention to adequate nutrition may have contributed much to the fall in mortality and perhaps to a lesser extent to the lowering of handicap rates.

Techniques for respiratory support have been developing steadily since the mid-1960s, but until very recently they have been of little certain advantage to those of lowest weight. Their use however has proved invaluable to much greater numbers of larger and more mature babies, and has significantly contributed to lowered mortality in hyaline membrane disease, a principal cause of death previously. There is a suggestion however that in the early 1970s some of the difficulties associated with respiratory support in the smallest babies are being overcome. Some ethical problems may now start to play an increasing role, for there is slim but slowly accumulating evidence to suggest that some brain-damaged children who would previously have died are now being kept alive. These problems will need very careful consideration by paediatricians, especially because many very low birth weight infants come from a background of social and economic disadvantage which can least support handicapping conditions. In saying this, however, it must be emphasised that the outlook for the majority of very low birth weight infants is now very good, a situation which could not have been envisaged 20 years ago. The benefit to individual children and their families is immeasurable in human terms and thoroughly justifies the pioneering spirit of those who introduced intensive perinatal care with such energy and skill. As already stated, in tackling the problems posed by this minority a very much larger number of children have benefited, and will continue to do so. Neonatal intensive care must be closely and constantly monitored for safety by skilled personnel. Since harmful effects may not be immediately apparent and may even be long delayed, follow-up studies provided on a continuing basis must constitute an essential part of a neonatal intensive care service.

REFERENCES

Abitbol, C. L., Feldman, D. B., Ahmann, P. & Rudman, D. (1975) Plasma amino acid patterns during supplemental intravenous nutrition of low-birth-weight infants. *Journal of Pediatrics*, **86,** 766–772.

Ackerman, B. D., Dyer, G. Y. & Leydorf, M. M. (1970) Hyperbilirubinemia and kernicterus in small premature infants. *Pediatrics*, **45,** 918–925.

Alberman, E. (1974) Stillbirths and neonatal mortality in England and Wales by birthweight, 1953–71. *Health Trends*, **6,** 14–17.

Alden, E. R., Mandelkorn, T., Woodrum, D. E., Wennberg, R. P., Parks, C. R. & Hodson, A. (1972) Morbidity and mortality of infants weighing less than 1000 g in an intensive care nursery. *Pediatrics*, **50,** 40–49.

Allen, L. P., Blake, A. M., Durbin, G. M., Ingram, D., Reynolds, E. O. R. & Wimberley, P. D. (1975) *British Medical Journal*, **4,** 137–139.

Aranda, J. V. & Sweet, A. Y. (1974) Sustained hyperoxemia without cicatricial retrolental fibroplasia. *Pediatrics*, **54,** 434–437.

Auld, P. A. M., Bhangananda, P. & Mehta, S. (1966) The influence of an early caloric intake with I–V glucose on catabolism of premature infants. *Pediatrics*, **37,** 592–596.

Avery, M. E. (1975) Pharmacological approaches to the acceleration of fetal lung maturation. *British Medical Bulletin*, **31,** 13–17.

Babson, S. G. & Henderson, N. B. (1974) Fetal undergrowth: relation of head growth to later intellectual performance. *Pediatrics*, **53,** 890–894.

Babson, S. G. & Phillips, D. S. (1973) Growth and development of twins dissimilar in size at birth. *New England Journal of Medicine*, **289,** 937–940.

Babson, S. G., Kangas, J., Young, N. & Bramhall, J. L. (1964) Growth and development of twins of dissimilar size at birth. *Pediatrics*, **33,** 327–333.

Baden, M., Bauer, C. R., Colle, E., Klein, G., Taeusch, H. W. & Stern, L. (1972) A controlled trial of hydrocortisone therapy in infants with respiratory distress syndrome. *Pediatrics*, **50,** 526–534.

Bancalari, E., Garcia, O. L. & Jesse, M. J. (1973) Effects of continuous negative pressure on lung mechanics in idiopathic respiratory distress syndrome. *Pediatrics*, **51,** 485–493.

Banerjee, C. K., Girling, D. J. & Wigglesworth, J. S. (1972) Pulmonary fibroplasia in newborn babies treated with oxygen and artificial ventilation. *Archives of Disease in Childhood*, **47,** 509–518.

Bard, H., Guy, A., Teasdale, F., Doray, B. & Martineau, B. (1973) Prophylactic antibiotics in chronic umbilical artery catheterisation in respiratory distress syndrome. *Archives of Disease in Childhood*, **48**, 630–635.

Barrie, H. (1973) Continuous positive airway pressure for respiratory-distress syndrome. (Letter). *Lancet*, **2**, 851.

Baum, J. D. & Roberton, N. R. C. (1974) Distending pressure in infants with respiratory distress syndrome. *Archives of Disease in Childhood*, **49**, 766–781.

Baum, J. D. & Roberton, N. R. C. (1975) Immediate effects of alkaline infusion in infants with respiratory distress syndrome. *Journal of Pediatrics*, **87**, 255–261.

Baum, J. D. & Searls, D. (1971) Head shape and size of pre-term low-birthweight infants. *Developmental Medicine and Child Neurology*, **13**, 576–581.

Baxter, R. J., Johnson, J. D., Goetzman, B. W. & Hackel, A. (1975) Cosmetic nasal deformities complicating prolonged nasotracheal intubation in critically ill newborn infants. *Pediatrics*, **55**, 884–887.

Baylen, B. G., Meyer, R. A., Kaplan, S., Ringenburg, W. E. & Korfhagen, J. (1975) The critically ill premature infant with patent ductus arteriosus and pulmonary disease—an echocardiographic assessment. *Journal of Pediatrics*, **86**, 423–432.

Beard, A. G., Panos, T. C., Burroughs, J. C., Marasigan, B. V. & Oztalay, A. G. (1963) Perinatal stress and the premature neonate. 1. Effect of fluid and caloric deprivation. *Journal of Pediatrics*, **63**, 361–385.

Behrman, R. E. (1974) Preliminary report of the committee on phototherapy in the newborn infant. *Journal of Pediatrics*, **84**, 135–147.

Behrman, R. E. & Fisher, D. E. (1970) Phenobarbital for neonatal jaundice. *Journal of Pediatrics*, **76**, 945–948.

Belgaumkar, T. K. & Scott, K. E. (1975a) Effects of low humidity on small premature infants in servocontrol incubators. I. Decrease in rectal temperature. *Biology of the Neonate*, **26**, 337–347.

Belgaumkar, T. K. & Scott, K. E. (1975b) Effects of low humidity on small premature infants in servocontrol incubators. II. Increased severity of apnea. *Biology of the Neonate*, **26**, 348–352.

Berg, T. J., Pagtakhan, R. D., Reed, M. H., Langston, C. & Chernick, V. (1975) Bronchopulmonary dysplasia and lung rupture in hyaline membrane disease. Influence of continuous distending pressure. *Pediatrics*, **55**, 51–54.

Berry, F. A., Blankenbaker, W. L. & Ball, C. G. (1973) A comparison of bacteremia occurring with nasotracheal and orotracheal intubation. *Anesthesia and Analgesia Current Researches*, **52**, 873–876.

Bhakoo, O. N. & Scopes, J. W. (1974) Minimum rates of oxygen consumption in small-for-dates babies during the first week of life. *Archives of Disease in Childhood*, **49**, 583–585.

Birch, H. G. & Gussow, J. D. (1970) *Disadvantaged Children. Health, Nutrition and School Failure*, pp. 46–80. New York and London: Grune & Stratton.

Blackburn, M. G., Orzalesi, M. M. & Pigram, P. (1972) Effect of light on fetal red blood cells in vivo. *Journal of Pediatrics*, **80**, 641–643.

Boggs, T. R., Hardy, J. B. & Frazier, T. M. (1967) Correlation of neonatal serum total bilirubin concentrations and developmental status at age eight months. A preliminary report from the Collaborative Project. *Journal of Pediatrics*, **71**, 553–560.

Bolton, D. P. G. & Cross, K. W. (1974) Further observations on cost of preventing retrolental fibroplasia. *Lancet*, **1**, 445–448.

Boros, S. J. & Reynolds, J. W. (1974) Duodenal perforation: a complication of neonatal nasojejunal feeding. *Journal of Pediatrics*, **85**, 107–108.

Boros, S. J. & Reynolds, J. W. (1975) Hyaline membrane disease treated with early nasal end-expiratory pressure: one year's experience. *Pediatrics*, **56**, 218–221.

Brandt, I. & Schroder, R. (1974) Postnataler Entwicklungsausgleich bei Fruhgeborenen mit pranataler dystrophie. *Monatsschrift für Kinderheilkunde*, **122**, 697–700.

Brans, Y. W., Sumners, J. E., Dweck, H. S. & Cassady, G. (1974) Feeding the low birth weight infant: orally or parenterally? Preliminary results of a comparative study. *Pediatrics*, **54**, 15–22.

Bray, P. F., Shields, W. D., Wolcott, G. J. & Madsen, J. A. (1969) Occipito frontal head circumference—an accurate measure of intracranial volume. *Journal of Pediatrics*, **75**, 303–305.

Bryan, M. H., Wei, P., Hamilton, J. R., Chance, G. W. & Swyer, P. R. (1973) Supplemental intravenous alimentation in low-birth-weight infants. *Journal of Pediatrics*, **82**, 940–944.

Buckler, J. M. H. & Robinson, A. (1974) Matched development of a pair of monozygous twins of grossly different size at birth. *Archives of Disease in Childhood*, **49**, 472–476.

Caliumi-Pellegrini, G., Agostino, R., Orzalesi, M., Nodari, S., Marzetti, G., Savignoni, P. G. & Bucci, G. (1974) Twin nasal cannula for administration of continuous positive airway pressure to newborn infants. *Archives of Disease in Childhood*, **49**, 228–230.

Carswell, F., Kerr, M. M. & Dunsmore, I. R. (1972) Sequential trial of effect of phenobarbitone on serum bilirubin of preterm infants. *Archives of Disease in Childhood*, **47**, 621–625.

Chadd, M. A. & Gray, O. P. (1972) Hypothermia and coagulation defects in the newborn. *Archives of Disease in Childhood*, **47**, 819–821.

Churchill, J. A. (1965) The relationship between intelligence and birth weight in twins. *Neurology*, **15**, 341–347.

Churchill, J. A., Masland, R. S., Naylor, A. A. & Ashworth, M. R. (1974) The etiology of cerebral palsy in preterm infants. *Developmental Medicine and Child Neurology*, **16**, 143–149.

Clifford, S. H. (1947) Management of emergencies. *American Journal of Diseases of Children*, **73**, 706–712.

Corner, B. D. (1962) The premature infant's diet (Letter). *Lancet*, **1**, 321.

Cox, W. M. & Filer, L. J. (1969) Protein intake for low-birth-weight infants. *Journal of Pediatrics*, **74**, 1016–1020.

Cremer, R. J., Perryman, P. W. & Richards, D. H. (1958) Influence of light on the hyperbilirubinaemia of infants. *Lancet*, **1**, 1094–1097.

Cross, K. W. (1973) Cost of preventing retrolental fibroplasia? *Lancet*, **2**, 954–956.

Culley, P., Powell, J., Waterhouse, J. & Wood, B. (1970) Sequelae of neonatal jaundice. *British Medical Journal*, **3**, 383–386.

Cumarasamy, N., Nüssli, R., Vischer, D., Dangel, P. H. & Duc, G. V. (1973) Artificial ventilation in hyaline membrane disease: the use of positive end-expiratory pressure and continuous positive airway pressure. *Pediatrics*, **51**, 629–640.

Dahm, L. S. & James, L. S. (1972) Newborn temperature and calculated heat loss in the delivery room. *Pediatrics*, **49**, 504–513.

Dailey, K. M., Sturtevant, A. B. & Feary, T. W. (1972) Incidence of antibiotic resistance and R factors among Gram-negative bacteria isolated from the neonatal intestine. *Journal of Pediatrics*, **80**, 198–203.

Davie, R., Butler, N. & Goldstein, H. (1972) *From Birth to Seven. A Report of the National Child Development Study*, pp. 81–86. London: Longman.

Davies, P. A. (1975) Perinatal nutrition of infants of very low birth weight and their later progress. In *Modern Problems in Paediatrics*, ed. Falkner, F., Kretchmer, N. & Rossi, E., Vol. 14, pp. 119–133. Basel: Karger.

Davies, P. A. & Davis, J. P. (1970) Very low birthweight and subsequent head growth. *Lancet*, **2**, 1216–1219.

Davies, P. A. & Stewart, A. (1975) Low-birth-weight infants: neurological sequelae and later intelligence. *British Medical Bulletin*, **31**, 85–91.

Davies, P. A. & Tizard, J. P. M. (1975) Very low birthweight and subsequent neurological defect (with special reference to spastic diplegia). *Developmental Medicine and Child Neurology*, **17**, 3–17.

Davies, P. A., Darrell, J. H., Chandran, K. R. & Waterworth, P. M. (1970) The efficacy of antibiotics in the neonatal period. In *The Control of Chemotherapy*, ed. Watt, P. J., pp. 49–68. Edinburgh and London: Livingstone.

Davies, P. A., Robinson, R. J., Scopes, J. W., Tizard, J. P. M. & Wigglesworth, J. S. (1972) Medical care of newborn babies. *Clinics in Developmental Medicine*, No. 44/45. London: SIMP with Heinemann Medical.

Dobbing, J. (1968) Vulnerable periods in developing brain. In *Applied Neurochemistry*, ed. Davison, A. N. & Dobbing, J., pp. 287–316. Oxford: Blackwell.

Dobbing, J. (1970) Undernutrition and the developing brain. The relevance of animal models to the human problem. *American Journal of Diseases of Children*, **124**, 411–415.

Dobbing, J. (1972) Vulnerable periods of brain development. In *Lipids, Malnutrition and the Developing Brain*, ed. Elliott, K. & Knight, J., pp. 9–29. Amsterdam: Associated Scientific Publishers.

Dobbing, J. (1974) The later development of the brain and its vulnerability. In *Scientific Foundations of Paediatrics*, ed. Davis, J. A. and Dobbing, J., pp. 565–577. London: Heinemann Medical.

Dobbing, J. & Sands, J. (1970) Timing of neuroblast multiplication in developing human brain. *Nature*, **226**, 639–640.

Dobbing, J. & Sands, J. (1973) Quantitative growth and development of human brain. *Archives of Disease in Childhood*, **48**, 757–767.

Dobson, V., Riggs, L. A. & Siqueland, E. R. (1974) Electroretinographic determination of dark adaptation functions of children exposed to phototherapy as infants. *Journal of Pediatrics*, **85**, 25–29.

Drillien, C. M. (1964) *The Growth and Development of the Prematurely Born Infant*. Edinburgh and London: Livingstone.

Drillien, C. M. (1972) Aetiology and outcome in low-birthweight infants. *Developmental Medicine and Child Neurology*, **14**, 563–574.

Dunn, P. M. (1974) Continuous positive airway pressure (CPAP) using the Gregory box. *Proceedings of the Royal Society of Medicine*, **67**, 245–247.

Fanaroff, A. A., Wald, M., Gruber, H. S. & Klaus, M. H. (1972) Insensible water loss in low birth weight infants. *Pediatrics*, **50**, 236–245.

Fanaroff, A. A., Cha, C. C., Sosa, R., Crumrine, R. S. & Klaus, M. H. (1973) Controlled trial of continuous negative external pressure in the treatment of severe respiratory distress syndrome. *Journal of Pediatrics*, **82**, 921–928.

Farmer, K. (1968) The influence of hospital environment and antibiotics on the bacterial flora of the upper respiratory tract of the newborn. *New Zealand Medical Journal*, **67**, 541–544.

Fitzhardinge, P. M. (1975) Early growth and development in low-birthweight infants following treatment in an intensive care nursery. *Pediatrics*, **56**, 162–172.

Fitzhardinge, P. M. & Ramsay, M. (1973) The improving outlook for the small prematurely born infant. *Developmental Medicine and Child Neurology*, **15**, 447–459.

Fitzhardinge, P. M., Pape, K., Arstikaitis, M., Boyle, M., Ashby, S., Rowley, A., Netley, C. & Swyer, P. R. (1976) Mechanical ventilation of infants of less than 1501 g birthweight: health, growth and neurological sequelae (in press).

Francis-Williams, J. & Davies, P. A. (1974) Very low birthweight and later intelligence. *Developmental Medicine and Child Neurology*, **16**, 709–728.

Fujikura, T. & Froehlich, L. A. (1974) Mental and motor development in monozygotic co-twins with dissimilar birth weights. *Pediatrics*, **53**, 884–889.

Gaisford, W. (1950) Delayed feeding in premature neonates. *Archives of Diseases in Childhood*, **25**, 209–210 (Abstract).

Gartner, L. M., Snyder, R. N., Chabon, R. S. & Bernstein, J. (1970) Kernicterus: high incidence in premature infants with low serum bilirubin concentrations. *Pediatrics*, **45**, 906–917.

Gerard, P., Fox, W. W., Outerbridge, E. W., Beaudry, P. H. & Stern, L. (1975) Early versus late introduction of continuous negative pressure in the management of the idiopathic respiratory distress syndrome. *Journal of Pediatrics*, **87**, 591–595.

Girling, D. J. (1972) Changes in heart rate, blood pressure, and pulse pressure during apnoeic attacks in newborn babies. *Archives of Disease in Childhood*, **47**, 405–410.

Glass, L., Lala, R. V., Jaiswal, V. & Nigam, S. K. (1975) Effect of thermal environment and caloric intake on head growth of low birthweight infants during late neonatal period. *Archives of Disease in Childhood*, **50**, 571–573.

Gleiss, von J. (1955) Zum Frühgeborenenproblem der Gegenwart. IX Mitteilung. Über futterungs-und umwelthedingte Atemstorungen bei Fruhgeborenen. *Zeitschrift für Kinderheilkunde*, **76**, 261–268.

Goddard, P., Keith, I., Marcovitch, H., Roberton, N. R. C., Rolfe, P. & Scopes, J. W. (1974) Use of a continuously recording intravascular electrode in the newborn. *Archives of Disease in Childhood*, **49**, 853–860.

Gordon, H. H., Levine, S. Z. & McNamara, H. (1947) Feeding of premature infants. A comparison of human and cow's milk. *American Journal of Diseases of Children*, **73**, 442–452.

Graham, J. M. (1975) *An investigation into the aerobic and anaerobic bacterial flora of normal and ill/low birth weight newborn babies*. Ph.D. thesis, University of London.

Gregory, G. A., Kitterman, J. A., Phibbs, R. H., Tooley, W. H. & Hamilton, W. K. (1971) Treatment of the idiopathic respiratory distress syndrome with continuous positive airway pressure. *New England Journal of Medicine*, **284**, 1333–1340.

Gustafson, A., Kjellmer, I., Olegard, R. & Victorin, L. H. (1974) Nutrition in low-birth-weight infants. II. Repeated intravenous injections of fat emulsion. *Acta paediatrica scandinavica*, **63**, 177–182.

Hagberg, B., Hagberg, G. & Olow, I. (1975a) The changing panorama of cerebral palsy in Sweden 1954–1970. I. Analysis of the general changes. *Acta paediatrica scandinavica*, **64**, 187–192.

Hagberg, B., Hagberg, G. & Olow, I. (1975b) The changing panorama of cerebral palsy in Sweden 1954–1970. II. Analysis of the various syndromes. *Acta paediatrica scandinavica*, **64**, 193–200.

Harries, J. (1971) Intravenous feeding in infants. *Archives of Disease in Childhood*, **46**, 855–863.

Harris, H., Wirtschafter, D. & Cassady, G. (1975) Endotracheal intubation and infection. *Pediatric Research*, **9**, 341 (Abstract).

Heird, W. C. & Winters, R. W. (1973) Total intravenous alimentation. *American Journal o; Diseases of Children*, **126**, 287–289.

Hess, J. H., Mohr, G. J. & Bartelme, P. F. (1934) *The Physical and Mental Growth of Prematurely Born Children*. Chicago: University of Chicago Press.

Hey, E. (1971) The care of babies in incubators. In *Recent Advances in Paediatrics*, 4th edn, ed. Gairdner, D. & Hull, D., pp. 171–216. London: Churchill.

Hey, E. N. (1972) Thermal regulation in the newborn. *British Journal of Hospital Medicine*, **8**, 51–64.

Hey, E. (1975) Thermal neutrality. *British Medical Bulletin*, **31**, 69–74.

Hey, E. N. & Mount, L. E. (1967) Heat loss from babies in incubators. *Archives of Disease in Childhood*, **42**, 75–84.

Hillman, L. S., Goodwin, S. L. & Sherman, W. R. (1975) Identification and measurement of plasticizer in neonatal tissues after umbilical catheters and blood products. *New England Journal of Medicine*, **292**, 381–386.

Hohenauer, L. (1971) Studien zur intrauterinen Dystrophie. II. Folgen intrauteriner Mangelernahrung beim Menschen. Eine vergleichende Studie von Zwillingspaaren mit unter schiedlichem geburtsgewicht. *Pädiatrie und Pädologie*, **6**, 17–30.

Kamper, I., Baekgaard, P., Peitersen, B., Marstrand, P., Tygstrup, I. & Friis-Hansen, B. (1974) Artificial ventilation of neonates with respiratory distress. *Acta paediatrica scandinavica*, **63**, 636–637.

Kattwinkel, J., Nearman, H. S., Fanaroff, A. A., Katona, P. C. & Klaus, M. H. (1975) Apnea of prematurity. Comparative therapeutic effects of cutaneous stimulation and nasal continuous positive airway pressure. *Journal of Pediatrics*, **86**, 588–592.

Keenan, W. J., Perlstein, P. H., Light, I. J. & Sutherland, J. M. (1972) Kernicterus in small sick premature infants receiving phototherapy. *Pediatrics*, **49**, 652–655.

Kildeberg, P. (1964) Disturbances of hydrogen ion balance occurring in premature infants. II. Late metabolic acidosis. *Acta paediatrica scandinavica*, **53**, 517–526.

Koch, C. A. (1964) Hyperbilirubinemia in premature infants. A follow-up study. II. *Journal of Pediatrics*, **65**, 1–11.

Kopelman, A. E., Brown, R. S. & Odell, G. B. (1972) The 'bronze' baby syndrome: a complication of phototherapy. *Journal of Pediatrics*, **81**, 466–472.

Korner, A. F., Kraemer, H. C., Haffner, E. & Cosper, L. M. (1975) Effects of waterbed flotation on premature infants: a pilot study. *Pediatrics*, **56**, 361–367.

Krauss, A. N. & Auld, P. A. M. (1969) Metabolic requirements of low-birth-weight infants. *Journal of Pediatrics*, **75**, 952–956.

Krauss, A. N. & Marshall, R. E. (1975) Severe neck ulceration from CPAP head box. *Journal of Pediatrics*, **86**, 286–287.

Krauss, A. N., Klain, D. B. & Auld, P. A. M. (1975) Chronic pulmonary insufficiency of prematurity (CPIP). *Pediatrics*, **55**, 55–58.

Krouskop, R. W., Brown, E. G. & Sweet, A. Y. (1975) The early use of continuous positive airway pressure in the treatment of idiopathic respiratory distress syndrome. *Journal of Pediatrics*, **87**, 263–267.

Kuzemko, J. A. & Paala, J. (1973) Apnoeic attacks in the newborn treated with aminophylline. *Archives of Disease in Childhood*, **48**, 404–406.

Laurance, B. M. & Smith, B. H. (1962) The premature baby's diet (Letter). *Lancet*, **1,** 589–590.

Leonidas, J. C., Hall, R. T., Rhodes, P. G. & Amoury, R. A. (1974) Pneumoperitoneum in ventilated newborns. *American Journal of Diseases of Children*, **128,** 677–680.

Lewis, A. F. (1974) Cost of preventing retrolental fibroplasia (Letter). *Lancet*, **1,** 746–747.

Lubchenco, L. O., Horner, F. A., Reed, L. H., Hix, I. E., Metcalf, D., Cohig, R., Elliott, H. C. & Bourg, M. (1963) Sequelae of premature birth. Evaluation of premature infants of low birth weights at ten years of age. *American Journal of Diseases of Children*, **106,** 101–115.

Lucey, J. F. (1972) Neonatal phototherapy: uses, problems and questions. *Seminars in Hematology*, **9,** 127–135.

Lund, H. T. & Jacobsen, J. (1974) Influence of phototherapy on the biliary bilirubin excretion pattern in newborn infants with hyperbilirubinemia. *Journal of Pediatrics*, **85,** 262–267.

Machin, G. A. (1975) A perinatal mortality survey in south-east London, 1970–73: the pathological findings in 726 necropsies. *Journal of Clinical Pathology*, **28,** 428–434.

Marriage, K. & Davies, P. A. (1976) Neurological sequelae following mechanical ventilation in the neonatal period (in preparation).

McCaffree, M. A., Fletcher, A. B. & Avery, G. B. (1975) Prophylactic oral antibiotics in necrotising enterocolitis. *Pediatric Research*, **9,** 307.

McCracken, G. H., Sarff, L. D., Glode, M. P., Mize, S. G., Schiffer, M. S., Robbins, J. B., Gotschlich, E. C., Ørskov, I. & Ørskov, F. (1974) Relation between *Escherichia coli* K1 capsular polysaccharide antigen and clinical outcome in neonatal meningitis. *Lancet*, **2,** 246–250.

McDonald, A. (1967) *Children of very low birth weight.* MEIU Research Monograph No. 1. London: Heinemann.

Menkes, J. H., Welcher, D. W., Levi, H. S., Dallas, J. & Gretsky, N. E. (1972) Relationship of elevated blood tyrosine to the ultimate intellectual performance of premature infants. *Pediatrics*, **49,** 218–224.

Mockrin, L. D. & Bancalari, E. H. (1975) Early versus delayed initiation of continuous negative pressure in infants with hyaline membrane disease. *Journal of Pediatrics*, **87,** 596–600.

Murdock, A. I., Linsao, L., Reid, M. McC., Sutton, M. D., Tilak, K. S., Ulan, O. A. & Swyer, P. R. (1970) Mechanical ventilation in the respiratory distress syndrome: a controlled trial. *Archives of Disease in Childhood*, **45,** 624–633.

Mushin, A. S. (1974) Retinopathy of prematurity—a disease of increasing incidence? *Transactions of the Ophthalmological Society of the United Kingdom*, **94,** 251–257.

Nelson, K. B. & Deutschberger, J. (1970) Head size at one year as a predictor of four-year IQ. *Developmental Medicine and Child Neurology*, **12,** 487–495.

Newcombe, H. B. & McGregor, J. F. (1971) Childhood cancer following obstetric radiography (Letter). *Lancet*, **2,** 1151–1152.

Northway, W. H., Rosan, R. C. & Porter, D. Y. (1967) Pulmonary disease following respirator therapy of hyaline-membrane disease. Bronchopulmonary dysplasia. *New England Journal of Medicine*, **276,** 357–368.

Odell, G. B., Storey, G. N. B. & Rosenberg, L. A. (1970) Studies in kernicterus. III. The saturation of serum proteins with bilirubin during neonatal life and its relationship to brain damage at five years. *Journal of Pediatrics*, **76,** 12–21.

Oh, W. & Karecki, H. (1972) Phototherapy and insensible water loss in the newborn infant. *American Journal of Diseases of Children*, **124,** 230–232.

Oh, W., Yao, A. C., Hawson, J. S. & Lind, J. (1973) Peripheral circulatory response to phototherapy in newborn infants. *Acta padediatrica scandinavica*, **62,** 49–54.

Olegard, R., Gustafson, A., Kjellmer, I. & Victorin, L. (1975) Nutrition in low-birth-weight infants. III. Lipolysis and free fatty acid elimination after intravenous administration of fat emulsion. *Acta paediatrica scandinavica*, **64,** 745–751.

Omer, M. I. A., Robson, E. & Neligan, G. A. (1974) Can initial resuscitation of preterm babies reduce the death rate from hyaline membrane disease? *Archives of Disease in Childhood*, **49,** 219–221.

Ørskov, F. & Sorensen, K. B. (1975) *Escherichia coli* serogroups in breast-fed and bottle-fed infants. *Acta pathologica et microbiologica scandinavica*, section B, **83,** 25–30.

Ostrea, E. M. & Odell, G. B. (1974) Photosensitised shift in the O_2 dissociation curve of fetal blood. *Acta paediatrica scandinavica*, **63**, 341–346.

Ostrow, J. D. (1972) Mechanisms of bilirubin photodegradation. *Seminars in Hematology*, **9**, 113–125.

Pape, K., Armstrong, D. & Fitzhardinge, P. M. (1975) Intracerebellar haemorrhage as a possible complication of mask applied mechanical ventilation in the low birth weight infant. *Pediatric Research*, **9**, 383 (Abstract).

Perlstein, P. H., Edwards, N. K. & Sutherland, J. M. (1970) Apnea in premature infants and incubator-air-temperature changes. *New England Journal of Medicine*, **282**, 461–466.

Philip, A. G. S. (1975) Oxygen plus pressure plus time: the etiology of bronchopulmonary dysplasia. *Pediatrics*, **55**, 44–50.

Pildes, R. S., Ramamurthy, R. S., Cordero, G. V. & Wong, P. W. K. (1973) Intravenous supplementation of L-amino acids and dextrose in low-birth-weight infants. *Journal of Pediatrics*, **82**, 945–950.

Rasche, R. F. H. & Kuhns, L. R. (1972) Histopathologic changes in airway mucosa of infants after endotracheal intubation. *Pediatrics*, **50**, 632–637.

Reid, D. H. S., Tunstall, M. E. & Mitchell, R. G. (1967) A controlled trial of artificial respiration in the respiratory distress syndrome of the newborn. *Lancet*, **1**, 532–533.

Reynolds, E. O. R. (1975) Management of hyaline membrane disease. *British Medical Bulletin*, **31**, 18–24.

Reynolds, E. O. R. & Taghizadeh, A. (1974) Improved prognosis of infants mechanically ventilated for hyaline membrane disease. *Archives of Disease in Childhood*, **49**, 505–515.

Rhea, J. W., Ghazzawi, O. & Weidman, W. (1973) Nasojejunal feedings: an improved device and intubation technique. *Journal of Pediatrics*, **82**, 951–954.

Rhea, J. W., Ahmad, M. S. & Mange, M. S. (1975) Nasojejunal (transpyloric) feeding: a commentary. *Journal of Pediatrics*, **86**, 451–452.

Rhodes, P. G. & Hall, R. T. (1973) Continuous positive airway pressure delivered by face mask in infants with the idiopathic respiratory distress syndrome: a controlled study. *Pediatrics*, **52**, 1–6.

Rigatto, H. & Brady, J. P. (1972a) Periodic breathing and apnea in preterm infants. I. Evidence for hypoventilation possibly due to central respiratory depression. *Pediatrics*, **50**, 202–218.

Rigatto, H. & Brady, J. P. (1972b) Periodic breathing and apnea in preterm infants. II. Hypoxia as a primary event. *Pediatrics*, **50**, 219–228.

Rigatto, H., Brady, J. P. & Verduzco, R. de la T. (1975a) Chemoreceptor reflexes in preterm infants. I. The effect of gestational and postnatal age on the ventilatory response to inhalation of 100 per cent and 15 per cent oxygen. *Pediatrics*, **55**, 604–613.

Rigatto, H., Brady, J. P. & Verduzco, R. de la T. (1975b) Chemoreceptor reflexes in preterm infats. II. The effect of gestational and postnatal age on the ventilatory response to inhaled carbon dioxide. *Pediatrics*, **55**, 614–620.

Roberton, N. R. C. & Tizard, J. P. M. (1975) Prognosis for infants with idiopathic respiratory distress syndrome. *British Medical Journal*, **3**, 271–274.

Robillard, E., Alarie, Y., Dagenais-Perusse, P., Baril, E. & Guilbeault, A. (1964) Microaerosal administration of synthetic β-γ-dipalmitoyl-L-α-lecithin in the respiratory distress syndrome: a preliminary report. *Canadian Medical Association Journal*, **90**, 55–57.

Rubaltelli, F. F. & Largojolli, G. (1973) Effect of light exposure on gut transit time in jaundiced newborns. *Acta paediatrica scandinavica*, **62**, 146–148.

Rudoy, R. C. & Nelson, J. D. (1975) Enteroinvasive and enterotoxigenic *Escherichia coli*. *American Journal of Diseases of Children*, **129**, 668–672.

Sarff, L. D., McCracken, G. H., Schiffer, M. S., Glode, M. P., Robbins, J. S., Ørskov, I. & Ørskov, F. (1975) Epidemiology of *Escherichia coli* K1 in healthy and diseased newborns. *Lancet*, **1**, 1099–1104.

Scopes, J. W. (1970) Control of body temperatures in newborn babies. *Scientific Basis of Medicine Annual Reviews*, pp. 31–50.

Scopes, J. (1971) Respiratory distress syndrome. In *Recent Advances in Paediatrics*, 4th edn, ed. Gairdner, D. & Hull, D., pp. 89–117. London: Churchill.

Shannon, D. C., Gotay, F., Stein, I. M., Rogers, M. C., Todres, D. & Moylan, F. M. B. (1975) Prevention of apnea and bradycardia in low-birthweight infants. *Pediatrics*, **55**, 589–594.

Shaw, J. C. (1973) Parenteral nutrition in the management of sick low birthweight infants. *Pediatric Clinics of North America*, **20**, 333–358.

Simmons, M. A., Adcock, E. W., Bard, H. & Battaglia, F. L. (1974) Hypernatremia and intracranial hemorrhage in neonates. *New England Journal of Medicine*, **291**, 6–10.

Sinclair, J. C., Driscoll, J. M., Heird, W. C. & Winters, R. W. (1970) Supportive management of the sick neonate. *Paediatric Clinics of North America*, **17**, 863–893.

Smallpeice, V. & Davies, P. A. (1964) Immediate feeding of premature infants with undiluted breast milk. *Lancet*, **2**, 1349–1352.

Smith, C. A., Yudkin, S., Young, W., Minkowski, A. & Cushman, M. (1949) Adjustment of electrolytes and water following premature birth. *Pediatrics*, **3**, 34–48.

Stahlman, M. & Cotton, R. B. (1975) Commentary. *Journal of Pediatrics*, **87**, 601.

Stern, L. & Denton, R. L. (1965) Kernicterus in small premature infants. *Pediatrics*, **35**, 483–485.

Stevens, L. H. (1969) The first kilogram: 2. The protein content of breast milk of mothers of babies of low birth weight. *Medical Journal of Australia*, **2**, 555–557.

Stevenson, J. K., Oliver, T. K., Graham, C. B., Bell, R. S. & Gould, V. E. (1971) Aggressive treatment of neonatal necrotising enterocolitis. *Journal of Pediatric Surgery*, **6**, 28–33.

Stewart, A. & Kneale, G. W. (1970) Radiation dose effects in relation to obstetric x-rays and childhood cancers. *Lancet*, **1**, 1185–1188.

Stewart, A., Webb, J. & Hewitt, D. (1958) A survey of childhood malignancies. *British Medical Journal*, **1**, 1495–1508.

Stewart, A. (1972) The risk of handicap due to birth defect in infants of very low birthweight. *Developmental Medicine and Child Neurology*, **14**, 585–591.

Stewart, A. L. & Reynolds, E. O. R. (1974) Improved prognosis for infants of very low birthweight. *Pediatrics*, **54**, 724–735.

Stocks, J. & Godfrey, S. (1976) The role of artificial ventilation, O_2 and CPAP in the pathogenesis of lung damage in neonates, assessed by serial measurements of lung function. *Pediatrics* (in press).

Storrs, C. N. & Taylor, M. R. H. (1970) Transport of sick newborn babies. *Lancet*, **3**, 328–331.

Sun, S. C., Samuels, S., Lee, J. & Marquis, J. R. (1975) Duodenal perforation: a rare complication of neonatal nasojejunal tube feeding. *Pediatrics*, **55**, 371–375.

Svedbergh, B. & Lindstedt, E. (1973) Retrolental fibroplasia in Sweden. General survey and selected study on patients born in 1960–1966. *Acta paediatrica scandinavica*, **62**, 458–464.

Svenningsen, N. W. (1974) Renal acid–base titration studies in infants with and without metabolic acidosis in the postneonatal period. *Pediatric Research*, **8**, 659–672.

Svenningsen, N. W. & Blennow, G. (1973) Continuous positive airway pressure and noise level (Letter). *Lancet*, **2**, 623.

Svenningsen, N. W. & Lindquist, B. (1974) Postnatal development of renal hydrogen ion excretion capacity in relation to age and protein intake. *Acta paediatrica scandinavica*, **63**, 721–731.

Tsang, R. C., Light, I. J., Sutherland, J. M. & Kleinman, L. I. (1973) Possible pathogenetic factors in neonatal hypocalcemia of prematurity. *Journal of Pediatrics*, **82**, 423–429.

Tsang, R. C., Chen, I., Hayes, W., Atkinson, W., Atherton, H. & Edwards, N. (1974) Neonatal hypocalcemia in infants with birth asphyxia. *Journal of Pediatrics*, **84**, 428–433.

Turner, T., Evans, J. & Brown, J. K. (1975) Monoparesis. Complication of constant positive airways pressure. *Archives of Disease in Childhood*, **50**, 128–129.

Uauy, R., Shapiro, D. L., Smith, B. & Warshaw, J. B. (1975) Treatment of severe apnea in prematures with orally administered theophylline. *Pediatrics*, **55**, 589–594.

Valdes, O. S., Maurer, H. M., Shumway, C. N., Draper, D. A. & Hossaini, A. A. (1971) Controlled clinical trial of phenobarbital and/or light in reducing neonatal hyperbilirubinemia in a predominantly Negro population. *Journal of Pediatrics*, **79**, 1015–1017.

Valman, H. B., Heath, C. D. & Brown, R. J. K. (1972) Continuous intragastric milk feeds in infants of low birth weight. *British Medical Journal*, **3**, 547–550.

Vert, P., Andre, M. & Sibout, M. (1973) Continuous positive airway pressure and hydrocephalus (Letter). *Lancet*, **2**, 319.

Vidyasagar, D. & Chernick, V. (1971) Continuous positive transpulmonary pressure in hyaline membrane disease: a simple device. *Pediatrics*, **48**, 296–299.

van Vliet, P. K. J. & Gupta, J. M. (1973) Prophylactic antibiotics in umbilical artery catheterisation in the newborn. *Archives of Disease in Childhood*, **48**, 296–300.

von Bernuth, H. & Janssen, G. (1974) Behavioural changes in fototherapy. A polygraphic study. *Neuropädiatrie*, **5**, 369–375.

Vuchovich, D. M., Haimowitz, N., Bowers, N. D., Cosbey, J. & Hsia, D. T.-Y. (1965) The influence of serum bilirubin levels upon the ultimate development of low birthweight infants. *Journal of Mental Deficiency Research*, **9**, 51–60.

Washington, J. C., Brown, A. W. & Starrett, A. L. (1972) The question of diarrhea and phototherapy. *Pediatrics*, **49**, 279–280.

Weinberg, W. A., Dietz, S. G., Penick, E. C. & McAlister, W. H. (1974) Intelligence, reading achievement, physical size, and social class. *Journal of Pediatrics*, **85**, 482–489.

Widdowson, E. M. & Kennedy, G. C. (1962) Rate of growth, mature weight and life-span. *Proceedings of the Royal Society, B*, **156**, 96–108.

Wigglesworth, J. S., Keith, I. H., Girling, D. J. & Slade, S. A. (1976) Hyaline membrane disease, alkali and intraventricular haemorrhage. *Archives of Disease in Childhood*, in press.

Wilson, J. T. (1969) Phenobarbital in the perinatal period. *Pediatrics*, **43**, 324–327.

Wilkinson, A. & Yu, V. Y. H. (1974) Immediate effects of feeding on blood-gases and some cardiorespiratory functions in ill newborn infants. *Lancet*, **1**, 1083–1084.

Winick, M. & Noble, A. (1966) Cellular response during malnutrition at various ages. *Journal of Nutrition*, **89**, 300–306.

Winick, M. & Noble, A. (1967) Cellular response with increased feeding in neonatal rats. *Journal of Nutrition*, **91**, 179–182.

Winick, M. & Rosso, P. (1969) The effect of severe early malnutrition on cellular growth of human brain. *Pediatric Research*, **3**, 181–184.

Wishingrad, L., Cornblath, M., Takakuwa, T., Rozenfeld, I. M., Elegant, L. D., Kaufman, A., Lassers, E. & Klein, R. I. (1965) Studies of non-hemolytic hyperbilirubinemia in premature infants. 1. Prospective randomised selection for exchange transfusion with observations on the levels of serum bilirubin with and without exchange transfusion and neurologic evaluation one year after birth. *Pediatrics*, **36**, 162–172.

Woody, N. C. & Brodkey, M. J. (1973) Tanning from phototherapy for neonatal jaundice. *Journal of Pediatrics*, **82**, 1042–1043.

Wortis, H. & Freedman, A. (1965) The contribution of social environment to the development of premature children. *American Journal of Orthopsychiatry*, **35**, 57–68.

Wright, F. H., Blough, R. R., Chamberlin, A., Ernest, T., Halstead, W. C., Meier, P., Moore, R. Y., Naunton, R. F. & Newell, F. W. (1972) A controlled follow-up study of small prematures born from 1952 through 1956. *American Journal of Diseases of Children*, **124**, 506–521.

Wu, P. Y. K. & Hodgman, J. E. (1974) Insensible water loss in preterm infants: changes with postnatal development and non-ionising radiant energy. *Pediatrics*, **54**, 704–712.

Wu, P. Y. K., Teilmann, P., Gambler, M., Vaughan, M. & Metcoff, J. (1967) 'Early' versus 'late' feeding of low birth weight neonates: effect on serum bilirubin, blood sugar and responses to glucagon and epinephrine tolerance tests. *Pediatrics*, **39**, 733–739.

Wu, P. Y. K., Wong, W. H., Hodgman, J. E. & Levan, N. (1974) Changes in blood flow in the skin and muscle with phototherapy. *Pediatric Research*, **8**, 257–262.

Yllpo, A. (1954) Premature children. Should they fast or be fed in the first days of life? *Annales paediatriae Fenniae*, **1**, 99–104.

Yu, V. Y. H. (1975) Effect of body position on gastric emptying in the neonate. *Archives of Disease in Childhood*, **50**, 500–504.

5

PARENT-TO-INFANT ATTACHMENT

Marshall H. Klaus   John H. Kennell

Over the past 40 years, investigators from a wide variety of disciplines have painstakingly elaborated the process by which the human infant becomes attached to his[1] mother (Bowlby, 1958; Spitz, 1965). They have described the disastrous effects on the infant of long-term maternal separation in terms of his motor, mental, and affective development. This chapter describes the development of attachment in the opposite direction, from parent to infant— how it grows, develops and matures, and what distorts, disturbs or enhances it. This attachment is crucial to the survival and development of the infant. Its power is so great that it enables the mother or father to make unusual sacrifices necessary for the care of their infant, day after day, night after night, responding to his cry and protecting him from danger. Throughout his lifetime, the strength and character of this attachment will probably influence the quality of all future bonds and links to other individuals.

An 'attachment' can be defined as a unique relationship between two people which is specific and endures through time. Although it is difficult to define this lasting relationship operationally, we have taken as indicators of this attachment, behaviours such as fondling, kissing, cuddling, and prolonged gazing, behaviours which serve both to maintain contact and exhibit affection to the particular individual. While this definition is useful in experimental observations, it is important to distinguish between attachment and attachment behaviours. Close attachment can persist during long separations of time and distance even though there may at times be no visible sign of its existence. A call for help even after 40 years may bring a mother to her child and evoke attachment behaviours equal in strength to those of the first year.

The impetus to intensively study the mother-to-infant bond occurred 10 to 15 years ago when staffs of intensive care nurseries observed that sometimes, after all extraordinary efforts had been taken to save small premature infants, they would return to emergency rooms battered and partially destroyed by their parents even though they had been sent home intact and thriving. More careful studies of this phenomenon have consistently shown that battering and failure-to-thrive without organic cause appear in a disproportionate number of infants who were premature or hospitalised for other reasons during

[1] The pronouns 'he', 'him', 'his' are used in their generic sense in this chapter to refer to both male and female infants.

the newborn period. (Failure-to-thrive without organic disease is a syndrome in which the infant does not grow, gain or develop normally at home during the early months of life, and yet shows leaps in development and weight gain with routine hospital care.) Table 5.1 presents observations on the incidence of infant battering and failure-to-thrive without organic disease and its relationship to separation in the early days of life. Re-analysis of a number of these studies has shown an association between early separation and these disastrous conditions. The occurrence of these and other mothering disorders has provided a continuing stimulus to unravel the process of parental attachment.

Table 5.1   Separation in the days following delivery and the incidence of battering and failure-to-thrive without organic cause

	Authors	n	Number affected	Percentage affected
Failure to thrive	1. Ambuel and Harris, 1963	100	27 prematures	27
	2. Shaheen et al, 1968	44	16 prematures	36
	3. Evans, Reinhart and Succop, 1972	40	9 prematures	22.5
Battering	4. Elmer and Gregg, 1967	20	6 prematures	30
	5. Skinner and Castle, 1969	78	10 prematures	13
	6. Klein and Stern, 1971	51	12 low birth weight infants	23.5
	7. Oliver et al, 1974	38	8 prematures	21

Had we read closely the first text on neonatology by Budin (1907), we could have foreseen these tragic consequences of early separation. In this book, *The Nursling* published in 1907, he wrote, 'Unfortunately, ... a certain number of mothers abandon the babies whose needs they had not had to meet and in whom they had lost all interest. The life of the little one has been saved it is true but at the cost of the mother.' He recommended that mothers be encouraged to breast feed their premature babies and advised them to nurse full terms as well, to increase their milk production. He designed and promoted glass incubators which allowed a mother to look at her infant easily and permitted mothers to visit and care for their infants since they seemed to be so much more attentive to the infant's needs than were the hospital staff. Sadly, his original recommendations were not heeded.

Over the last six years, however, more and more mothers have been allowed to enter premature nurseries in the United States. None the less, in a recent survey of 1400 nurseries in the US done in 1970 by Barnett and Grobstein (1974), only 30 per cent of mothers were permitted to enter nurseries and of these, only 40 per cent allowed the mother to touch her baby in the first days of life. It is apparent from the data and definition of deprivation (Barnett et al, 1970) that most normal deliveries in the US are followed by several days of deprivation for the mother (Tables 5.2 and 5.3). A woman who delivers a premature infant suffers complete deprivation from the first day if she can only see her infant through a glass window for eight weeks. Only mothers who deliver at home and room in with their infants from the moment of birth experience no deprivation.

This report describes recent studies of the process by which a parent becomes attached to the infant and suggests applications of these findings to the care of the parents of a normal infant, a premature infant, and a malformed infant.

Table 5.2   Levels of interactional deprivation and component variables

Levels of deprivation	Duration of interaction	Sensory modalities of interaction	Caretaking nature of interaction
I. No deprivation	Full time	All senses	Complete
II. Partial deprivation	Part time	All senses	Partial
III. Moderate deprivation	Part time	All senses	None
IV. Severe deprivation	Part time	Visual only	None
V. Complete deprivation	None	None	None

Barnett et al (1970), Neonatal separation: the maternal side of interactional deprivation. *Pediatrics*, **45**, 197

BASIC CONSIDERATIONS

It has been difficult to assess the factors which determine the parenting behaviour of an adult human who has lived for 20 to 30 years. A mother and father's actions and responses towards their infant are derived from a complex combination of their own genetic endowment, the way the baby responds to them, a long history of interpersonal relations with their own families and with each other, past experiences with this or previous pregnancies, the absorption of the practices and values of their cultures, and probably most importantly how each was raised by his own mother and father. The mothering or fathering behaviour of each woman and man, his or her ability to tolerate stresses, and his or her need for special attention differ greatly and depend upon a mixture of these factors. Figure 5.1 is a schematic diagram of the major influences on paternal and maternal behaviour and the resulting disturbances which we hypothesise may arise from them. At the time the infant is born, some of these determinants (framed with a solid line) are ingrained and unchangeable. Other determinants (framed with a dotted line) can be altered, such as the attitudes, statements and practices of the doctor in the hospital, whether or not there is separation from the infant in the first days of life, the nature of the infant himself, his temperament, as well as whether he is healthy, sick or malformed.

Table 5.3   Deprivation levels over time, related to birth situations

Birth situation	Deprivation levels, days and weeks postpartum							
	Day 0	Day 1	Day 3	Day 7	Week 8	Week 9
Home, full term	II. No deprivation	I. No deprivation	I. No deprivation	I. No deprivation	I. No deprivation	I. No deprivation
Hospital, full term, rooming-in	III. Moderate deprivation	I. No deprivation	I. No deprivation	I. No deprivation	I. No deprivation	I. No deprivation
Hospital, full term, regular care	III. Moderate deprivation	II. Partial deprivation	II. Partial deprivation	I. No deprivation	I. No deprivation	I. No deprivation
Premature, mother allowed into nursery	V. Complete deprivation	IV. Severe deprivation	III. Moderate deprivation	II. Partial deprivation	II. Partial deprivation (discharge nursery)	I. No deprivation (home)
Premature, regular care (separated)	V. Complete deprivation	IV. Severe deprivation	IV. Severe deprivation	IV. Severe deprivation	II. Partial deprivation (discharge nursery)	I. No deprivation (home)
Unwed mother, refuses contact	V. Complete deprivation	V. Complete deprivation	V. Complete deprivation	V. Complete deprivation	V. Complete deprivation	V. Complete deprivation

Barnett et al (1970) Neonatal separation: the maternal side of interactional deprivation. *Pediatrics*, **45**, 197

Shown also on the schematic diagram are a series of mothering disorders ranging from mild anxiety (such as persistent concerns about a baby following a minor problem which has been completely resolved in the nursery) to the most severe manifestation—the battered child syndrome. It is our hypothesis that this entire range of problems may result, in part, from separation and other unusual circumstances that occur in the early newborn period as a consequence of present hospital care policies. The most easily manipulated variables in this scheme are the separation of the infant from his mother and the practices in the hospital during the first hours and days of life. It is here, during this period, that recent studies have in part clarified some of the steps

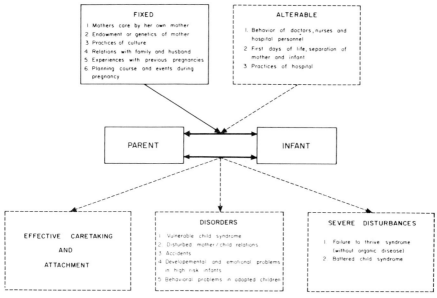

Figure 5.1 Disorders of mothering: a hypothesis of their aetiology. Solid lines indicate determinants that are ingrained; dashed lines indicate factors that may be altered or changed

in mother–infant attachment. The development of mother-to-infant rather than father-to-infant attachment will be the central focus of this chapter since more data from both clinical observations and controlled studies is available for mothers. Information relating to the father–infant bond will be presented parenthetically.

During the first stage of pregnancy, a woman must come to terms with the knowledge that she will be a mother. The second stage involves a growing awareness of the baby in the uterus as a separate individual, usually starting with the sensation of fetal movement (quickening), a remarkably powerful event. During this period, the woman must begin to change her concept of the fetus from a part of herself to a living baby who will soon be a separate individual.

After quickening, a woman will usually begin to have fantasies about what the baby will be like, attributing some human personality characteristics to him and developing a feeling of attachment. Unplanned, unwanted infants may now seem more acceptable. Objectively, there will usually be some outward evidence of the mother's preparation in such actions as the purchase of clothes or a crib, the selection of a name, and the rearrangement of space to accommodate the baby (nest building). Mothers who remain relaxed during labour and who cooperate and have good rapport with those caring for them are more apt to be pleased with their infants at the first sight (Newton and Newton, 1962). Unconsciousness during delivery does not cause the mother to reject her infant in an obvious manner as has been observed in some animals. However, early unconfirmed reports suggest that there may be a tenfold increase in child abuse after delivery by Caesarean section when compared with vaginal deliveries.

SPECIES-SPECIFIC BEHAVIOUR

Detailed observations of many species have shown that adaptive species-specific patterns of behaviour, including nesting, exploring, grooming and retrieving, before, during and after parturition have evolved to meet the needs of the young.

For example, the domestic cat, whether in the United States or England, behaves in a characteristic way at the time of delivery. Towards the end of her pregnancy, she finds a warm dark place, preferably with a soft surface, in which to give birth. Throughout labour and delivery, she spends increasingly more time licking her genital region. After delivery, she continues licking, but with the newborn kitten as her object. The placenta is usually promptly eaten. After the birth of the last kitten, the mother lies down encircling her kittens, and rests with them for about 12 h (Schneirla, Rosenblatt and Tobach, 1963). Each mammalian species studied has its own characteristic behavioural sequence around the time of delivery and following the birth (Hersher, Richmond and Moore, 1963).

We have searched for similar specific behaviour in the human mother in the hope that close observations of very early interaction between mother and infant might provide clues or principles that may not be evident at other times. If humans exhibit such specific patterns of behaviour, knowledge of the sequence might be clinically applicable in situations where mothers and infants are at present separated early, such as prematurity or sickness during the neonatal period. In addition, it is our hypothesis that there is an immediate interlocking, and a reciprocal set of behaviours for attachment which must quickly operate because of the infant's precarious state after delivery.

Filmed observations made after delivery in a hospital show that a mother presented with her nude, full-term infant (Fig. 5.2) begins with fingertip touching of the infant's extremities and within a few minutes proceeds to massaging, encompassing palm contact of the trunk (Klaus et al, 1970). Mothers of premature infants in incubators also follow a small portion of this sequence but proceed at a much slower rate. According to Rubin (1963), when mothers are given their infants fully clothed, it takes several days for them to move to palmar stroking of the trunk. We have observed that fathers go through some of the same routines.

In sharp contrast to the woman who gives birth in the hospital, a woman delivering at home with a midwife appears to be in control. She chooses both the room in the house and the location within the room where she would like the birth to take place as well as the close friends who will be present to share

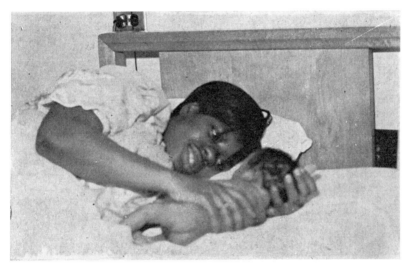

Figure 5.2   Mother's first contact with her nude full-term infant. (Klaus et al (1970) Human maternal behaviour at the first contact with her young. *Pediatrics*, **46,** 187)

this experience with her. She is an active participant rather than a passive patient during her labour and delivery. Immediately after delivery, she appears to be in a remarkable state of ecstasy. In fact many mothers have reported they had sensations similar to orgasm at the time of delivery (Lang, 1974). The exuberance is contagious and the observers share the festive mood of unreserved elation after the delivery. Striking in films is the observers' intense interest in the infant, especially in the first 15 to 20 min of life. Although controlled studies have not yet been done to test the effects of this experience on the mother–infant relationship, it seems clear that the conditions surrounding delivery greatly affect the mother's initial mood and interaction with her infant.

In the observed home deliveries, the mother cradles her infant in her arms immediately after his birth and begins touching his face with her fingertips.

Thus, we have fragmentary evidence that human mothers engage in a species-specific sequence of touching behaviours when first meeting their infants even though the speed and pattern of this sequence may be modified by environmental conditions.

In early contacts, a strong interest in eye-to-eye contact has been expressed by mothers of both full-term and premature infants. When the words of mothers who had been presented with their infants in privacy were taped, 70 per cent of the statements referred to the eyes. The mothers said, 'Let me see your eyes', and 'Open your eyes and I'll know you love me'. Robson (1967) has suggested that eye-to-eye contact appears to elicit maternal caregiving responses. Mothers seem to try hard to look 'en face' at their

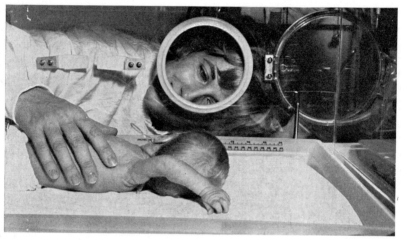

Figure 5.3   Mother and her premature infant in the 'en face' position. (Klaus et al (1970) Human maternal behaviour at the first contact with her young. *Pediatrics*, **46**, 187)

infants, that is, to keep their faces aligned so that their eyes are in the same vertical plane of rotation as their babies', as shown by the mother in Figure 5.3. Complementing the mother's interest in the infant's eyes is the early functional development of his visual pathways. The infant is alert, active, and able to follow during the first hour of life (Brazelton, Scholl and Robey, 1966) if maternal sedation has been limited and the administration of silver nitrate delayed.

This area has been greatly augmented by the recent explosion of information in a closely related field. Detailed studies of the amazing behavioural capacities of the normal neonate have shown that the infant sees, hears and moves in rhythm to his mother's voice in the first minutes and hours of life and that there may be a beautiful linking and synchronised dance between the mother and infant.

Recent exciting observations by Condon and Sander (1974) reveal that newborns move in with the structure of adult speech. '. . . When the infant is already in movement, points of change in the configuration of his moving body parts become coordinated with points of change in sound patterns characterising speech . . .' In other words, as the speaker pauses for breath or accents a syllable, the infant almost imperceptibly raises an eyebrow or lowers a foot. The investigators demonstrated that live speech is particularly effective in entraining infant movement by showing that neonate movement did not show correspondence with either tapping noises or disconnected vowel sounds as is noted with natural, rhythmic speech. Interestingly, synchronous movements were found at 16 h of age with both of the two natural languages tested, English and Chinese. As the authors note,

This study reveals a complex interaction system in which the organisation of the neonate's motor behaviour is entrained by and synchronised with the organised speech behaviour of adults in his environment. If the infant, from the beginning, moves in precise, shared rhythm with the organisation of the speech structure of his culture, then he participates developmentally through complex, socio-biological entrainment he later uses in speaking and communicating.

Thus it appears that the normal neonate is equipped in the first hours of life to follow his mother with his eyes and to move in time with her words. The appearance of the infant and its broad array of sensory and motor abilities evoke responses from the mother and provide several channels of communication which are essential in the process of attachment and the initiation of a series of reciprocal interactions. Lang (1974) noted that immediately after a home delivery, most mothers suckle their infants. The infants she observed did not suck but licked the area around the nipple.

MacFarlane (1975) has shown that six days after birth the infant will have the ability with significant reliability to identify by scent his own mother's breast pad from the breast pads of other women. The mother has an intense interest in looking at her newborn baby's open eyes. In the first 45 min of life, the infant is awake and alert and will follow his mother for 180 degrees with his own eyes. The licking of the nipple will induce a marked increase in prolactin secretion in the mother and at the same time oxytocin to contract the uterus and decrease bleeding. With the mother's strong desire to touch and see her child, nature has provided for the immediate and essential union of the two. The alert newborn rewards his mother for her efforts by following her with his eyes, thus maintaining their interaction, and kindling the tired mother's fascination with her baby.

Lind and his associates in Stockholm have shown that a surprising increase in blood flow to the breast occurs when a mother hears the cries of her own infant (Lind, Vuorenkoski and Wasz-Hoeckert, 1972). These intricate interactions have focused our attention on the cascade of interlocking sensory patterns that quickly develop between mother and infant in the first hours of life.

There is suggestive evidence that many of these early interactions also take place between the father and his newborn child. Parke (1974) in particular has demonstrated that when fathers are given the opportunity to be alone with their newborns, they spend almost exactly the same amount of time as mothers holding, touching, and looking at them.

In his work with a mother and her three month old twins, Stern (1971) observed that the pattern of interaction between a mother and her child has a characteristic rhythm. Intricate interchanges occur within a period of a few seconds. And when these interactions are repeatedly out of phase, for example if one partner looks away just as the other looks at him, many aspects of the relationship between the two individuals are disturbed. Our observations suggest that this dance of mother and infant, which may or may not be in rhythm, is first initiated in the immediate postpartum period. As Brazelton and his colleagues have stated, 'This interdependency of rhythms seems to be at the root of their "attachment" as well as communication' (Brazelton, Koslowski and Main, 1974). Thus, it seems important that the family have privacy in the first hours of life, in which the new and older members may become attuned to each other.

On the basis of our observations and the reports of parents, we believe that every parent has a task to perform during the postpartum period. She must look and 'take in' her real live baby and reconcile the fantasy of the infant she imagined with the one she actually delivered. Many cultures recognise this need by providing the mother with a *doula*, or 'aunt' who mothers her and relieves her of other responsibilities so that she can devote herself completely to this task (Raphael, 1973).

A SENSITIVE PERIOD

It has been found that in a large number of animal species, separation of mother and baby immediately after birth can severely distort mothering behaviour. For example, if the goat is separated for 1 h from her kid immediately after delivery, she is likely to butt it away when it is returned. However, if a separation of similar duration begins 10 min after delivery, the dam will re-accept her kid upon reunion and allow it to nurse (Klopfer, 1971). Thus, there appears to be a sensitive period in the first minutes of life in which any alteration in the normal pattern of interaction can result in aberrant subsequent mothering behaviour.

In monkeys, a separation immediately after birth for 1 h does not seem to affect the female's interest in being near her neonate. However, if the separation begins at birth and is for as long as 24 h, the mother's preference for neonates seems to have disappeared. Lab-reared females separated at birth for a couple of hours will not re-accept their infants, whereas feral females will do so within two days. The fact that feral females will not immediately accept their infants suggests that separation at birth is a stressful experience. Even after living with their infants for several months before being separated, some monkey mothers show markedly altered behaviour at the time of reunion (Meier, 1965; Sackett and Ruppenthal, 1974).

There is evidence that when human mothers are separated from their babies during the first hours and days after delivery, they may have difficulty forming an attachment. Studies of mothers of premature infants who spent their first weeks of life in neonatal intensive care nurseries highlight this problem. In those nurseries where the mothers are not allowed to visit, doctors find that mothers temporarily forget they have babies and find reasons to put off taking them home.

A small number of studies have focused on the possibility of an early sensitive period in the human mother. Observations at Stanford and in our own unit have been made with mothers of prematures, half of whom were permitted into the nursery in the first hours and half of whom could not come in until the twentieth day. At Case Western Reserve University, mothers who had early contact with their infants looked at them significantly more than late contact mothers during a filmed feeding at the time of discharge. Furthermore, preliminary data on the IQs of these two groups of children at 42 months indicate that children in the early contact group scored significantly higher (mean = 99) than did children in the late contact group (mean = 85). Strikingly, a significant correlation was found between IQ at 42 months and the amount of time women looked at their babies during the one month filmed feeding ($r = 0.71$). This is consistent with our hypothesis that early contact affects aspects of maternal behaviour which may have significance for the child's later development. At Stanford, when mothers separated from their premature babies from 3 to 12 weeks were compared with those of prematures permitted early contact, there were more divorces (five compared to one) and more infants relinquished (two compared to none) in the group of mothers with prolonged separation (Leifer et al, 1972). It should be noted that these were all middle-class families and they all had initially planned on keeping their infant.

During the past five years, six studies of the sensitive period of mothers and their full-term infants have either been completed or are underway.

In a tightly controlled study of 28 primiparous mothers and their full-term infants, half the mothers were given 1 h in the first 3 h and 15 more hours of contact with their infants in the first three days of life than were the controls. The mothers who had early and extended contact were more likely to stand near their infants and watch during the physical examination, showed significantly more soothing behaviour, engaged in more eye-to-eye contact and fondling during feeding, and were more reluctant to leave their infants with someone else at one month than were mothers not given the extended contact experience (Klaus et al, 1972). At one year the two groups of mothers were still significantly different. Extended contact mothers spent more time near the table assisting the physician and soothing their infant while he was being examined, and reported themselves to be more preoccupied with the baby when they went out (Kennell et al, 1974). At two years, when the linguistic behaviours of the two groups of mothers while speaking to their children were compared, extended contact mothers asked twice as many questions, and used more words per proposition, fewer content words, more adjectives and fewer commands than did the controls (Ringler et al, 1975). It is impressive evidence for a sensitive maternal period that just 16 extra hours of contact in the first three days of life had such far-reaching effects.

In a small but carefully controlled study, Winters (1973) gave six mothers in one group their babies to suckle shortly after birth and compared these with six mothers who did not have contact with their babies until approximately 16 h later. All had originally intended to breast feed and none stopped because of physical problems. When checked two months later, all six mothers who had suckled their babies on the delivery table were still breast feeding, whereas only one of the other six was still nursing.

Recently, Drs Kennell, Klaus, Mata, Sosa, and Urrutia started a long-term study in two hospitals in Guatemala. In the Social Security Hospital, one group of 19 mothers was given their babies on the delivery table during the episiotomy repair period, then allowed to stay with them in privacy for 45 min. Each mother–infant pair was nude under a heat panel. The other group of mothers was separated from their babies shortly after delivery, in the routine for both hospitals. Except for this difference in initial contact, the care of the two groups was identical. The infants were discharged with free milk at two days, as is the practice of the hospital.

When the babies were checked at 35 and 90 days after birth, the mean weight of those in the early contact group was significantly greater than that of the control group. The socio-economic, marital, housing, and income status of the mothers in the two groups were not significantly different.

In Roosevelt Hospital, a similar study was carried out and at 35 days there were no significant differences in weight gain. Other data are not yet available to help account for these discrepant findings.

In Pelotis, Brazil, Sousa et al (1974) recently compared the success of breast feeding during the first two months of life in two groups of 100 women who delivered normal full-term babies in a 20-bed maternity ward. In the study group, the newborn baby was put to breast immediately after birth and continuous contact between the mother and baby was maintained during the lying-in period. The baby lay in a cot beside his mother's bed. The control group had the traditional contact with their infants—a glimpse shortly after birth and then visits for approximately 30 min every 3 h, starting 12 to 14 h after birth. The babies were kept in a separate nursery. Successful breast feeding was defined as the mother's not using complementary feedings other than tea, water, or small amounts of fruit juice until two months after birth. At two months of age, 77 per cent of the early contact mothers were successfully breast feeding in contrast to only 27 per cent of the controls.

A weakness in this design which limits the strength of the findings is that during the experimental period there was a special nurse working in the unit to stimulate and encourage breast feeding. Although not definitive in itself, this study adds weight to our hypothesis.

In a third study in 1974 at Roosevelt Hospital in Guatemala, a different group of nine mothers was given their babies nude under a heat panel after they had left the delivery room. A second group of 10 was separated according to the usual routine. The babies in both groups were sent to the newborn nursery for the next 12 h, after which they went to the mother in a seven-bed

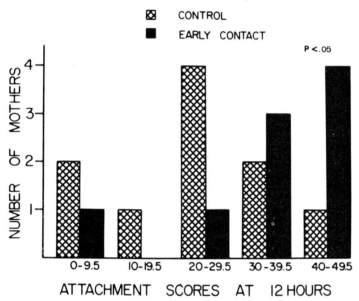

Figure 5.4   Attachment behaviour (fondling, kissing, looking 'en face', holding baby close) at 12 h postpartum in two groups of mothers. Experimental mothers received their infants for 45 min after delivery; control mothers did not have this additional contact

room for the first breast feeding. At 12 h, each mother's interactions with her infant were noted by an observer who did not know to which group they belonged. Observations of the mother's fondling, kissing, looking 'en face', gazing at, and holding her baby close were made for 15 s of every minute for 15 min (Fig. 5.4). The group with early contact showed significantly increased attachment behaviours.

Studies of the effects of rooming-in have also confirmed the importance of the early postnatal period. At Duke University a number of years ago, an increase in breast feeding and a reduction in anxious phone calls was noted when rooming-in was instituted (McBryde, 1951). In Sweden, mothers randomly assigned to rooming-in arrangements were more confident and felt more competent in caregiving. They also appeared to be more sensitive to the crying of their own infants than were mothers who did not have the rooming-in experience (Greenberg, Rosenberg and Lind, 1973). In an interesting and significant observation of fathers, Lind (1973) noted that paternal caregiving was markedly increased in the first three months of life when the father was asked to undress the infant twice and establish eye-to-eye contact with him for 1 h during the first three days of life.

It is our own belief that other principles also govern the attachment process. Though solid evidence is scanty, the following additional rules appear to be important.

1. The process of attachment is structured so that the father and mother will become attached optimally to only one infant at a time. In 1958, Bowlby stated this principle for the attachment process in the other direction (infant to mother) and termed it 'monotropy' (Bowlby, 1958).
2. During the early process of the mother's attachment to her infant, it is necessary that the infant respond to the mother by some signal such as body or eye movements.
3. People who witness the birth process become strongly attached to the infant.
4. It is difficult and possibly mutually incompatible for some people to both become attached and detached at the same time as in simultaneously attempting to go through the processes of attachment to one person while mourning the loss or threatened loss of the same or another person.
5. Early events have long-lasting effects. Anxieties in the first day about the well-being of a baby with a temporary disorder may result in long-lasting concerns that may adversely shape the development of the child (Kennell and Rolnick, 1960).

Practical Considerations

Up until 100 years ago, events surrounding the delivery had changed little over the centuries. Elaborate customs of the society helped parents through this time. In the last century, however, increasing emphasis has been placed on the medical and scientific aspects of delivery but less attention has been paid to the equally valid psychological considerations. A question may be raised: has the enormous improvement in medical management, which has lessened the physical dangers, contributed to a waning concern about the many other problems a mother faces during pregnancy? In 1959, Bibring wrote, 'What was once a crisis with carefully worked-out traditional customs of giving support to the woman passing through this crisis-period has become at this time a crisis with no mechanisms within the society for helping the woman involved in this profound change of conflict-solutions and adjustive tasks'. This deficiency accounts for the development of the many support systems in our society. The wide assortment of childbirth classes which attempt to continue previous customs are good examples. These groups help the mother through the delivery period as well as aiding her in later infant and child care. They also lessen the tensions, fears, and fantasies that occur during normal pregnancies. By joining a group of mothers, with whom she can chat and share her feelings, a woman can alleviate the many emotional upsets that occur during normal pregnancy. We therefore believe that these courses, particularly those in which mothers participate actively, have a valuable supportive role during pregnancy.

To minimise the number of unknowns for a mother while she is in the hospital, she and her husband should visit the maternity unit to see where labour and delivery will take place. She should also learn about the anaesthetic (if she is to receive one), delivery routines and all the procedures and medication she will receive before, during, and after delivery. By reducing the possibility of surprise, such advance preparation will increase confidence during labour and delivery. For an adult, just as for a child entering the hospital for surgery, the more meticulously every step and event is detailed in advance, the less the subsequent anxiety. The less anxiety the mother experiences while delivering and becoming attached to her baby, the better will be her immediate relationship with him.

The mother must have continuing support and reassurance during her labour and delivery, whether from her husband, a midwife, or a nurse. She also must be satisfied with the arrangements that have been made to maintain her home during her hospitalisation. In Holland, when the mothers deliver at home, mother-helpers come into the home at the time of delivery and take over the care of the family. The mother-helper helps the midwife to deliver the infant. This gives the mother the freedom to concentrate on the needs of the baby and to enjoy her family in the process, and it relieves pressure on the father, reserving his energies for the family.

In an effort to reduce the amount of tension on the mother, she should labour and deliver in the same room, preventing the necessity of rushing to a delivery room in the last minutes of labour. Once the delivery is completed and the mother has had a quick glance at the infant, it is important for her to have a few seconds to regain her composure and, in a sense, catch her breath before she proceeds to the next task—taking on the infant. This breath-catching usually occurs during the period when the placenta is being delivered, while the mother is being cleansed and is having any necessary suturing. It has been our experience that it is best not to give a mother her baby until she indicates that she is ready to take it on. It should be her decision.

In many hospitals it is customary to put the baby on the mother's chest for 1 or 2 min shortly after delivery. This is helpful, but coupled with the lack of privacy, the narrow table and the short time period does not allow sufficient opportunity for the mother to touch and explore her baby. Although it is a reasonable procedure, it is not sufficient to optimise maternal attachment.

After delivery, it is extremely valuable for the father, mother, and baby to have a period alone in either the delivery room or an adjacent room (i.e. a recovery room). Obviously, this is only possible if the infant is normal and the mother is well. The mother should have the infant with her on the bed so she can hold him. The infant should not be off in a bassinet where she can only see his face. She should be given the baby nude and allowed to examine him completely. We have found it valuable to encourage the mother to move over in her regular hospital bed, so that she only takes up about half of it, leaving the other half for her partially dressed or nude infant. A heat panel easily maintains or, if need be, increases the body temperature of the infant (Fig. 5.5 shows how we manage this situation). Several mothers have told us of the unforgettable experience of holding their nude baby against their

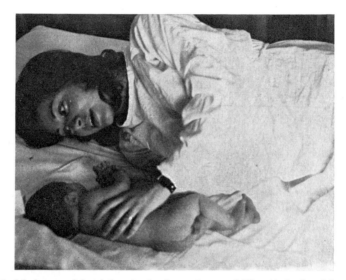

Figure 5.5   Mother receiving infant in the first minutes of life with husband in the room. (Klaus and Fanaroff (1973) *Care of the High-Risk Neonate*. W. B. Saunders)

own bare chest, so we recommend skin-to-skin contact. The father sits or stands at the side of the bed by the infant. This allows the parents and infant to become acquainted. Because the eyes are so important for both the parents and baby, we withhold the application of silver nitrate ($AgNO_3$) to the eyes until after this rendezvous.

We have found it valuable for the mother, father, and infant to be together for about 30 min. After 10 to 15 min, the mother and baby often fall into a deep sleep. In Guatemalan hospitals, where drugs and anaesthesia are used more sparingly, most mothers were usually awake after 45 min of privacy with their infants. The mother and father never forget this significant and stimulating shared experience. It helps to firmly bond the actual, real infant to both parents. We must emphasise that this should be a private session.

Affectional bonds are further consolidated in the succeeding four to five days through continued close association of baby and mother, particularly when she cares for him. Close contact with her husband and other children is also obviously important.

IMMATURE OR SICK NEONATES

We recommend the following procedures:

1. We have found it useful and safe when a premature weighing 1.5 to 2.5 kg is delivered, and appears to be doing well without grunting and retractions, for the mother to have the baby placed in her bed in the first hour of life with a heat panel above them. We do not recommend this unless the physician feels relaxed about the health of the infant.

2. A mother and her infant should be kept near each other in the same hospital, ideally on the same floor. When the long-term significance of early mother–infant contact is kept in mind a modification of restrictions and territorial traditions can usually be arranged.

3. We have found it helpful if the baby does have to be moved to a hospital with an intensive care unit, to give the mother a chance to see and touch her infant, even if he has respiratory distress and is in an oxygen hood. The house officer or the attending physician stops in the mother's room with the transport incubator and encourages her to touch her baby and look at him at close hand. A comment about the baby's strength and healthy features may be long remembered and appreciated.

4. We encourage the father to follow the transport team to our hospital so he can see what is happening with his baby. He uses his own transportation so that he can stay in the premature unit for 3 to 4 h. This extra time allows him to get to know the nurses and physicians in the unit, to find out how the infant is being treated, and to talk with the physicians in a relaxed fashion about what we expect will happen with the baby and his treatment in the succeeding days. We allow him to come into the nursery and explain in detail everything that is going on with the infant, often offering him a cup of coffee. We ask him to help act as a link between us and his family by carrying information back to his wife, and request that he come to our unit before he visits his wife so that he can let her know how the baby is doing. We suggest that he take a polaroid picture, even if the infant is on a respirator, so that he can describe to his wife in detail how the baby is being cared for. The mothers often tell us how valuable the picture is in keeping some contact with their infant, even while physically separated.

5. A mother should be permitted to enter the premature nursery as soon as she is able to manoeuvre easily. When she makes her first visit it is important to anticipate that she may become faint or dizzy when she looks at her infant. We always have a stool nearby so that she can sit down, and a nurse stays at her side during most of the visit describing in detail the procedures being carried out, such as the monitoring of respiration and heart rate, the umbilical catheter,

the feeding through the various infusion lines, and the functioning of the incubator.

6. We also encourage grandparents, brothers, sisters and other relatives to view the infant through the glass window of the nursery so that they will begin to feel attached to the infant.

7. It is necessary to find out what the mother believes is going to happen or what she has read about the problem. We try to move at her pace during any discussion to ensure that she understands.

8. In discussing the infant's condition by telephone with the mother who is still in the referring hospital, we ask the father to stand nearby so that we can talk to them both at the same time and they can hear the same message. This group communication reduces misunderstandings and usually is helpful in assuring the mother that we are telling her the whole story.

9. If there is any chance that the infant will survive, we are optimistic in our talks with the parents from the beginning. There is no evidence that if a favourable prediction proves to be incorrect and the baby expires, the parents will be harmed by the early optimism. There is almost always time to prepare them before the baby actually dies. If the infant lives and the physician has been pessimistic, it is almost impossible for parents to become closely attached after they have figuratively dug a few shovelfuls of earth. We recognise that this recommendation goes contrary to many old customs and places a heavy burden on the physician. It is our belief that if the infant does expire, we must still work with the mother and help her with the mourning period.

10. Once the possibility that a baby has brain damage has been mentioned, the parents will not forget it. Therefore, unless we are 100 per cent sure that the baby is damaged, we do not mention the possibility of any brain damage or retardation to the parents. On many occasions we have had neonates who have appeared to be brain damaged but who later were obviously perfectly normal.

11. It is important to emphasise that if we have a clear objective finding, such as a cardiac abnormality or a specific congenital malformation, we see no reason to hide this from the parents. We would never lie to a parent.

12. As soon as possible we describe to both the father and the mother the value of touching the infant in helping them get to know him, in reducing the number of apnoeic episodes (if this is a problem), in increasing weight gain, and in hastening his discharge from the unit.

13. It is important to remember that feelings of love for the baby are often elicited through eye-to-eye contact. Therefore if an infant is under bilirubin lights, we turn them off and remove the eye patches so that the mother and her infant can really see each other.

14. From our previous observations, we have found that keeping a book in which to record parental phone calls and visits is useful in determining which mothers are likely to require additional help from a social worker or extra discussions about the health of their infant. If a mother visits less than three

times in two weeks, in the nursery, the chance of her developing some sort of mothering disorder such as failure-to-thrive, battering, or giving up the baby, increases. Therefore, if the visiting pattern of the mother is less than most mothers, the mother is given extra help in adapting to the hospitalisation (Fanaroff, 1972).

CONGENITAL MALFORMATIONS

The birth of an infant with a congenital malformation presents complex challenges to the physician who will care for the affected child and his family (Johns, 1971; National Association for Mental Health, 1971). Despite the relatively large number of infants with congenital anomalies our understanding of how parents develop an attachment to a malformed child remains incomplete. Although previous investigators agree that the child's birth often precipitates major family stress (Johns, 1971; National Association for Mental Health, 1971; Roskies, 1972), relatively few have described the process of family adaptation (Hare et al, 1966; Johns, 1971; Roskies, 1972) during the infant's first year of life. A major advance was Solnit and Stark's conceptualisation of parental reactions (Solnit and Stark, 1961) They emphasised that a significant aspect of adaptation is the necessity for parents to mourn the loss of the normal child they had expected. Other observers (Waterman, 1948; Zuk, 1959; Michaels and Shucman, 1962) have noted the pathological aspects of family reactions including the chronic sorrow which envelops the family of a defective child (Olshansky, 1962). Less attention has been given to the more adaptive aspects of parental attachment to children with malformations.

Parental reactions to the birth of a child with a congenital malformation appear to follow a predictable course. For most parents, initial shock, disbelief, and a period of intense emotional upset (including sadness, anger, and anxiety) are followed by a period of gradual adaptation, which is marked by a lessening of intense anxiety and emotional reaction (Fig. 5.6). This adaptation is characterised by an increased satisfaction with and ability to care for the baby. These stages in parental reactions are similar to those reported in other crisis situations, such as terminally ill children (Friedman et al, 1963). The shock, disbelief, and denial reported by many parents seem to be an understandable attempt to escape the traumatic news of the baby's malformation, so discrepant with usual parental expectations for a newborn that it is impossible to register except gradually (Geleerd, 1965).

The intense emotional turmoil described by parents who have given birth to a child with a congenital malformation corresponds to a period of crisis, defined as 'upset in a state of equilibrium caused by a hazardous event which creates a threat, a loss, or a challenge for the individual' (Bloom, 1963; Rappoport, 1965). A crisis includes a period of impact, a rise in tension associated with stress, and finally a return to equilibrium. During such crisis periods a person is at least temporarily unable to respond with his usual problem-solving activities to solve the crisis. Roskies (1972) noted a similar 'birth crisis' in her observations of mothers who had given birth to children with birth defects caused by thalidomide.

Solnit and Stark (1961) have likened the crisis of the birth of a child with a malformation to the emotional crisis following the death of a child, in that the mother must mourn the loss of her expected, normal infant. In addition she must become attached to her actual living, damaged child. However, the

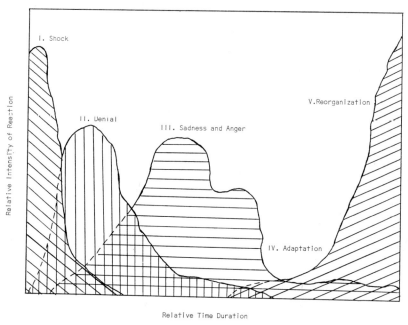

Figure 5.6 Hypothetical model of a normal sequence of parental reactions to the birth of a malformed infant

sequence of parental reactions to the birth of a baby with a malformation differs from that following the death of a child in yet another respect. The mourning or grief work appears not to take place in the usual manner because of the complex issues raised by continuation of the child's life and the demands of his physical care. The parents' sadness, which is important initially in their relationship with their child, diminishes in most instances once the parents take over the physical care. Most parents reach a point at which they are able to care adequately for their children and cope effectively with disrupting feelings of sadness and anger. The mother's initiation of the relationship with her child is a major step in the reduction of anxiety and emotional upset associated with the trauma of the birth. As with normal children, the parents' initial experience with their infant seems to release positive feelings which aid the mother–child relationship following the stresses associated with the news of the child's anomaly and, in many instances, the separation of mother and child in the hospital (Zuk, 1959).

Practical Suggestions for Parents of Malformed Infants

1. We have come to believe that it is far better to leave the infant with the mother for the first two to three days, if medically feasible. If the child is rushed to the hospital where special surgery will eventually be done, the mother will not have enough opportunity to become attached to him. Even if the surgery is required immediately, as for bowel obstruction, it is best to bring the baby to the mother first, allowing her to touch and handle him, and point out to her how normal he is in all other respects.

2. It is our impression that the parents' mental picture of the anomaly is often far more alarming than the actual problem. Any delay during which the parents suspect that there may be a problem greatly heightens their anxiety and causes their imaginations to run wild. Thefore, we suggest that it is helpful to bring the baby to both parents when they are together as soon after delivery as possible.

3. We believe that parents should not be given tranquillisers. This tends to blunt their responses and slows their adaptation to the problem. However, a small dose of Seconal at night is often helpful.

4. It has been our clinical experience that parents who are adapting reasonably well initially often ask many questions and at times appear to be almost over involved in clinical care. In our unit we are pleased by this and more concerned about parents who ask few questions and who appear stunned and overwhelmed by the problem. Parents who become involved in trying to find out what the best procedures are, who ask many questions about care— why this, why that—are sometimes very bothersome but often make the best adaptation in the end.

5. Many anomalies are very frustrating not only to the parents but to the physicians and nurses as well. There is a temptation for the physician to withdraw from the parents and their infant. The many questions asked by the parent who is trying to understand the problem are often very frustrating for the physician. The parent often appears to forget and asks the same questions over and over again.

6. We have found it best to move at the parents' pace. If we move too quickly, we run the risk of losing the parents along the way. It is beneficial to ask the parents how they view their infant. 'Maybe you could tell me how you see the infant?'

7. Each parent may move through the process of shock, denial, anger, guilt and adaptation at a different pace so the two parents may not be synchronised with one another. If they are unable to talk with each other about the baby,

there may be a marked disruption in their own relationship. Therefore, we use the process of early crisis intervention, meeting several times with the parents. During these discussions, we ask the mother how she's doing, how she feels her husband is doing, and how he feels about the infant. We then reverse the questions and ask the father how he's doing and how he thinks his wife is progressing. The hope is that they will think not only about their own reactions, but will begin to consider each other's as well.

SUMMARY

The hospital now determines the events surrounding birth and death. These two most important events in the life of an individual have been stripped of all the long-established traditions and support systems which were established over centuries to help families through these transitions that have such long-lasting effects on everyone involved.

Since the newborn baby is utterly dependent upon his parents for his survival and optimal development, it is essential to understand the process of attachment as it develops from the first moments after the child is born. Although we have only a beginning understanding of this complex phenomenon, those responsible for the care of mothers and infants would be wise to re-evaluate hospital procedures that interfere with early, sustained mother–infant contact, to consider measures which promote a mother's contact with her nude infant and to help her appreciate the wide range of sensory and motor responses of her neonate.

REFERENCES

Ambuel, J. & Harris, B. (1963) Failure to thrive: a study of failure to grow in height or weight. *Ohio Medical Journal*, **59,** 997.

Barnett, C. R., Leiderman, P. H., Grobstein, R. & Klaus, M. (1970) Neonatal separation: the maternal side of interactional deprivation. *Pediatrics*, **45,** 197–205.

Barnett, C. R. & Grobstein, R. (1974) Personal communication.

Bibring, G. (1959) Some considerations of the psychological processes in pregnancy. *Psychoanalytic Study of the Child*, **14,** 113.

Bloom, B. (1963) Definitional concepts of the crisis concept. *Journal of Consulting Psychology*, **27,** 42.

Bowlby, J. (1958) Nature of a child's tie to his mother. *International Journal of Psychoanalysis*, **39,** 350–373.

Brazelton, T. B., Scholl, M. & Robey, J. (1966) Visual responses in the newborn. *Pediatrics*, **37,** 284–290.

Brazelton, T. B., Koslowski, B. & Main, M. (1974) The origins of reciprocity—the early infant interaction. In *The Effect of the Infant on its Caregiver*, ed. Lewis, M. and Rosenblum, L., Vol. 1, Ch. 3. New York: John Wiley & Sons.

Budin, P. (1907) *The Nursling*. London: Caxton Publishing Co.

Condon, W. S. & Sander, L. W. (1974) Neonate movement is synchronised with adult speech: interactional participation and language acquisition. *Science*, **183,** 99–101.

Elmer, E. & Gregg, D. (1967) Developmental characteristics of abused children. *Pediatrics*, **40,** 596.

Evans, S., Reinhart, J. & Succop, R. (1972) A study of 45 children and their families. *The Journal of the American Academy of Child Psychiatry*, **11,** 440–454.

Fanaroff, A. A., Kennell, J. H. & Klaus, M. H. (1972) Follow-up of low birth-weight infants—the predictive value of maternal visiting patterns. *Pediatrics*, **49**, 288–290.

Friedman, S. B., Chodoff, P., Mason, J. W. & Hamburg, D. A. (1963) Behavioral observations on parents anticipating the death of a child. *Pediatrics*, **32**, 610.

Geleerd, E. R. (1965) Two kinds of denial. Neurotic denial and denial in the service of the need to survive. In *Drives, Affects and Behavior*, ed. Schur, M., Vol. 2. New York: International Universities Press.

Greenberg, M., Rosenberg, I. & Lind, J. (1973) First mothers rooming-in with their newborns: its impact upon the mother. *American Journal of Orthopsychiatry*, **43**, 783–788.

Hare, E. H., Lawrence, K. M., Paynes, H. & Rawnsley, K. (1966) Spina bifida cystica and family stress. *British Medical Journal*, **2**, 757.

Hersher, L., Richmond, J. & Moore, A. (1963) Mernal behavior in sheep and goats. In *Maternal Behavior in Mammals*, ed. Rheingold, H. New York: John Wiley & Sons.

Johns, N. (1971) Family reactions to the birth of a child with a congenital abnormality. *Medical Journal of Australia*, **7**, 277.

Kennell, J. & Rolnick, A. (1960) Discussing problems in newborn babies with their parents. *Pediatrics*, **26**, 832–838.

Kennell, J. H., Jerauld, R., Wolfe, H., Chesler, D., Kreger, N., McAlpine, W., Steffa, M. & Klaus, M. H. (1974) Maternal behavior one year after early and extended post-partum contact. *Developmental Medicine and Child Neurology*, **16**, 172–179.

Klaus, M. & Fanaroff, A. (1973) *Care of the High-risk Neonate*. Philadelphia: W. B. Saunders.

Klaus, M. H., Kennell, J. H., Plumb, N. & Zuehlke, S. (1970) Human maternal behavior at the first contact with her young. *Pediatrics*, **46**, 187–192.

Klaus, M. H., Jerauld, R., Kreger, N., McAalpine, W., Steffa, M. & Kennell, J. H. (1972) Maternal attachment—importance of the first post-partum days. *New England Journal of Medicine*, **286**, 460–463.

Klein, M. & Stern, L. (1971) Low birth weight and the battered child syndrome. *American Journal of Diseases of Children*, **122**, 15.

Klopfer, P. (1971) Mother love! What turns it on? *American Scientist*, **49**, 404–407.

Lang, R. (1972) *Birth Book*. Ben Lomond: Genesis Press.

Lang, R. (1974) Personal communication.

Leifer, A., Leiderman, P., Barnett, C. & Williams, J. (1972) Effects of mother–infant separation on maternal attachment behavior. *Child Development*, **43**, 1203–1218.

Lind, J., Vuorenkoski, V. & Wasz-Hoeckert, O. (1973) The effect of cry stimulus on the temperature of the lactating breast primipara: a thermagraphic study. In *Psychosomatic Medicine in Obstetrics and Gynaecology*, ed. Morris, N. Basel: S. Karger.

Lind, J. (1973) Personal communication.

MacFarlane J. A. (1975) Olfaction in the development of social preferences in the human neonate. In *The Parent–Infant Relationship*, Ciba Foundation. Amsterdam: Elsevier.

McBryde, A. (1951) Compulsory rooming-in in the ward and private newborn service at Duke Hospital. *Journal of the American Medical Association*, **45**(a), 625.

Meier, G. W. (1965) Maternal behavior of feral- and laboratory-reared monkeys following the surgical delivery of their infants. *Nature*, **206**, 492–493.

Michaels, J. & Shucman, H. (1962) Observations on the psychodynamics of parents of retarded children. *American Journal of Mental Deficiency*, **66**, 568.

National Association for Mental Health Working Party (1971) The birth of an abnormal child: telling the parents. *Lancet*, **2**, 1075.

Newton, N. & Newton, M. (1962) Mother's reactions to their newborn babies. *Journal of the American Medical Association*, **181**, 206–211.

Oliver, J. E., Cox, J., Taylor, A. & Baldwin, J. (1974) Severely ill-treated young children in North-East Wiltshire. Research Report No. 4. Oxford University Unit of Clinical Epidemiology.

Olshansky, S. (1962) Chronic sorrow: a response to having a mentally defective child. *Social Casework*, **43**, 190.

Parke, R. (1974) Family interactions in the newborn period: some findings, some observations, and some unresolved issues. In *Proceedings of the International Society for Study of Behavior Development*, ed. Riegel, K. & Meacham, J.

Raphael, D. (1973) *The Tender Gift: Breastfeeding*. Englewood Cliffs: Prentice-Hall, Inc.

Rappoport, L. (1965) The state of crisis: some theoretical considerations. In *Crisis Intervention*, ed. Parad, H. J., p. 22. New York: Family Service Association.

Ringler, N. M., Kennell, J. H., Jarvella, R., Navojosky, B. & Klaus, M. H. (1975) Mother-to-child speech at two years—effects of early postnatal contacts. *Behavioral Pediatrics*, **86**, 141–144.

Robson, K. (1967) The role of eye-to-eye contact in maternal–infant attachment. *Journal of Child Psychology and Psychiatry*, **8**, 13–25.

Roskies, E. (1972) *Abnormality and Normality: the Mothering of Thalidomide Children.* New York: Cornell University Press.

Rubin, R. (1963) Maternal touch. *Nursing Outlook*, November, 828–831.

Sackett, G. P. & Ruppenthal, G. G. (1974) Some factors influencing the attraction of adult female macaque monkeys to neonates. In *The Effect of the Infant on its Caregiver*, ed. Lewis, M. & Rosenblum, L. New York: John Wiley & Sons.

Schneirla, T., Rosenblatt, J. & Tobach, E. (1963) Maternal behavior in the cat. In *Maternal Behavior in Mammals*, ed. Rheingold, J. New York: John Wiley & Sons.

Shaheen, E., Alexander, D., Truskowsky, M. & Barbero, G. (1968) Failure to thrive—a retrospective profile. *Clinical Pediatrics*, **7**, 225.

Skinner, A. & Castle, R. (1969) Seventy-eight battered children: a retrospective study. Report by the National Society for the Prevention of Cruelty to Children.

Solnit, A. J. & Stark, M. H. (1961) Mourning and the birth of a defective child. *Psychoanalytic Study of the Child*, **16**, 523.

Sousa, P. I. R., Baros, F. C., Cazalle, R. V., Begéres, R. M., Pinheiro, G. N., Menezes, S. T. & Arruda, L. A. (1974) Attachment and lactation. Presented at *Pediatria XIV: Nutrition, Toxicology and Pharmacology*, Buenos Aires, Argentina.

Spitz, R. (1965) *The First Year of Life.* New York: International Universities Press.

Stern, D. (1971) A micro-analysis of mother–infant interaction. *Journal of the American Academy of Child Psychiatry*, **10**, 510–517.

Waterman, J. H. (1948) Psychogenic factors in parental acceptance of feeble-minded children. *Diseases of the Nervous System*, **9**, 184.

Winters, M. (1973) The relationship of time of initial breastfeeding to success of breastfeeding. Submitted thesis (nursing master's), University of Washington.

Zuk, G. H. (1959) Religious factor and the role of guilt in parental acceptance of the retarded child. *American Journal of Mental Deficiency*, **64**, 145.

6

SCREENING AND MANAGEMENT OF INFANTS WITH AMINO ACID DISORDERS

Barbara E. Clayton

SCREENING

It is a traumatic experience for a new mother when she becomes aware that doctors and nurses are interested in her infant because a positive result has been given by a screening test. Her infant appears to her to be healthy and thriving, and suddenly she is filled with apprehension. Screening raises many ethical problems since people are easily harmed if they become aware that an abnormality has been found, or if treatment which may be at best unnecessary and at worst harmful, is initiated. If it is to be of high standard it requires excellent organisation, close collaboration between clinicians and laboratories and, most important, a very clear idea of its purpose. The ethics of screening have been discussed by the Institute of Society, Ethics and Life Sciences in 1972, and they also emphasised the need to be clear about the goals served and the benefits to be obtained by the individuals and their families. They emphasised that there was need to protect the subject when relatively untried screening procedures were used and to provide counselling.

Principles of Screening

The principles for screening on a service basis, as opposed to research, have been given recently by Whitby (1974) and Holland (1974). They include

1. As much as possible should be known about the natural history of the disease;
2. The condition must be an important health problem if screening is to be justified;
3. It is important not to screen for conditions which cannot be treated; this would not of course be a necessary criterion in a research project;
4. There must be facilities for diagnosis and treatment;
5. Tests used in screening must be acceptable to those who undergo them and must satisfy criteria of sensitivity, precision and specificity (Wilson, 1973);
6. the whole process must be economically justifiable in the context of the rest of the claims on limited Health Service finance.

It is essential, therefore, that screening programmes of a service nature should be clearly differentiated from those which are research projects· Sometimes there will be a national programme for screening for certain disorders, e.g. for phenylketonuria in the United Kingdom, but in other instances screening may have been initiated by laboratory workers as a result of techniques which they have developed. When looking for abnormalities of amino acid disorders it is necessary to distinguish between those of proven clinical significance and those which may be biochemical abnormalities only.

The laboratory technique used in a screening programme determines which biochemical abnormalities or clinical disorders (not necessarily synonymous) will be detected. With respect to amino acid disorders the test may be reasonably specific, e.g. the bacterial inhibition test of Guthrie (1961) may be set up to detect raised phenylalanine in blood and thus enable phenylketonuria to be found in infants. Alternatively, techniques employing chromatography of various kinds detect a whole range of biochemical abnormalities. For example, using the Scriver technique (Scriver, Davies and Cullen, 1964) it is potentially possible to detect up to 20 amino acid disorders (Raine et al, 1972). This raises many problems. Laboratory and clinical staff require a clear policy on how to deal with the results obtained, bearing in mind that some of the findings may in fact have no clinical relevance for the individual.

Cost–Benefit of Screening

There have been few reports on the cost–benefit arising from newborn screening. A comprehensive scheme for detecting inborn errors of metabolism and transport has been described by Levy (1974) for Massachusetts, USA, and the Massachusetts Department of Public Health has recently published (1974) an important cost–benefit analysis of this programme. It was found that when all discernable costs were considered, even when potential contributions to society by successfully treated individuals were excluded there was a substantial net saving resulting from the programme. The study emphasised that the expense of collecting specimens was substantial.

The Massachusetts programme is particularly comprehensive. At birth, cord blood is tested for 'classical' galactosaemia and maternal phenylketonuria, and capillary blood collected at three to five days of age is used for screening for phenylketonuria, maple syrup urine disease, homocystinuria, tyrosinosis and galactosaemia. Urine is collected when the infant is three to four weeks old and paper chromatography enables a variety of other biochemical abnormalities concerned with amino acids to be detected. These may or may not be of clinical significance, and in the Massachusetts programme Levy (1974) suggested that 40 per cent are probably benign. He listed the following as of immediate significance: phenylketonuria, hyperphenylalaninaemia (high variant), maple syrup urine disease, homocystinuria (certain types), arginosuccinic acidaemia (certain types), hyperglycinaemia (non-ketotic) and propionic acidaemia. He considered cystinuria and the Fanconi syndrome to be of delayed significance. The following conditions were considered to be benign: hyperphenylalaninaemia (mild), histidinaemia, cystathioninaemia, iminoglycinuria and Hartnup disease.

PHENYLKETONURIA

Need for treatment
There is no doubt that infants should be screened for phenylketonuria since this is one of the few causes of mental retardation for which effective medical treatment is available. Although the efficiency of treatment has been questioned in the past (Bessman, 1966; Birch and Tizard, 1967), paediatricians who have had the care of infants from early life and undertaken dietary treatment have no doubt that this is worthwhile. Adequate intellectual development takes place, the children attend normal schools and they differ strikingly from untreated or late-treated phenylketonuric children whose mean intelligence is about 50 (Clayton, Moncrieff and Roberts, 1967; Baumeister, 1967; Fuller and Shuman, 1969; Hudson, Mordaunt and Leahy, 1970; Kang, Sollee and Gerald, 1970; Koch et al, 1973). Although it has been suggested that absolute scientific proof of the efficacy of treatment could only be provided from a control trial of diet, it would be unethical to undertake such a study now since the results of good treatment are so striking.

A critical appraisal of the natural history of the disease and the influence of early treatment has been made recently by Smith and Wolff (1974) who studied eight sibling pairs with phenylketonuria in which the index case presented because of retarded development. In 16 pairs, there was a second sibling in the family when the index case was diagnosed and their study suggested that one in six or seven patients with untreated classical phenylketonuria would achieve an IQ above 70, although there would be evidence of intellectual impairment. The outcome was very different in the second siblings born after diagnosis of the index case in 12 pairs, the beneficial effects of early treatment being striking. Smith and Wolff (1974) have pointed out that if their estimated frequency of one in six or seven for normal intelligence in the untreated subject is correct, then in the general adult population there should be one person with phenylketonuria per 80 000. This estimate agrees with that actually found by Levy et al (1970) amongst adults in Massachusetts (where the incidence of phenylketonuria is similar to that in South-east England). They found three affected adults, all with educationally subnormal levels of intelligence but able to lead independent lives in the community.

An additional piece of evidence for the efficacy of treatment has been given by Webb, Khazen and Hanley (1973) and MacCready (1974), who compared the number of patients with phenylketonuria admitted to residential institutions before and after the advent of screening programmes in Canada and the USA. They observed a reduction in the admissions, coinciding closely with the particular times the screening programmes were actually begun in the localities where the children were born. The authors recognised that it was still early days to make such a study, but their findings did support the views of paediatricians on the effectiveness of treatment.

Screening for phenylketonuria

In phenylketonuria the concentration of phenylalanine in the blood is high and abnormal metabolites are present in the urine. Early screening programmes relied on the detection of metabolites in urine; either phenyl-pyruvic acid (Woolf et al, 1958) initially using ferric chloride but in later years Phenistix (Ames Co. Ltd), or orthohydroxyphenylacetic acid (Woolf, 1967). Concern about the number of infants missed with the Phenistix test (Stephenson and McBean, 1967) led the Medical Research Council to convene a working party to review screening methods. It was concluded that the screening test should rely on the detection of raised levels of phenylalanine in the blood and that the Guthrie test would be the most satisfactory for routine mass screening of infants (Medical Research Council Working Party, 1968), although other blood tests should be studied too. The Department of Health and Social Security then issued a memorandum (HM(69)72) recommending the establishment of a screening programme using a blood sample.

The subsequent screening programme for phenylketonuria in the United Kingdom has been successful, and has been described by Hawcroft and Hudson (1974) who work at the Phenylketonuria Office established by the Medical Research Council and the Department of Health and Social Security in Liverpool for the purpose of collecting information about the diagnosis and treatment of phenylketonuria in the United Kingdom. In the MRC/DHSS Phenylketonuria Register Newsletter No. 3 (Hudson and Hawcroft, 1975) it was shown that 93 to 99 per cent of all infants born in the United Kingdom were being tested. One patient reported to have a negative Guthrie test was found two years later to be mentally retarded and the original test card gave a positive result on retesting, so presumably there had been a human error in reading the original result. This is the only known missed case since screening of blood was introduced in the UK. Table 6.1 shows the age when diagnosis was confirmed in patients with phenylketonuria in the United Kingdom (Hudson and Hawcroft, 1974).

Personal experience with setting up a screening service using the Guthrie test for phenylketonuria for about 110000 infants per year has emphasised the importance of a number of practical points.

The collection of capillary samples of blood on to the Guthrie cards. It is important that the midwives and health visitors should perform this properly. With poor technique the infant's heel may be bruised and the collection may be inadequate. This necessitates a further collection, causing distress to the mother and extra work for all the staff involved. Adequate teaching is thus essential. Detailed instructions (Clayton and Jenkins, 1970) and an illustrative set of colour slides are available.[1] Visits to the screening laboratory by the community staff are helpful, and in the early days of setting up the service the laboratory staff should visit centres in the community to demonstrate the technique.

Timing of the blood collection. HM(69)72 recommended that blood should be collected between the sixth and fourteenth days of life. A practical rule is 'add six days to the baby's date of birth and collect as soon after that as possible'. Collection before this time leads to an increased number of false positive tests. On repeating these will have become normal and this causes extra work and anxiety. More seriously, it also leads to infants with phenylketonuria being missed as the screening test may give a false negative result owing to a slower rise in the phenylalanine level. This is a problem in the

Table 6.1 Age when diagnosis of phenylketonuria confirmed

Year of birth	Under 4 months	4–12 months	Over 1 year	Total
1964	22	3	10	35
1965	23	4	11	38
1966	29	4	6	39
1967	35	4	7	46
1968	35	1	8	44
1969	46	1	5	52
1970	66	2	0	68
1971	60	–	–	60
1972	68	–	–	68
1973	51	–	–	51

(From Hudson and Hawcroft, 1974)

United States (Holtzman, Meek and Mellits, 1974; Holtzman, Mellits and Kallman, 1974).

Information about phenylketonuria. To maintain the interest of medical and nursing staff in the community and enable them to answer questions put to them by mothers, it is helpful to provide a brief account of the condition. Stencilled sheets are adequate and they must be available continuously as staff change.

Liaison. There must be a close relationship between the screening laboratory and the community services. This is necessary for dealing with poor blood collections and positive results.

Positive screening tests. The majority of these will not be due to phenylketonuria. If the screening test shows a positive result but the concentration of phenylalanine is less than 8 mg/dl blood, a further blood collection should be requested one week later. The majority will then give a negative test.

[1] From the Department of Medical Illustration, Institute of Child Health, 30 Guilford Street, London WC1N 1EH.

If still positive but not more than 8 mg/dl, the health visitor and general practitioner should be advised to reduce the infant's intake of protein if this is excessive and to prescribe 50 mg ascorbic acid daily. Blood should be collected after another week and if the result is still positive the infant should be referred to the hospital for further study although he will not have phenylketonuria. If the original Guthrie test shows a positive result with a phenylalanine concentration higher than 8 mg/dl a further blood collection should be requested immediately. In the meantime one of the spots of blood on the Guthrie card should be eluted with acetone and examined by thin-layer chromatography (Ersser, 1971) or a similar technique, so that the amino acid pattern can be studied in detail. In practice if the screening laboratory is also responsible for monitoring patients with phenylketonuria who are being treated, there will be so many phenylalanine standards incorporated in the agar plates used in the Guthrie test that the high concentration of phenylalanine present in an infant with phenylketonuria will be immediately apparent (Lemag Working Party, 1971).

Close cooperation between the screening laboratory and the biochemist. Actual biochemical diagnosis requires more sophisticated techniques, including analysis of urine for metabolites of phenylalanine.

Problems of diagnosis

With the introduction of more sensitive screening procedures, not only are infants with classical phenylketonuria detected, but also a whole spectrum of children with hyperphenylalaninaemia, the significance of which is largely unknown (Bickel, 1970). Although figures for the birth frequency of classical phenylketonuria are quoted in the literature (e.g. for the United Kingdom see Carter, 1973), they should be interpreted with caution in view of the increasing realisation of the genetic heterogeneity of the condition. It may be only after several months of treatment that it becomes apparent that an infant is not behaving like a classical case of phenylketonuria. The enzymic system for the conversion of phenylalanine to tyrosine is complex involving a pteridine cofactor and dihydropteridine reductase as well as phenylalanine *p*-hydroxylase. In addition, tyrosine:alpha-ketoglutarate and phenylalanine:pyruvate aminotransferases and aromatic alpha-ketoacid reductase are involved in the metabolism of phenylalanine and tyrosine (McLean, Marwick and Clayton, 1973). It is therefore not surprising that variants occur. Recently a rare form with severe progressive neurological disease, chemical phenylketonuria and failure to respond to a low phenylalanine diet in spite of satisfactory control of phenylalanine levels has been observed (Smith, 1974; Smith, Clayton and Wolff, 1975a, b). It was postulated that the disorder was due to a defect in the metabolism of biopterin, the natural cofactor for phenylalanine *p*-hydroxylase. Butler et al (1975) have demonstrated deficient activity of dihydropteridine reductase in cultured fibroblasts from such a patient.

Treatment

There is no general agreement about the level of phenylalanine for which treatment is required since the cause of mental retardation in phenylketonuria is not understood. There is incomplete myelination of the central nervous system. The aim of treatment is to lower the circulating level of phenylalanine to a concentration similar to, and a little higher than, that found in normal subjects. Patients with concentrations below 10 mg/dl blood, plasma or serum are not usually treated, and the clinician may or may not decide to treat an infant with concentrations between 10 and 15 mg/dl. If the phenyl-alanine level is persistently between 15 and 20 mg/dl, the clinician may try to reduce the concentration by using a low protein diet (2.0–3.0 g protein with total calories exceeding 115 ± 15/kg body weight daily during the neonatal period) or he may use a synthetic diet and reassess the infant after three to six months. The team at the Hospital for Sick Children in London treats the infant only if the phenylalanine concentration is persistently greater than 15 mg/dl and abnormal metabolites are present in the urine when the infant is on a normal diet.

For good results, these children should be treated in centres where there is a team comprising not only the paediatrician, but a paediatric dietitian, biochemist, psychiatrist and psychologist. The advantages of a centre in my view far outweigh the disadvantage of the journey to the centre. The family doctor will also be intimately involved in the care and he will require infor-mation and support from the centre since he may never have seen this rare disorder. The local paediatrician may wish to be concerned also and it is essential to be absolutely certain about the role of each individual in decision-making as it affects the patient and his family. Such centralisation accords with the views given by the Department of Health and Social Security in England and Wales in HM(69)72 and by many others, including Wamberg (1973), who has described a special treatment home and research centre in Denmark.

The phenylalanine intake is reduced by using a synthetic substitute for much of the protein in the diet. This may be based on either a hydrolysate of protein from which most of the phenylalanine has been removed or on a mixture of amino acids excluding phenylalanine. Since phenylalanine is an essential amino acid, it is necessary to provide a small amount of natural protein, the amount varying from time to time and patient to patient. Regular monitoring of the phenylalanine concentration in the patient's blood is thus essential and a microprocedure using capillary blood from heel or finger should be employed. It is unnecessary and cruel to employ femoral puncture for collecting blood in order to control the diet. Details of the diet have been given by Clayton (1975) and Francis (1975).

The patient with phenylketonuria still poses many problems. The optimal age at which the low phenylalanine diet may be stopped is not known and opinions vary so that some workers feel it is safe at three years, others that it is never safe and yet others who compromise at some age in between. As Parker (1973) has pointed out, even within the same clinic at Los Angeles, clinicians hold differing views! Dobbing and Sands (1973) have concluded that the growth-spurt complex of the human brain may possibly continue into the fourth or fifth postnatal year, and it is likely that deposition of myelin continues until the age of 15 to 20 years (Davison, 1970). In the light of available knowledge older children and adolescents should probably limit their intake of natural protein so that the blood phenylalanine concentration does not rise above 20 to 25 mg but this is speculative.

In due course, pregnancy in the treated phenylketonuric woman will become more common. The children of mothers with untreated phenylketonuria have a very high incidence of congenital abnormalities (Leader, 1970) including mental retardation, intrauterine and postnatal retardation of growth, microcephaly, skeletal, cardiac and ocular malformations. It has therefore been suggested (Yu and O'Halloran, 1970) that a planned pregnancy with dietary restriction during the period of conception and throughout the pregnancy will be necessary to avoid the teratogenic effect of phenylalanine. A low phenylalanine diet has been used successfully in several pregnancies in women with phenylketonuria (Allan and Brown, 1968) but is potentially hazardous since undernutrition and malnutrition in the prenatal period can affect brain development.

TYROSINE DISORDERS

Abnormalities of tyrosine metabolism in infants occur for a number of reasons. Transient rises in the tyrosine concentration in blood and associated tyrosyluria are frequent in premature babies and to a less extent in full-term babies, and do not appear to cause problems (La Du and Gjessing, 1972). In a small number of patients these findings have persisted and they have presented with mental retardation (Holston et al, 1971). Danks, Tippett and Rogers (1975) have described a patient with a prolonged transient rise in tyrosine, associated with severe metabolic acidosis. An inherited form of abnormal tyrosine metabolism with involvement of the liver has been found in a few communities especially in certain French Canadians (Larochelle et al, 1967) and concentrations of phenylalanine, tyrosine and methionine are raised in the blood. Such patients have occurred rarely and sporadically in the United Kingdom and the prognosis, even with early treatment, is very poor. Other variants have been described including patients with liver involvement and elevated phenylalanine and tyrosine but not methionine in the blood and sometimes the condition is transient (Harries et al, 1969). Although disorders of tyrosine metabolism should be considered in sick babies, there does not seem to be any justification for screening all infants for them on a service basis in the United Kingdom at present.

HOMOCYSTINURIA

Several inherited disorders of sulphur metabolism have been described and of these homocystinuria is particularly important. In classical homocystinuria during the first two years of life the child frequently appears normal and gradually develops the characteristic features (Carson et al, 1963) comprising ectopia lentis, malar flush, skeletal abnormalities which may include severe osteoporosus of the spine, abnormal gait and muscle weakness. Thromboembolic attacks are common and thrombosis is especially likely in the coronary, renal and cerebral arteries. About two-thirds of the patients are mentally retarded and even those of normal intelligence have swings of mood and other behaviour abnormalities. Patients with the classical form of the disorder have a deficient activity of cystathionine synthase in various sites including liver (Mudd et al, 1964), brain (Mudd et al, 1967), cultured skin fibroblasts and amniotic fluid cells (Uhlendorf and Mudd, 1968).

Patients can be detected by screening for raised methionine in blood and the Guthrie test is suitable. The majority of positive screening tests will not be due to the condition since raised methionine can result from delayed enzymatic maturation and high protein intakes (Gaull, Sturman and Raiha, 1972). Detailed biochemical studies are essential for accurate diagnosis. Worldwide results of routine newborn screening give an incidence for homocystinuria of 1 in 230000 births (Levy, 1974) but the incidence in the United Kingdom appears to be about 1 in 100000 births. It should be noted that in the variant type with a defect in the biosynthesis of a folate coenzyme (see below), hypomethioninaemia is present in association with homocystine in urine and thus would not be detected when screening blood.

Treatment has included: diets restricted in methionine and supplemented with cystine (Komrower et al, 1966; Komrower and Sardharwalla, 1971), administration of large doses of pyridoxine (Barber and Spaeth, 1967; Seashore, Durant and Rosenberg, 1972), a combination of pyridoxine and a low protein diet. Additional folate may be necessary as well as pyridoxine (Morrow and Barness, 1972). Details have been given by Carson (1975). It is too early to predict the final outcome of treatment, although reports so far are hopeful (for a summary, see Carson, 1975).

Variants of homocystinuria have been described including a form due to deficiency of 5-methyltetrahydrofolate methyltransferase (Mudd et al, 1970) and another due to deficiency of 5,10-methylene tetrahydrofolate reductase (Mudd et al, 1972). Reports on treatment of these variants are not available.

Since treatment appears likely to be beneficial and prenatal diagnosis is possible, there is need for more research on this condition. Screening, treatment and research should be undertaken by interested teams, but screening of every newborn in the United Kingdom at this stage could not be justified.

MAPLE SYRUP URINE DISEASE

Classical maple syrup urine disease was first described in 1954 (Menkes, Hurst and Craig, 1954) and several variants of it are now known. It appears to be a rare disorder with an incidence of 1 in 340000 births (Seakins et al, 1972). The first symptoms appear at three to five days of age in the classical form, the infant appearing normal until then. The infant may be difficult to feed, is listless, has attacks of hyponuria and hypertonicity, progresses to convulsions and then to coma and slow respiration with periods of apnoea, and a fatal outcome. The infant develops a characteristic odour, specially noticeable in the urine. In the intermittent types the usual presentation is an attack of severe metabolic acidosis associated with a trivial infection. The initial symptoms may not occur until the child is several years old (Kiil and Rokkones, 1964; Valman et al, 1973) or may occur only with a normal protein intake (Snyderman, 1972). The branched chain amino acids, leucine, valine and isoleucine, are raised in the blood and urine, as is alloisoleucine. Abnormal excretion of the keto acid derivatives of the branched chain amino acids occurs and hence there is a positive response to 2,4-dinitrophenylhydrazine and ferric chloride. Impaired oxidative decarboxylation of the keto acids can be demonstrated in peripheral leucocytes with no detectable activity in the classical form of the disease, but significant activity in the intermittent forms.

Treatment of severe forms requires the use of a synthetic diet based on the replacement of most of the protein by amino acids. It is necessary to supply the three branched chain amino acids, the amount of each having to be varied individually. The diet is exceedingly difficult and details have been given by Francis (1975) and Snyderman (1975). Occasionally acute episodes in early life may best be treated by exchange transfusion or peritoneal dialysis although modification of diet is usually sufficient later. In the variant forms diet may be necessary during infections only and Scriver et al (1971) have described a form which responds to thiamine.

The best 'screening test' for maple syrup urine disease is a heightened awareness by the clinician that this is a possible diagnosis in severe metabolic acidosis. By the sixth day of life it may be too late for detecting the classical form because the infant may already be very ill or dead, and variant forms might easily not be detectable.

HISTIDINAEMIA

There are inherited conditions with definite biochemical abnormalities, the clinical significance of which is not understood and histidinaemia (Ghadimi, Partington and Hunter, 1961) is a good example. The subjects show increased histidine in plasma and urine, raised urinary excretion of metabolites of histidine, marked reduction in histidine ammonia lyase (histidase) activity and urocanic acid content in the skin, and an abnormal histidine tolerance curve.

Apart from screening programmes, biochemical changes have usually been discovered during the investigation of a mentally retarded patient (e.g. Gatfield et al, 1969) and this has led to studies on other members of the family whether retarded or not. Even with this bias to selection, Neville et al in 1972 found that amongst their own subjects and those in the literature, 28 of 42 with the typical biochemical findings had intelligence within the normal range (IQ > 80). Neville et al (1972) were unable to demonstrate any biochemical difference between retarded subjects and those of normal intelligence and their frequent coexistence in one family would be against a genetic explanation.

When 'biochemical histidinaemia' is detected during the screening of new-borns a complex ethical problem arises. Although it is possible to lower the histidine level in the blood with diet, there are two problems. Firstly, the relationship of the biochemical findings to retardation is unknown. Secondly, if dietary treatment is given then it appears that, at best, in more than half the infants, it would be used unnecessarily. Neville et al (1972) concluded from their study that there was little justification for the use of the diet in infancy and they suggested that careful follow-up of neonates detected by screening would help to solve this difficult problem. Neville, Clayton and Lilly (unpublished observations) began to screen for histidinaemia by the Guthrie test in June 1971. So far, 30 infants have been detected giving an incidence of 1 in 11 000 births. The infants have been seen approximately every six months and so far (and the eldest is now aged four years) no major developmental problems have arisen. These findings are similar to those in the more extensive series of untreated patients reported by Levy, Shih and Madigan in 1974. I would agree with Levy et al that it is premature to state unequivocally that histidinaemia is a totally benign disorder, and that only long-term follow-up will show whether any changes occur late in childhood or in adult life. However, with the information so far available there is no justification for instituting dietary therapy or for screening on a national basis but further research is required.

SCREENING AND THE SICK INFANT

For reasons already presented, I have no doubt that it is correct to screen for phenylketonuria on a service basis, but I regard screening for other amino acid disorders to fall within the realm of research. This view accords with that of Holland (1974) and Raine (1974). Further research on maple syrup urine disease, homocystinuria and histidinaemia would appear to be of particular interest.

The problem is very different in the sick infant and it is essential for the paediatrician to consider metabolic disorders amongst possible diagnoses. Many of them have similar presenting features: lethargy, failure to feed, vomiting and then seizures or coma. There may be a family history of unexplained death in infancy and the patient may have a smell. A careful history will reveal that the symptoms began after feeding with protein had begun. Since such disorders may present early in life even a sophisticated research screening programme with close cooperation between clinicians and the laboratory may fail to provide an answer before the infant succumbs or is severely damaged. The sick infant with a possible metabolic disorder should be considered, therefore, as a specific problem for which more extensive biochemical facilities are essential. Several classes of amino acids or their organic acid derivatives are involved and include branched chain amino acids, urea cycle compounds, sulphur-containing amino acids, glycine, aromatic amino acids, β-amino compounds and dipeptides. The problem has been considered by O'Brien and Goodman (1970) and Rosenberg (1974).

If the paediatrician suspects such a disorder it would seem wise to restrict the infant's protein intake and prevent catabolism of his own tissues by providing a high calorie intake from carbohydrate. Francis (1975) has described such an infant feed based on glucose, sucrose, Caloreen (Scientific Hospital Supplies), Prosparol (British Drug Houses), electrolytes and water.

GENETICS AND PRENATAL DIAGNOSIS

The management of an amino acid disorder includes genetic counselling. Additionally, prenatal detection of some metabolic disorders in families known to be at risk for a second affected child is possible. Significant progress has been made already in the field of lipid storage disorders, e.g. Tay–Sachs disease, and advances in the prenatal diagnosis of aminoacidopathies are likely in the future. So far the prenatal diagnosis of phenylketonuria has proved impossible, but has been successfully performed for maple syrup urine disease (e.g. Dancis, 1972), homocystinuria (Bittles and Carson, 1973) and cystinosis (Schneider et al, 1974).

ORGANISATION OF SCREENING

Amino acid disorders are only one group in a vast spectrum of inherited metabolic disease. Many metabolic disorders are very rare, but cystic fibrosis has an incidence of about 1 in 2000 births in the United Kingdom and of course in some parts of the world, the haemoglobinopathies are common. For disorders which are rare, centralisation offers the best means of detection and care. This is not easy to achieve. Although HM(69)72 suggested centralisation for screening for phenylketonuria, Hawcroft and Hudson pointed out in 1974 that in England and Wales no less than 34 laboratories were screening for the condition. They considered this was too many but refrained from suggesting the ideal size and location of regional screening centres because so much depends on personal involvement and interest, local geography and the new organisation of the Health Service. It has been suggested (Notes and News

1975) that one centre could screen the whole of England and Wales for phenyl-ketonuria. I agree strongly with Komrower (1975) that this would be disastrous for the good communication necessary between the community, the laboratory and the hospital unit providing experienced clinical and biochemical back-up for the confirmation of diagnosis and the supervision of treatment. Komrower (1975) suggested that the United Kingdom could be served by perhaps 10 biochemical genetics laboratories which would have further responsibilities in addition to screening, and I would agree with this view. Raine (1972) also suggested specialist centres, about five for a population of 50 million for the management of inherited metabolic disease so that prenatal detection, neonatal screening, heterozygote detection, diagnosis and treatment could be coordinated. In a field which is developing so rapidly centres are bound to work closely with many research workers who have an expertise in one or two disorders only. Provided the system is flexible centralisation offers the best care for the patient.

It is essential that no one should lose sight of the fact that the aim of screening is to help the individual, his family and the community. The psychological aspects of screening are very important and continuing thought must be given to the fact that biochemical abnormalities do not necessarily equate with disease.

REFERENCES

Allan, J. D. & Brown, J. K. (1968) Maternal phenylketonuria and foetal brain damage. An attempt at prevention by dietary control. In *Some Recent Advances in Inborn Errors of Metabolism*, ed. Holt, K. S. & Coffey, V. P., pp. 14–38. London and Edinburgh: Livingstone.

Barber, G. W. & Spaeth, G. L. (1967) Pyridoxine therapy in homocystinuria. *Lancet*, **1**, 337.

Baumeister, A. A. (1967) The effects of dietary control on intelligence in phenylketonuria. *American Journal of Mental Deficiency*, **71**, 840–847.

Bessman, S. P. (1966) Legislation and advances in medical knowledge—acceleration or inhibition? *Journal of Pediatrics*, **69**, 334–338.

Bickel, H. (1970) Phenylalaninaemia or classical phenylketonuria (PKU). *Neuropadiatrie*, **1**, 379–382.

Birch, H. G. & Tizard, J. (1967) The dietary treatment of phenylketonuria: not proven? *Developmental Medicine and Child Neurology*, **9**, 9–12.

Bittles, A. H. & Carson, N. A. J. (1973) Tissue culture techniques as an aid to prenatal diagnosis and genetic counselling in homocystinuria. *Journal of Medical Genetics*, **10**, 120–121.

Butler, I. J., Holtzman, N. A., Kaufman, S., Koslow, S. H., Krumholz, A. & Milstien, S. (1975) Phenylketonuria due to deficiency of dihydropteridine reductase. *Pediatric Research*, **9**, 348.

Carson, N. A. J. (1975) Homocystinuria. In *The Treatment of Inherited Metabolic Disease*, ed. Raine, D. N., pp. 33–69, Lancaster: Medical & Technical Publishing Co. Ltd.

Carson, N. A. J., Cusworth, D. C., Dent, C. E., Field, C. M. B. & Gaull, G. E. (1963) Homocystinuria: a new inborn error of metabolism associated with mental deficiency. *Archive of Disease in Childhood*, **38**, 425–436.

Carter, C. O. (1973) Nature and distribution of genetic abnormalities. *Journal of Biosocial Science*, **5**, 261–272.

Clayton, B. E. (1975) The principles of treatment by dietary restriction as illustrated by phenylketonuria. In *The Treatment of Inherited Metabolic Disease*, ed. Raine, D. N., pp. 1–32. Lancaster: Medical and Technical Publishing Co. Ltd.

Clayton, B. E. & Jenkins, P. (1970) Collection of blood for the Guthrie test. *Midwife and Health Visitor*, **6**, 170–176.

Clayton, B. E., Moncrieff, A. & Roberts, G. E. (1967) Dietetic treatment of phenylketonuria: a follow-up study. *British Medical Journal*, **3**, 133–136.

Dancis, J. (1972) Maple syrup urine disease. In *Antenatal Diagnosis*, ed. Dorfman, A., pp. 123–125. Chicago: University of Chicago Press.

Danks, D. M., Tippett, P. & Rogers, J. (1975) A new form of prolonged transient tyrosinemia presenting with severe metabolic acidosis. *Acta paediatrica scandinavica*, **64**, 209–214.

Davison, A. N. (1970) *Myelination*, pp. 100–143. Illinois: Charles C. Thomas.

Dobbing, J. & Sands, J. (1973) Quantitative growth and development of human brain. *Archives of Disease in Childhood*, **48**, 757–767.

Ersser, R. (1971) *Chromatography in Clinical Biochemistry using Flexible Thin-layers*. Koch-Light Laboratories Ltd, England.

Francis, D. E. M. (1975) *Diets for Sick Children*, 3rd edn. London: Blackwell Scientific Publications.

Fuller, R. N. & Shuman, J. B. (1969) Phenylketonuria and intelligence: trimodal response to dietary treatment. *Nature (London)*, **221**, 639–642.

Gatfield, P. D., Knights, R. M., Devereux, M. & Pozsonyi, J. P. (1969) Histidinaemia: report of four new cases in one family, and the effect of low-histidine diets. *Canadian Medical Association Journal*, **101**, 465–469.

Gaull, G. E., Sturman, J. A. & Raiha, N. C. R. (1972) Development of mammalian sulphur metabolism: absence of cystathionase in human foetal tissue. *Pediatric Research*, **6**, 538–547.

Ghadimi, H., Partington, M. W. & Hunter, A. (1961) A familial disturbance of histidine metabolism. *New England Journal of Medicine*, **265**, 221–224.

Guthrie, R. (1961) Blood screening for phenylketonuria (Letter). *Journal of the American Medical Association*, **178**, 863.

Harries, J. T., Seakins, J. W. T., Ersser, R. S. & Lloyd, J. K. (1969) Recovery after dietary treatment of an infant with features of tyrosinosis. *Archives of Disease in Childhood*, **44**, 258–267.

Hawcroft, J. & Hudson, F. P. (1974) Screening for phenylketonuria in the United Kingdom. *Health Trends*, **6**, 72–74.

HM(69)72 National Health Service. Screening for early detection of phenylketonuria.

Holland, W. W. (1974) Screening for disease. Taking stock. *Lancet*, **2**, 1494–1497.

Holston, J. L., Levy, H. L., Tomlin, G. A., Atkins, B. J., Patton, T. H. & Hosty, T. S. (1971) Tyrosinosis. A patient without liver or renal disease. *Pediatrics*, **48**, 393–400.

Holtzman, N. A., Meek, A. G. & Mellits, E. D. (1974) Neonatal screening for phenylketonuria. *Journal of the American Medical Association*, **229**, 667–670.

Holtzman, N. A., Mellits, E. D. & Kallman, C. H. (1974) Neonatal screening for phenylketonuria: II. Age dependence of initial phenylalanine in infants with PKU. *Pediatrics*, **53**, 353–357.

Hudson, F. P. & Hawcroft, J. (1974) MRC/DHSS Phenylketonuria Register, Newsletter No. 2.

Hudson, F. P. & Hawcroft, J. (1975) MRC/DHSS Phenylketonuria Register, Newsletter No. 3.

Hudson, F. P., Mordaunt, V. L. & Leahy, I. (1970) Evaluation of treatment begun in first three months of life in 164 cases of phenylketonuria. *Archives of Disease in Childhood*, **45**, 5–12.

Institute of Society, Ethics and Life Sciences (1972) Ethical and social issues in screening for genetic disease. *New England Journal of Medicine*, **286**, 1129–1132.

Kang, E. S., Sollec, N. D. & Gerald, P. S. (1970) Results of treatment and termination of the diet in phenylketonuria (PKU). *Pediatrics*, **46**, 881–890.

Kiil, R. & Rokkones, T. (1964) Late manifesting variant of branched-chain ketoaciduria (maple syrup urine disease). *Acta paediatrica scandinavica*, **53**, 356–364.

Koch, R., Dobson, J. C., Blaskovics, M., Williamson, L., Ernest, A. E., Friedman, E. G. & Parker, C. E. (1973) Collaborative study of children treated for phenylketonuria. In *Treatment of Inborn Errors of Metabolism*, ed Seakins, J. W. T., Saunders, R. A. & Toothill, C., pp. 3–8. Edinburgh: Churchill Livingstone.

Komrower, G. (1975) Screening for phenylketonuria. *Lancet*, **1**, 328.

Komrower, G. M., Lambert, A. M., Cusworth, D. C. & Westall, R. G. (1966) Dietary treatment of homocystinuria. *Archives of Disease in Childhood*, **41**, 666–671.

Komrower, G. M. & Sardharwalla, I. B. (1971) The dietary treatment of homocystinuria. In *Inherited Disorders of Sulphur Metabolism*, ed. Carson, N. A. J. & Raine, D. N. pp. 254–263. Edinburgh and London: Churchill Livingstone.

La Du, B. N. & Gjessing, L. R. (1972) Tyrosinosis and tyrosinaemia. In *The Metabolic Basis of Inherited Disease*, ed. Stanbury, J. B., Wyngaarden, J. B. & Fredrickson, D. S., pp. 296–307. New York: McGraw-Hill.

Larochelle, J., Mortezai, A., Belanger, M., Tremblay, M., Claveau, J. C. & Aubin, G. (1967) Experience with 37 infants with tyrosinemia. *Canadian Medical Association Journal*, **97**, 1051–1054.

Leader (1970) Maternal phenylketonuria. *British Medical Journal*, **4**, 192.

Lemag Working Party (1971) Estimation of blood phenylalanine from a dried blood spot using the Guthrie test. *Journal of Clinical Pathology*, **24**, 576–578.

Levy, H. L. (1974) Neonatal screening for inborn errors of amino acid metabolism. *Clinics in Endocrinology and Metabolism*, **3**, 153–166.

Levy, H. L., Karolkewicz, V., Houghton, S. A. & MacCready, R. A. (1970) Screening the normal population in Massachusetts for phenylketonuria. *New England Journal of Medicine*, **282**, 1455–1458.

Levy, H. L., Shih, V. E. & Madigan, P. M. (1974) Routine newborn screening for histidinaemia. *New England Journal of Medicine*, **291**, 1214–1219.

MacCready, R. (1974) Admissions of phenylketonuric patients to residential institutions before and after screening programs of the newborn infant. *Journal of Pediatrics*, **85**, 383–385.

Massachusetts Department of Public Health (1974) Cost–benefit analysis of newborn screening for metabolic disorders. *New England Journal of Medicine*, **291**, 1414–1416.

McLean, A., Marwick, M. J. & Clayton, B. E. (1973) Enzymes involved in phenylalanine metabolism in the human foetus and child. *Journal of Clinical Pathology*, **26**, 678–683.

Medical Research Council Working Party (1968) Present status of different mass screening procedures for phenylketonuria. *British Medical Journal*, **4**, 7–13.

Menkes, J. H., Hurst, P. L. & Craig, J. M. (1954) A new syndrome: progressive familial infantile dysfunction associated with an unusual urinary substance. *Pediatrics*, **14**, 462–466.

Morrow, G. III & Barness, L. A. (1972) Combined vitamin responsiveness in homocystinuria. *Journal of Pediatrics*, **81**, 946–954.

Mudd, S. H., Finkelstein, J. D., Irreverre, F. & Laster, L. (1964) Homocystinuria: an enzymatic defect. *Science*, **143**, 1443–1445.

Mudd, S. H., Laster, L., Finkelstein, J. D. & Irreverre, F. (1967) Studies in homocystinuria. In *Amines and Schizophrenia*, ed. Himwich, H. E., Kety, S. S. & Smythies, J. R., pp. 247–256. London: Pergamon Press.

Mudd, S. H., Uhlendorf, B. W., Hinds, K. R. & Levy, H. L. (1970) Deranged B$_{12}$ metabolism: studies of fibroblasts grown in tissue culture. *Biochemical Medicine*, **4**, 215–239.

Mudd, S. H., Uhlendorf, B. W., Freeman, J. M., Finkelstein, J. D. & Shih, V. E. (1972) Homocystinuria associated with decreased methylene-tetrahydrofolate reductase deficiency. *Biochemical and Biophysical Research Communications*, **46**, 905–912.

Neville, B. G. R., Bentovim, A., Clayton, B. E. & Shepherd, J. (1972) Histidinaemia: study of relation between clinical and biological findings in 7 subjects. *Archives of Disease in Childhood*, **47**, 190–200.

Notes and News (1975) The Phenylketonuria Register. *Lancet*, **1**, 178.

O'Brien, D. & Goodman, S. I. (1970) The critically ill child: acute metabolic disease in infancy and early childhood. *Pediatrics*, **46**, 620–626.

Parker, C. E. (1973) Remarks on the longterm aspects of phenylketonuria. In *Treatment of Inborn Errors of Metabolism*, ed. Seakins, J. W. T., Saunders, R. A. & Toothill, C., pp. 19–21. London: Churchill Livingstone.

Raine, D. N. (1972) Management of inherited metabolic disease. *British Medical Journal*, **2**, 329–336.

Raine, D. N. (1974) Screening for disease. Inherited metabolic disease. *Lancet*, **2**, 996–998.

Raine, D. N., Cooke, J. R., Andrews, W. A. & Mahon, D. F. (1972) Screening for inherited metabolic disease by plasma chromatography (Scriver) in a large city. *British Medical Journal*, **3**, 7–13.

Rosenberg, L. E. (1974) Diagnosis and management of inherited aminoacidopathies in the newborn and unborn. *Clinics in Endocrinology and Metabolism*, **3**, 145–152.

Schneider, J. A., Verroust, F. M., Kroll, W. A., Garvin, A. J., Horger, E. O. III, Wong, V. G., Spear, G. S., Jacobson, C., Pellett, O. L. & Becker, F. L. A. (1974) The prenatal diagnosis of cystinosis. *New England Journal of Medicine*, **290**, 878–882.

Scriver, C. R., Davies, E. & Cullen, A. M. (1964) Application of a simple micromethod to the screening of plasma for a variety of aminoacidopathies, *Lancet*, **2**, 230–232.

Scriver, C. R., Mackenzie, S., Clow, C. L. & Delvin, E. (1971) Thiamine-responsive maple syrup urine disease. *Lancet*, **1**, 310–312.

Seakins, J. W. T., Haktan, M., Andrew, B. C. & Ersser, R. S. (1972) Screening for inherited metabolic disorders: a new look at metabolic screening tests. *Annals of Clinical Biochemistry* **9**, 103–108.

Seashore, M. R., Durant, J. L. & Rosenberg, L. E. (1972) Studies of the mechanism of pyridoxine-responsive homocystinuria. *Pediatric Research*, **6**, 187–196.

Smith, I. (1974) Atypical phenylketonuria accompanied by a severe progressive neurological illness unresponsive to dietary treatment. *Archives of Disease in Childhood*, **49**, 245.

Smith, I., Clayton, B. E. & Wolff, O. H. (1975a) A variant of phenylketonuria. *Lancet*, **1**, 328–329.

Smith, I., Clayton, B. E. & Wolff, O. H. (1975b) New variant of phenylkeotnuria with progressive neurological illness unresponsive to phenylalanine restriction. *Lancet*, **1**, 1108–1111.

Smith, I. & Wolff, O. H. (1974) Natural history of phenylketonuria and influence of early treatment. *Lancet*, **2**, 540–544.

Snyderman, S. E. (1972) A variant of branched-chain ketoaciduria. In *Organic Acidurias*, ed. Stern, J. & Toothill, C., pp. 87–98. Edinburgh and London: Churchill Livingstone.

Snyderman, S. E. (1975) Maple syrup urine disease. In *The Treatment of Inherited Metabolic Disease*, ed. Raine, D. N., pp. 71–90. Lancaster: Medical and Technical Publishing Co. Ltd.

Stephenson, J. B. P. & McLean, M. S. (1967) Phenylketonuria: a reassessment of mass infant screening by napkin test. *British Medical Journal*, **3**, 582.

Uhlendorf, B. W. & Mudd, S. H. (1968) Cystathionine synthase in tissue culture derived from human skin: enzyme defect in homocystinuria. *Science*, **160**, 1007–1009.

Valman, H. B., Patrick, A. D., Seakins, J. W. T., Platt, J. W. & Gompertz, D. (1973) Family with intermittent maple syrup urine disease. *Archives of Disease in Childhood*, **48**, 225–228.

Wamberg, E. (1973) A survey of centralised treatment of phenylketonuria in Denmark. In *Treatment of Inborn Errors of Metabolism*, ed. Seakins, J. W. T., Saunders, R. A. & Toothill, C., pp. 35–40. London: Churchill Livingstone.

Webb, J. F., Khazen, R. S. & Hanley, W. B. (1973) PKU Screening—is it worth it? *Canadian Medical Association Journal*, **108**, 328–329.

Whitby, L. G. (1974) Screening for disease. Definitions and criteria. *Lancet*, **2**, 819–822.

Wilson, J. M. G. (1973) Current trends and problems in health screening. *Journal of Clinical Pathology*, **26**, 555–563.

Woolf, L. I. (1967) In *Phenylketonuria and Allied Metabolic Diseases*, ed. Anderson, J. A. & Swaiman, K. F., p. 50. Washington: US Government Printing Office.

Woolf, L. I., Griffiths, R., Moncrieff, A., Coates, S. & Dillistone, F. (1958) The dietary treatment of phenylketonuria. *Archives of Disease in Childhood*, **33**, 31–45.

Yu, J. & O'Halloran, M. (1970) Children of mothers with phenylketonuria. *Lancet*, **1**, 210–212.

7
IMMUNISING PROCEDURES
IN CHILDHOOD

J. A. Dudgeon

'It is generally recognised that immunisation is one of the best and most effective investments which any government can make towards the health of its citizens.'

This statement came from the opening paragraph of the recommendations of a Conference on 'Immunisation in Africa' held in Kampala in December 1971 under the auspices of the Centre Internationale de l'Enfance (Seminar, 1971). Although it is undoubtedly true that, in many circumstances, immunisation is the best and most effective method of prevention, as exemplified by the control of smallpox, tetanus, diphtheria and poliomyelitis, at the same time, it must be recognised that immunisation alone cannot control all forms of communicable disease. General public health measures, which include sanitation, hygiene, medical, social and educational services, and legislative powers to put recommendations into force, are all necessary elements of the overall plan to control communicable disease. But even more important than these general measures is the provision of finance to enable preventive measures to be implemented and, above all, to be maintained, a fact which was also clearly recognised at the Kampala Conference.

Although the principal problem of the Kampala Conference was related to immunisation in the continent of Africa, what was discussed there and the recommendations which were made hold true for every nation in the world, irrespective of its size and economic position. Every nation, however rich, never has enough resources to meet *all* the needs for *all* health care. Every government has its own problems to invest and distribute what financial resources it has available to the best of its ability to meet the local need for the maximum benefit of its peoples. Immunisation programmes can be extremely costly to implement in purely financial terms, but whenever they are implemented, whether in the developed or in the developing areas of the world, it is essential to ensure that provision is made for them in the annual budget for health programmes to be maintained, and where necessary, extended. Once a nation has embarked upon a campaign to control a disease by immunisation, be it smallpox, diphtheria, poliomyelitis or measles, there is no going back. Immunisation programmes must be continued unless complete eradication of the disease can be assured, or unless some other form of prevention can be instituted, otherwise the risk must be faced that epidemic disease, brought under control by immunisation will recur, affecting a wider population of susceptible individuals and more harm than good may have been done.

Much has been achieved by the development of immunisation procedures in the past 50 years and a generation of doctors in practice today have seen, during their professional lifetime, many of the most severe and crippling of the communicable diseases brought under control, and the younger generation may not even have seen a case of diphtheria or poliomyelitis.' How has this been achieved and what are the problems which still confront us?

HISTORICAL ASPECTS

Throughout the history of medicine, and long before the concept of contagious disease was accepted, examples can be found in medical writings of preventive measures aimed at restricting the spread of disease by quarantine and of early methods of prophylaxis. The latter are of special interest based as they were in the belief that recovery from infection led to a state of resistance. The stimulus to do something about these epidemics scourges stemmed largely from fear, fear of smallpox and fear of measles, and even in modern times the development of poliomyelitis vaccines was to a great extent motivated by fear of paralytic disease.

Smallpox had been known in India and China from ancient times and in these early days, people accepted the risk of being artificially infected with smallpox in order to become immune and to avoid the gross disfigurement of those who survived. In China, the practice developed of taking dried smallpox crusts into the nose in the form of snuff. In Turkey, a method was developed of inserting variolous (smallpox) matter into a vein; this practice, known as 'variolation', was first introduced into England early in the eighteenth century by an Italian physician, Dr Emmanuel Timoni, but it was very largely due to the influence of Lady Mary Wortley Montagu, wife of the British Ambassador to Turkey, that variolation became an established practice in England. On return to England in 1725, she persuaded King George I to take an interest in the subject. The King must have been impressed, but clearly had some reservations as he first decided to carry out a 'trial' on six condemned prisoners held in Newgate Prison. Dr Richard Meade, the Royal Physician, inoculated them with variolous matter. The experiment proved successful in that all, not only survived the initial inoculation, but also resisted exposure to natural smallpox. The prisoners were freed and the King's children were then variolated with no apparent ill-effect. The method then caught on in London and spread to the rest of the country, to Europe and to the American colonies.

By this time an alternative procedure to variolation was being sought. The fact that individuals who contracted cowpox, a naturally occurring disease of cows, characterised by a pustular eruption on the udders, seldom developed smallpox, had been recognised in England early in the nineteenth century. A Dorsetshire farmer, Benjamin Jesty, in 1774, had infected his wife and two children with cowpox matter and they had remained free of smallpox, although his action caused much displeasure in the parish; but it was Edward Jenner (1747–1823), a practitioner in Berkeley, Gloucestershire, who recognised the significance of the cross-protection between cowpox and smallpox. In September 1796 Jenner introduced cowpox material taken from a milkmaid, Sarah Neames, into the arm of James Phipps, a healthy boy of eight years of age. Eight weeks later the boy withstood a 'challenge' inoculation with smallpox matter. Jenner's claim that cowpox conferred immunity to smallpox was rejected by the Royal Society of which he was a Fellow, and indeed he was admonished 'for presenting anything to the learned body which was at variance to accepted knowledge and was so incredible'.

Further vaccinations were performed and in 1797, Jenner published his findings entitled 'An Enquiry into the Causes and Effects of Variolae Vaccinae' (Jenner, 1798) followed a year later by his 'Further Enquiry' (Jenner, 1799). Jenner regarded cowpox as smallpox of the cow, hence the term variolae vaccinae (from the Latin vacca, a cow, and Latin derivative vaccinus, hence to 'vaccinate'). The immediate reaction in London to 'vaccination' or 'cowpoxing' was unenthusiastic except for one or two physicians, notably Mr Henry Cline of St Thomas's Hospital, and Dr Woodville, physician to the Smallpox and Inoculation Hospital in London. The House of Commons appointed a Select Committee in 1802 which voted Jenner the sum of £20000, and in 1806 the Chancellor of the Exchequer moved that a humble Address be presented to the King 'Praying that he be pleased to direct the Royal Colleges of Physicians of London, Edinburgh and Dublin to enquire into the state of vaccine inoculation in the Kingdom and to report progress'. The Colleges reported nine months later (1807) 'strongly recommending the practice of vaccination'. In 1808 the National Vaccine Establishment was set up in London under Royal Warrant from the Privy Council for the purpose of distributing vaccine lymph and for rendering vaccine inoculation generally beneficial to His Majesty's subjects (*Hansard*, 1808). Jenner's discovery aroused great interest in Europe and in the New World, but in England there was general apathy and fierce controversy between the advocates of variolation and those who advocated the new method of vaccination or cowpoxing. The first Vaccination Act (3 and 4, Victoria XXIX) was passed by Parliament 'making it lawful for the Guardians of every Parish to contract with the Medical Officer . . . for the vaccination of all persons in the Parish', and the same Act made variolation illegal. This did not work well in practice and in 1853 a second Vaccination Act (16 and 17, Victoria XXX) made vaccination compulsory. Objection to compulsory vaccination inevitably followed and the antivaccinationists grew even more vociferous (Bowers, 1973). Further Vaccination Acts were passed in 1853, 1874 and 1898, but it was not until 1947 that compulsory vaccination was finally abolished, although a conscience clause, allowing a parent to decline vaccination for his child had been introduced in the meantime.

The most important report on vaccination was made by a Royal Commission in 1898 which made a number of important recommendations. First, it was recommended that calf-lymph should be used wherever possible, except for those who preferred human lymph. Secondly, it was considered that safety would be increased by preserving lymph in tubes instead of on 'dry-points' (made from feather quills) and by the use of glycerine as a preservative of the lymph as recommended by Dr Copeman (Copeman, 1899; Royal Commission, 1898).

These early endeavours to prevent smallpox have been described in some detail (see reviews by Dudgeon, 1963; Bowers, 1973) as they demonstrate how many of the problems were tackled by a generation of physicians who had none of the knowledge of microbiology and immunology which is available to us today. Moreover, many of the terms used today to describe immunisation procedures emanated from those days. Timoni introduced the term 'inoculation' to describe the procedure for carrying out variolation. The term 'immunity', meaning sanctuary from danger (from the Latin immunis, immunitas), came to have a scientific meaning of resistance and hence the term immunisation or to immunise. Jenner introduced the terms 'vaccine' and also 'virus' of smallpox in the sense of a noxious poison of unknown cause some 100 years before microrganisms, bacteria and viruses had been identified. Nevertheless, in the circumstances it proved to be a most applicable term.

Even in those days, before the importance of biological control was recognised, problems of safety and potency were well recognised. The original source of the vaccine lymph (or seed virus as it would now be called) used by Jenner was cowpox material. It was the practice at the time to variolate those vaccinated to see if they were immune. In modern terms this would be called a 'challenge' inoculation. During the course of postvaccination variolation at the London Smallpox Hospital it is almost certain that the vaccine lymph became contaminated with smallpox virus. The method of arm to arm transfer of human lymph had other defects as well; one was the risk of contracting other infections such as erysipelas and syphilis, and secondly the loss of potency. In 1836, for example, it was estimated that one of the vaccine strains used in London had had over 2000 passages in human beings and the number of 'takes' had declined (Ballard, 1868) and a new strain of lymph had to be obtained (see review by Dudgeon, 1963).

Similar problems had been faced in the prevention of another severe epidemic disease—measles. Francis Home of Edinburgh wrote in 1758 as follows:

Considering how destructive this disease is, in some seasons; considering how many die, even in the mildest epidemical constitution; considering how it hurts the lungs and eyes; I thought I should do no small service to mankind, if I could render this disease more mild and safe, in the same way as the Turks have taught us to mitigate the small-pox. I suspect strongly, that the cough, often so harassing, even in the mildest kind, was produced by receiving the infection mostly by the lungs; and I hoped that this symptom would abate considerably, if I could find a method of communicating the infection by the skin alone. I could not find a sufficient quantity of scaly matter, after the measles were dried, to serve my purpose. I then applied directly to the magazine of all epidemic diseases, the blood. I chused to take it from the most feverish patients. It was applied to an incision in each arm as is done in the small-pox. It appears that the inoculated measles are a much milder disease than the natural as the former are not attended with that degree of fever which precedes the latter; nor with the cough, want of rest, and other inflammatory complaints. . . . Whence does this arise? (Home, 1758).

During the period 1866 to 1896 events of the greatest consequence were taking place on the Continent. The work of Louis Pasteur (1822–1895) and Robert Koch (1843–1911) clearly established the microbial theory of infectious disease and the benefits were soon to become apparent. The discovery that diphtheria and tetanus were caused by soluble exotoxins by Roux and Yersin at the Pasteur Institute in Paris and Kitasato and Betring in Berlin respectively was a major breakthrough in preventive medicine. This was made even more significant with the discovery that both diphtheria and tetanus could be prevented in animals by prior injection of antitoxin. Passive immunisation against diphtheria was first successfully achieved in 1894, but early attempts at active immunisation with toxin–antitoxin mixtures (TAM) were discontinued on grounds of safety (see review by Wilson, 1967). By the early 1920s the foundations of modern immunisation procedures had been finally established by the successful results of the use of antitetanus serum in the treatment of wounds in the British Army in the 1914 to 1918 War. In 1921, Ramon (1924) in Paris and Glenny and Südmersen (1921) in England showed that diphtheria toxin could be rendered atoxic by treatment with formaldehyde. Anatoxine, or toxoid as it is called in England, was the forerunner of a series of highly effective prophylactic agents for active immunisation against diphtheria. Formalin treatment of tetanus toxin led to the development of tetanus toxoid which was later to be found so successful in the active prophylaxis of wounds against tetanus in the Allied Forces in the 1939 to 1945 War.

In the field of viruses, progress had been slower. Although Pasteur had postulated that the cause of rabies was due to a microbe so small that it could not be seen under the microscope, it was not until 1892 that Ivanowski showed that tobacco mosaic disease was caused by an agent capable of passing through a bacteriological filter. A few years later Loeffler and Frosch showed that a filtrable agent was the cause of foot and mouth disease and thus the concept of a 'contagium vivum fluidum' being due to an ultramicroscopic and filtrable agent was established and the era of virology began, but it took some years before it was finally accepted that these small microbial agents were obligate intracellular parasites. Nevertheless, in the first decade of the twentieth century the viral aetiology of poliomyelitis, measles and yellow fever was established either by human volunteer experiments or inoculation of subhuman primates and by tissue culture and other techniques. The real breakthrough in virology came in 1949 following the discovery by Enders, Weller and Robbins (1949) that poliovirus could be grown in human tissue cell cultures. There can be no doubt that it was this discovery of Enders and his colleagues which completely revolutionised virological procedures and within the space of 15 years led to the development of vaccines against poliomyelitis, measles, rubella and mumps.

PRINCIPLES OF IMMUNISATION

Before embarking on the development of any immunological product, whether it be a vaccine, antiserum, or human immunoglobulin, certain basic requirements should be taken into consideration.

1. The need: is there a need for prevention? This has to be assessed in terms of morbidity, or mortality or both.
2. The method: how can this be achieved; by active immunisation with a killed inactivated or live attenuated vaccine, or by passive immunisation?
3. Safety: it goes without saying that all products must be safe, but safety is a relative term and cannot be considered as absolute. Requirements of safety are governed by regulation, putting responsibility on the manufacturer and the licensing authority that every safeguard has been taken to ensure that the product is safe, but there is also a responsibility on those who administered such products to ensure that the instructions for their use are carried out.
4. Potency: the antigenic potency and composition of vaccines are of prime importance in order to ensure protection.
5. Economy of production: immunological products are costly to produce both in regard to production costs and to safety tests. This fact is of special importance in the developing areas of the world.

Immunity

Immunisation procedures whether they are active or passive, or both, are based on the principle that recovery from infection is associated with immunity to reinfection. In some cases immunity is of long duration as in diphtheria, measles, rubella and poliomyelitis, and in others of short duration, as in influenza and the common cold. The fact that antitoxin or antibody to the infecting agent could be detected in the blood-stream following recovery, led to the belief that antibody was responsible for recovery. It now seems more probable that the presence of antibody is a consequence of infection rather than the factor responsible for recovery and is an important factor in conferring protection. The fact that the passive administration of antiserum or human immunoglobulin given at the appropriate time prior to, or very soon after exposure, and in the appropriate dosage will confer protection against a number of infections, is an indication that antitoxin or antibody by itself is protective. The effect is, however, of a temporary nature, as antibody does not stimulate the immune mechanisms of the body. Immunity from natural infection, or from active immunisation results from an integrated response in which macrophages, complement, thymus-derived lymphocytes and immunoglobulins all play a part, both in the elimination of the infecting agent and in recovery with immunity. Circulating lymphocytes derived from the thymus (T cells) are intimately concerned with cell mediated immunity, whereas 'B' cells (bone-marrow derived) are responsible for synthesis of immunoglobulins and antibodies. It is probable that cell-mediated immunity plays an important role in recovery from infection, and perhaps also in protection as well, but the relative importance of the two systems, humoral and cellular immunity may differ from one infection to another. This may explain the different response to a number of virus infections in individuals having a defect in humoral immunity, in cellular immunity or in combined immune-deficiency states.

Antibody can be found in the three main classes of immunoglobulins, IgM, IgG and IgA. The initial response to infection, and to administration of a vaccine, is production of IgM antibody followed soon after by production of IgG antibody. On subsequent contact with the antigen, the titre of antibody rises quickly and to a higher level and is also largely IgG. This state of altered reactivity, called 'immunological memory' is a function of both T and B lymphocytes. IgG antibody to many bacterial and viral antigens remains detectable for many years both after infection and immunisation. This overall phenomenon resulting from reinfection or a booster inoculation is a direct effect of the initial antigenic stimulus.

Immunisation Strategy

Although the value of immunisation procedures is well recognised, the means by which they are introduced are sometimes overlooked or not understood. A first requirement is for a national administrative organisation which has responsibility for making recommendations as to the need for immunisation and to keep such recommendations under review. Although the ultimate responsibility in this country is vested in the Secretary of State, responsibility is delegated to the Chief Medical Officers for England, Scotland, Wales and Northern Ireland, who receive advice from a Joint Standing Committee on Vaccination and Immunisation. This body, comprised of experts in many disciplines concerned with preventive medicine, is responsible for making recommendations, via the Central Health Services Council, to the Secretaries of State on all and every aspect of immunisation procedures. The Committee may make recommendations on the advice of its own members, or with information received from international organisations such as the World Health Organisation. For example, the decision taken in 1971 to recommend that *routine* vaccination of children in this country against smallpox be discontinued was taken in that light. It may also receive advice or request advice, via the Department of Health and Social Security, from scientific bodies such as the Medical Research Council, the Public Health Laboratory Service and the National Institute for Biological Standards and Control. These bodies have, over the years, carried out clinical field trials on the effect of immunisation against whooping-cough, tuberculosis, poliomyelitis, measles and rubella which have greatly assisted the Joint Committee in making recommendations. Similarly, the Committee on Development of Vaccines and Immunisation Procedures of the Medical Research Council considers the need for the development of new products and with the cooperation of experts and research workers, makes what recommendations is considers advisable. Such has been the case with rubella vaccines and methods of prevention of cytomegalovirus and respiratory syncytial virus infections are currently being studied.

Safety is another vital factor where coordination of responsibility is of paramount importance. The DHSS is the licensing authority for all immunological products and it receives advice on the one hand from the National Institute for Biological Standards and Control and the Committee on the Development of Vaccines of the MRC, and also from the Committee on Safety of Medicines on the other. This latter Committee, as far as immunological products are concerned, has a dual statutory role. The Biological Subcommittee considers applications for clinical trials certificates or product licence certificates for all biological products including vaccines, antisera and immunoglobulins. The Subcommittee on Adverse Reactions is responsible for monitoring adverse reactions to any product so licensed through the reporting system on yellow cards.

Communicable disease may be controlled in a number of different ways and the method employed will, to a great extent, depend on the natural history of the individual diseases. For example, the strategy behind the control and eventual eradication of smallpox is to block the chain of transmission from one human being to another by large scale vaccination with potent smallpox vaccines. Other factors play a vital part, such as financial provision for the enterprise, training of vaccinators, the use of simple and effective methods of vaccination and, above all, a system of surveillance to monitor the effect of vaccination. In 1967 smallpox was endemic in 42 countries, now it is endemic in only two (WHO, 1975), but one important provision, namely political stability, may have been underestimated in defining the target date for eradication. War is frequently followed by disease and the continued strife in the Indian subcontinent is adding to the difficulties in eradication of smallpox. Nevertheless, the control of the disease over a wide area of the world is a remarkable achievement of modern preventive medicine.

The control of tuberculosis required a different approach. The eradication of bovine tuberculosis was a necessary first step followed later by the detection and treatment of individuals with active disease by chemotherapy. Vaccination with BCG has also played a contributory part, particularly in the prevention of tuberculosis meningitis in the developing countries, but the extent to which routine administration of BCG vaccine to 10 to 13 year old children now contributes to the control of tuberculosis is open to question. Here again, reappraisal of immunisation is necessary because it is more important to concentrate on protecting those at special risk such as hospital personnel and children of immigrants and deciding upon the appropriate treatment of contacts of known cases of tuberculosis.

The control of poliomyelitis requires yet another approach. Paralytic poliomyelitis has been virtually eliminated from this country by means of immunisation with oral poliovaccine, but despite widespread use of vaccine in the developing countries, poliomyelitis continues to occur (WHO, 1974). Thus there is a risk to susceptible unvaccinated individuals travelling to endemic areas, or from contracting the disease from an imported case. Whenever a case of poliomyelitis is reported and confirmed, immunisation of contacts in the neighbourhood is strongly recommended (Smith, 1973). Likewise the control of measles could probably be achieved if a sufficient number of children were immunised. If small outbreaks occurred then the same procedure could be used as for poliomyelitis—immunisation of all close contacts in the neighbourhood. The use of rubella vaccines requires yet another approach in that the objective is to protect the fetus from damage from maternal rubella and this is achieved indirectly by ensuring that women are immune before their first pregnancy.

The final aspect of general strategy is the need for surveillance. Those responsible for immunisation should constantly ask the question—is immunisation proving effective and what is the evidence that it is? If not, a reappraisal of policy is called for.

The details of immunisation strategy, recommendations for immunisation, vaccine surveillance, as well as methods of production and safety testing described in this chapter refer, in the main, to those practised in the United Kingdom. It should be stressed, however, that essentially similar schemes are in operation in many other countries where the need for clear-cut recommendations and quality control are recognised as an essential part of immunisation procedures.

ACTIVE IMMUNISATION

Active immunisation, either with a killed, inactivated vaccine or a live attenuated vaccine, can now be achieved against a wide range of infectious diseases. Table 7.1 includes a list of the most important of these shown in three columns; (a) those diseases where major advances in control have been made as a result of immunisation; (b) those where problems still exist; and (c) those where vaccine development is either under consideration or is in the experimental stage.

Three factors play an important part in determining the efficacy of active immunisation. First, the natural history and pathogenesis of the disease; secondly, the serological types of the causative agents, and thirdly, the nature of the immune response to the natural infection. The importance of these factors can be gauged by comparing the effects of immunisation against the infections shown in columns 1 and 2 of Table 7.1. Control of diphtheria and tetanus has been achieved, both by the effectiveness of diphtheria and tetanus toxoids in inducing antitoxin formation as a means of neutralising toxin in the blood-stream, as well as the fact that both organisms consist of a

Table 7.1   Current status of bacterial and viral vaccines (listing diseases under advances, problems and future developments)

Advances	*Problems*	*Future developments*
Diphtheria	Influenza	Meningococcal infections
Tetanus	Acute respiratory disease complex	*H. influenzae* infections
Pertussis	Respiratory syncytial virus	Cytomegalovirus infections
Tuberculosis		Hepatitis B
Smallpox		Hepatitis A
Yellow fever		
Poliomyelitis		
Measles		
Rubella		
Mumps[a]		

[a] Limited information as yet available on protection

single antigenic type. The situation with pertussis is somewhat different as several serotypes of *Bordetella pertussis* exist and the selection of the correct serotypes in pertussis vaccines is necessary in order to achieve protection. Yellow fever, poliomyelitis, measles, rubella and mumps are all examples of diseases in which the virus invades via the blood-stream with the result that circulating antibody induced by immunisation can exert a protective effect; and moreover, the viruses consist of a single, or in the case of polio-virus, of three closely related antigenic types. In addition, local gut immunity provides an added degree of protection. Cell-mediated immunity is probably an important factor in protection against smallpox and tuberculosis following immunisation and here again, antigenic homogeneity between strains of variola virus and between strains of *Mycobacterium tuberculosis* contributes to the effectiveness of vaccines against these diseases.

In striking contrast the diseases listed in column 2 are caused by viruses consisting, in most cases with the exception of respiratory syncytial virus (RSV), of multiple serological types. In the case of influenza vaccine effectiveness is made even more complicated by the periodic antigenic variation which occurs particularly amongst the influenza A strains. The natural history of these infections is also markedly different from those shown in column 1 as the portal of entry of the respiratory viruses is the mucosa of the upper respiratory tract. The viruses either produce disease at that site or spread along the mucosal surfaces of the respiratory tract without entering the bloodstream. Prevention by means of circulating antibody is, on theoretical grounds, less likely to be effective than in those infections where viraemic spread is the rule.

Table 7.2 Schedules of vaccination and immunisation procedures in the United Kingdom

Schedule I		Schedule II	
Age	Vaccine	Age	Vaccine
3 months	DPT 1[a] OPV 1[b]	6 months	DPT 1 OPV 1
	Interval 4–6 weeks		
4–5 months	DPT 2 OPV 2	7–8 months	DPT 2 OPV 2
	Interval 4–6 months		
9–12 months	DPT 3 OPV 3	12–14 months	DPT 3 OPV 3
Second year of life	Measles vaccine		
5 years of age or school entry	DT OPV 4	5 years of age or school entry	DT OPV 4
10–13 years of age	BCG	10–13 years of age	BCG
11–13 years of age for girls	Rubella	11–13 years of age for girls	Rubella
15–19 years of age or on school-leaving	OPV 5 tetanus vaccine	15–19 years of age or on school-leaving	OPV 5 tetanus vaccine

[a] DPT = diphtheria–pertussis–tetanus vaccine
[b] OPV = trivalent oral poliovaccine containing types I, II and III attenuated strains of poliovirus
From 'Immunisation Against Infectious Disease' prepared by the Standing Medical Advisory Committee for the CHSC, DHSS and Secretary of State for Social Services and for Wales. Crown Copyright. Reproduced with permission of The Controller, Her Majesty's Stationery Office

The diseases listed in the right hand column of Table 7.1 are some of those where a need for prevention exists, but where there are practical difficulties in the development of a suitable prophylactic.

Routine Immunisation Procedures

Immunisation forms an essential part of primary health care and it is important, therefore, that those who administer vaccines and the parents of those who receive them should recognise the benefits which may accrue from an effective immunisation programme. Schedules of immunisation play a useful part in reaching this objective. They cannot satisfy all needs and will, to a great extent, depend on the priorities in different countries, but they can produce useful guidelines.

Table 7.3 Recommended schedule for active immunisation of normal infants and children in the United States of America

Age	Vaccine	
2 months	DTP[a]	TOPV[b]
4 months	DTP	TOPV
6 months	DTP	TOPV
1 year	Measles[c]	Tuberculin test[d]
	Rubella[c]	Mumps[c]
1½ years	DTP	TOPV
4–6 years	DTP	TOPV
14–16 years	Td[e] and thereafter every 10 years	

[a] DPT—diphtheria and tetanus toxoids combined with pertussis vaccine

[b] TOPV—trivalent oral poliovirus vaccine. This recommendation is suitable for breast-fed as well as bottle-fed infants

[c] May be given at one year as measles–rubella or measles–mumps–rubella combined vaccines

[d] Frequency of repeated tuberculin tests depends on risk of exposure of the child and on the prevalence of tuberculosis in the population group. The initial test should be at the time of, or preceding, the measles immunisation

[e] Td—combined tetanus and diphtheria toxoids (adult type) for those more than six years of age in contrast to diphtheria and tetanus (DT) which contains a larger amount of diphtheria antigen. Tetanus toxoid at time of injury: for clean, minor wounds, no booster dose is needed by a fully immunised child unless more than 10 years have elapsed since the last dose. For contaminated wounds, a booster dose should be given if more than five years have elapsed since the last dose

Quoted by permission of the American Academy of Pediatrics from the Report of the Committee on Infectious Diseases (1974), *The Red Book*, 17th edn, American Academy of Pediatrics, Evanston, Illinois

The schedules shown in Tables 7.2 and 7.3 set out the recommended schedules in the United Kingdom and in the United States (DHSS, 1972; American Academy of Pediatrics, 1974; Memorandum on Immunological Procedures, MOD, 1971). The basic plan is to introduce a primary course of immunisation in the first year of life against those infections which can cause severe disease in infancy and childhood, and thereafter to follow this up by reinforcing booster inoculations changing the composition of the vaccines and introducing additional vaccines at the appropriate age. The current practice in the United Kingdom and many other European countries and in the United States is to carry out primary immunisation against diphtheria, tetanus, pertussis and poliomyelitis in the first year of life (International Symposium, 1973). Pertussis is the only infection of any consequence in the first year as 60 per cent of deaths in the United Kingdom occur under six months of age. Nevertheless, it is convenient to immunise against all four infections at the same stage in life. The other differences between the UK and US schedules are concerned with the age at which immunisation is started, the spacing of injections and the composition of vaccines for reinforcing inoculations. In the UK immunisation against pertussis is usually discontinued after the third dose of triple vaccine with immunisation against measles, rubella and BCG being introduced at the ages shown in Table 7.2.

In the developing countries the priorities are different and every effort should be made to introduce comprehensive immunisation at the earliest possible age against diseases which are of the greatest importance in terms of mortality and morbidity (King, 1966; Morley, 1973). BCG vaccine (without prior tuberculin testing) and smallpox vaccine should be given at birth and triple antigen and oral polio vaccine at one, two and three months. An alternative schedule is to give triple antigen and oral polio vaccine at one, two and nine months. One of the main difficulties is deciding on the age of administration of measles vaccine. As the disease is so severe between 9 and 12 months of age early immunisation is recommended, but as the 'take rate' is likely to be lower than when administered in the second year of life, consideration has to be given to further immunisations. Booster doses of triple or diphtheria–tetanus vaccine may be given on school entry and revaccination against smallpox in areas where the disease is still endemic.

Spacing of injections

The earlier schedules in use in this country recommended three primary injections of diphtheria–pertussis–tetanus vaccine at four-week intervals with the fourth and booster dose at 18 months. The revised schedules have been worked out on the principle that, if sufficient time is allowed to elapse between the first and second injection (six to eight weeks) and an even longer interval (four to six months) between the second and third, the fourth dose is no longer required. It will be noticed that in the US three primary injections and a fourth dose in the second year are still recommended. In the event of these schedules being interrupted there is no need to start the series of injections again because immunity will be achieved despite long intervals between doses. If a child has had no immunisations by the time of school entry the recommended schedule is diphtheria–tetanus vaccine, and polio-vaccine and measles vaccine at the appropriate intervals.

Age of immunisation

Immunisation can start either at three months or at six months of age. Although it is stated in the 'additional notes' to the DHSS pamphlet on Immunisation against Infectious Diseases (1972) that the desirable age for starting is six months of age, rather than three months, the evidence that the infant's antibody-forming mechanism is less mature in the early months of life was certainly true when vaccines of lower potency were employed, but with more potent and adsorbed vaccines, as are now used, this presents less of a problem. Also the evidence that severe reactions to pertussis vaccine are less common in children over six is slender (Butler, 1972). There is much to be said for early immunisation, particularly in the developing countries, and in any case the schedules shown in Table 7.2 provide for individual doctors and authorities to select the age at which to start immunisation.

Administration of vaccines

The basic course of immunisation in the UK against diphtheria, tetanus and pertussis should be carried out with triple vaccine, unless contraindicated, and with simultaneous administration of oral poliovaccine. Three doses each of an adsorbed triple vaccine (Dip.Tet.Per. vac PTAH BP; (PTAH stands for purified toxoids with aluminum hydroxide; in the new *Pharmacopoeia*, diphtheria and tetanus toxoids are now referred to as vaccines)) should be given at the recommended intervals by the intramuscular or deep subcutaneous route. The route of administration is important when adjuvant vaccines are employed. Three drops of trivalent oral poliovaccine (Pol. vac oral trivalent BP) should be given at the same time.

If triple vaccine is contraindicated three doses, each of 0.5 ml of diphtheria–tetanus vaccine (Dip.Tet. vac PTAH BP) should be given by the intramuscular or deep subcutaneous route.

Measles vaccine is recommended in the second year of life, but can be given to any child up to the age of 15 years who has not had natural measles. Measles vaccine (Meas. vac live BP) is presented as a freeze-dried product; a single dose of the reconstituted vaccine, i.e. 0.5 ml, should be given by the intramuscular or deep subcutaneous route. It is most important to take great care in reconstituting live measles vaccine according to the instructions prepared by the manufacturer and to store the vaccine at the recommended temperature in a refrigerator at 2 to 10°C. (This temperature applies to ambient temperature conditions in this country. Vaccine should be used within 1 h of reconstitution.) Measles vaccine currently used in this country produces fewer general reactions than the earlier products; nevertheless, between 10 and 20 per cent of immunised children may develop some mild illness, fever, coryza, cough, and occasionally a rash between the first and second week after receiving the vaccine. Although they are generally mild it is advisable to mention the fact that these may occur to parents. Measles vaccine is especially recommended for children in institutions, with chronic lung disease such as cystic fibrosis or other physical disability. The use of measles vaccine in children who have previously had a convulsion, or where a febrile reaction is best avoided is discussed under a later section on immunisation in special circumstances.

Reinforcing doses against diphtheria and tetanus are carried out with diphtheria–tetanus vaccine at school entry or with plain tetanus vaccine (Tet. vac FT BP) on school leaving. The dose and route of administration is the same as for the primary course.

Rubella vaccine (Rub. vac live BP) is recommended for schoolgirls aged 11 to 13 years and for adult women known to be susceptible as a result of a blood-test. The dose is 0.5 ml by the intramuscular or deep subcutaneous route.

BCG vaccine is presented as a freeze-dried product prepared from the bacillus of Calmette and Guerin, a bovine strain of the tubercle bacillus attenuated by growth in culture. The dose is 0.1 ml of the reconstituted vaccine (BCG vac intradermal BP) by the intradermal route and 0.05 ml for neonates. Except for the newborn BCG vaccine should not be given to anyone without prior tuberculin testing carried out by the Mantoux test with 10 tuberculin units PPD per 0.1 ml, or by the Heaf or Tine tests. Special care should also be taken to ensure that vaccine is administered intradermally. An interval of at least three weeks should be allowed to elapse before administration of another live vaccine after BCG.

Natural measles infection and live vaccines such as measles, rubella and mumps vaccine cause a temporary suppression of tuberculin sensitivity. In the US (see Table 7.2) more use is made of combined viral vaccines, measles and rubella (MR), or measles, mumps and rubella (MMR). As measles and rubella vaccines are recommended at different ages in this country, combined vaccines are not used to any great extent in the UK, but can be made available on request. Live attenuated mumps vaccine can also be made available on request.

Contraindication to vaccination

Any procedure, medical or surgical, which includes immunisation carries a potential risk but these can be greatly reduced if careful attention is paid to known contraindications. Details for each vaccine which are agreed between the manufacturer and licensing authority, are set out in the leaflet accompanying each product. They should be read carefully *before* a vaccine is administered. Some general examples of well-recognised contraindications are set out in Table 7.4. Basically it depends on whether an inactivated or live attenuated vaccines is to be used as their mode of action is different. In most cases the contraindications are a matter of common sense. It is clearly unwise to immunise a child with a fever or febrile intercurrent infection; postponement of immunisation is called for in such circumstances. Special care has to be taken in immunising infants with pertussis or triple vaccine. Vaccines contain-

7

ing pertussis antigen should not be given to children with a personal or family history of convulsions, cerebral irritation in the neonatal period, epilepsy or other disorders of the central nervous system. Children with acute illness, particularly those with respiratory symptoms should not be immunised until they have recovered. If a child shows any local or general reaction to pertussis or triple vaccine its use should be discontinued and further vaccination carried out with diphtheria–tetanus vaccine.

There is also a danger from 'over-immunising' with tetanus vaccine, particularly in patients receiving treatment for a wound whose immune status is not known (Peebles et al, 1969; Edsall et al, 1967). Influenza and measles vaccines should not be given to patients with a recognised allergy to egg protein. The contraindications to live vaccines are as set out in Table 7.4 and should be carefully observed, and in particular, enquiry should be made

Table 7.4   Contraindications to immunisation

Inactivated vaccines	Attenuated vaccines
Febrile illness	Febrile illness
Intercurrent infections	Intercurrent infections
Specific contraindication to pertussis and DPT	Eczema (e.g. smallpox, BCG)
'Over-immunisation' with tetanus toxoid	Immunedeficiency
Allergy to egg protein (e.g. influenza vaccine)	Corticosteroid and/or immunosuppressive therapy (e.g. drugs, radiotherapy)
	Malignant conditions such as leukaemia
	Pregnancy
	Allergy to egg protein (e.g. measles vaccine)
	BCG in tuberculin positive patients

as to whether a woman is pregnant, or likely to be before administering smallpox or rubella vaccines. Children under one year of age should not be given yellow fever vaccine. The vaccine is not required for international travel at this age.

Hazards of immunisation

Many untoward reactions to immunisation can be avoided by recognising the known contraindications and attention to detail. Nevertheless, over the years incidents have occurred, some of them extremely serious, following the administration of immunological products and in many cases they were preventable. The subject has been reviewed in detail by Wilson (1967) and a summary of the more important hazards extracted from his review are shown in Table 7.5. As he says 'Immunological products do a great deal more good than harm. The complications and accidents for which they are, from time to time, responsible must be looked upon as the price we pay for protection these agents confer. Our business is to provide a greater and more compre-

Table 7.5   Hazards of immunisation

Probable cause	Complication	Product concerned
1. *Normal toxicity/reactivity*	Local/general reaction	TAB, plague vaccine, early live measles vaccines
2. *Faulty production:*		
Residual toxicity	Diphtheria	Diphtheria–antitoxin mixture (TAM)
	Tetanus	Tetanus toxoid
Toxin present	Tetanus	Diphtheria antitoxin
Bacterial contamination	Septicaemia (staphylococcal, streptococcal)	TAB vaccine, TAM, measles antiserum
Viral contamination	Hepatitis	Yellow fever vaccine
Incomplete inactivation	Poliomyelitis	Poliovaccine
	Rabies	Rabies vaccine
Wrong culture	Tuberculosis	BCG vaccine (Lübeck disaster)
3. *Non-sterile apparatus*	Tuberculous abscess	Diphtheria TAF, TAM and toxoid
	Septicaemia	
Contamination from operator	Tuberculosis	Diphtheria APT, pertussis vaccine
4. *Allergic reactions*	Cyst formation	Adjuvant vaccines
	Serum sickness	Tetanus antitoxin (ATS)
	Neuritis and encephalomyelitis	Rabies vaccine, pertussis and triple vaccine
	Arthus phenomenon	'Over-immunisation' with tetanus toxoid
	Anaphylaxis	Use of antisera containing foreign protein
5. *Abnormal sensitivity of patient*	Generalised vaccinia with eczema	Smallpox vaccine
	Immune deficiency	Smallpox vaccine
6. *Indirect effect:*		
Provoking effect	Provocation poliomyelitis	APT and diphtheria–tetanus vaccines with adjuvant
Fetal damage	Generalised fetal vaccinia Fetal death	Smallpox vaccine
	Fetal infection, damage death	Rubella vaccine

hensive insurance and to diminish the size of the premium.' The probable causes of the hazards shown in Table 7.5 are listed under six main headings. TAB and cholera vaccines or TAB/cholera vaccines are more reactogenic than most vaccines such as diphtheria and tetanus because they contain a suspension of the whole bacterial cell. Reactions can be considerably reduced, however, by the intradermal route of inoculation. The hazards listed under subheadings 2 and 3 in Table 7.5 were due to contamination, incomplete inactivation, the use of the wrong culture, or to the use of non-sterile apparatus. Such hazards by modern standards can be ascribed to negligence, carelessness or lack of knowledge of immunological procedures.

The allergic reactions (subheading 4) tend to occur with certain immunological products, but frequently there is a known contraindication to their use and their incidence can be reduced. Those shown under subheadings 5 and 6 are a result of an abnormal reaction on the part of the patient. The frequency of this occurrence can also be reduced by recognition of the risk.

Immunisation in special circumstances

Immunisation, particularly of children, should as far as possible be carried out as an elective procedure and not as an emergency operation. Nevertheless, there are circumstances in which children going overseas with their parents may require some immunisations which are not normally recommended. This still applies to children with eczema going to areas where smallpox is still endemic. Although smallpox vaccine is considered inadvisable for children with eczema, the presence of eczema is not an absolute contraindication. The decision as whether to vaccinate or not must depend on the circumstances of each individual case. It should be remembered that eczematous children are probably at greater risk from accidental vaccinia from a recently vaccinated member of the household than from deliberate vaccination. The following policy can be adopted for children with eczema going to endemic areas. If the eczema is extensive then a certificate of contraindication should be issued to the immigration authority of the country to which the child is going. The Ministry of Health Memorandum on Vaccination against Smallpox (Memo 312/MED Revised 1962) states:

It should be noted that vaccination is not obligatory if a medical contraindication exists. The following is a quotation from the *Official Records of the World Health Organisation*, **54,** 56. 'If a vaccinator is of the opinion that vaccination is contraindicated on medical grounds, he should provide the person with written reasons underlying that opinion, which the health authority of arrival may take into account. Decision on a claim for exemption from the requirement to be in possession of a certificate lies solely with the health authority of arrival'.

The vaccinator should supply such a certificate written in English or in French stating his qualifications and appointment. Most health authorities will accept such a certificate, but there is always the risk that despite this, vaccination will be carried out at the port of entry. As an additional safeguard it is advisable to check with the Office of the High Commission in the UK of the country concerned, that a certificate of contraindication will be accepted because the actual technique of vaccination of eczematous children is important, and it is desirable to avoid the risk of indiscriminate vaccination.

If the eczema is not extensive and is controlled by the use of topical steroid therapy, it is advisable to stop the steroid treatment for seven days; if there is no exacerbation of the eczema then vaccination can be carried out, selecting a suitable site of unaffected skin and giving simultaneous administration of vaccinial immunoglobulin into the opposite arm (see Table 7.6 for details). The parents should be given careful instructions, if necessary in writing, to keep the vaccination site covered with a sterile 'air-strip' dressing, replacing this every three days until the vaccination site has healed. The parents should be advised when removing the 'air-strip' cover not to contaminate the skin with any vesicle fluid which may be present. An alternative procedure which the author has found useful is to undertake primary vaccination with the Rivers attenuated CV1-78 strain of smallpox vaccine (Kempe et al, 1968), and then revaccinate six months to a year later with standard lymph. Although this procedure has worked well in the author's hands it has not been the experience of other workers in this country, notably Ducksbury et al (1972).

Measles vaccine for patients with convulsions and chronic chest and heart conditions

A single convulsion in a child should not necessarily be considered a contraindication to measles vaccine as the risk of severe convulsions is greater following the natural disease. Provided sufficient time has elapsed since the original episode measles vaccine can be administered, but it is recommended that simultaneous administration of human normal immunoglobulin (for use with measles vaccine) into the contralateral arm, details of which are also shown in Table 7.6. A similar procedure can be used for children with a chronic debilitating condition in whom a febrile reaction would be undesirable.

Measles vaccine can be extremely effective in preventing the spread of measles in susceptible children in an outbreak, for example, in a family or in a hospital ward. The incubation period of vaccine measles is several days shorter than in natural measles, so that if vaccine is given within three days of contact (provided that there is no contraindication), spread of infection can usually be controlled.

PASSIVE IMMUNISATION

Although active immunisation is recommended wherever possible because of the more durable effect compared with passive immunisation, this may not always be practicable. For example, a vaccine may not have been developed because the causative agents have either not yet been isolated, or in a form suitable for use in human beings. Such a situation at present applies to hepatitis A and B viruses. Another reason is that the immune status of the individual coming into contact with a case of potentially severe infection may not be known, or the administration of a live vaccine may be contraindicated.

Passive immunisation procedures are in the main used prophylactically, but in certain circumstances can be recommended for treatment, as for example, in the cases of generalised and progressive vaccinia. Originally, passive immunisation was achieved by administration of antisera prepared in animals (diphtheria and tetanus antisera), or by means of convalescent human plasma, but because of the risks of allergic reactions from foreign protein, or from hepatitis from icterogenic human plasma, there has been a progressive move towards the use of human immunoglobulin, derived either from pooled normal plasma or from hyperimmune individuals. Details as to the use of human immunoglobulin (IG) (immune serum globulin is the term used in the US) in prophylaxis can be found in an article on this subject by Pollock (1969). Since this was published further developments have taken place, details of which are summarised in Table 7.6 and the accompanying notes.

Table 7.6   Passive immunisation against certain infectious diseases

Disease	Reason for passive rather than active immunisation	Recommended preparation and dosage
Measles	(a) For prevention: live vaccine contraindicated	(a) Normal IG[a] 0.20 ml/kg; 0–1 years 250 mg; 1–2 years 500 mg; >3 years 750 mg
	(b) With live vaccine to modify reaction	(b) Human normal IG for use with measles vaccine 0.6 mg/kg standard dose in 0.5 ml
Rubella	Contact with rubella in pregnancy (adults only)	Normal IG 2×1500 mg[b]
Vaccinia	(a) With smallpox vaccine for patients with eczema	(a) Hyperimmune VIG 0.3 ml/kg; 0–1 years 500 mg; 1–6 years 1000 mg; 7–14 years 1500 mg
	(b) Treatment of generalised or accidental vaccinia	(b) As above
Varicella zoster	For patients with leukaemia and those on immunosuppressive therapy	Hyperimmune ZIG[c] (0.17–0.66 ml/kg) 0–1 years 500 mg; 1–6 years 1000 mg
Hepatitis A	For contacts in outbreaks	Normal IG 250 mg; 0.02–0.04 ml/kg
Hepatitis B	Prevention of congenital infection	Hyperimmune hepatitis, type B IG 500 mg in 5 ml
Mumps	Rarely needed except for children on immunosuppressive therapy	Hyperimmune IG, dose as for varicella
Tetanus	Treatment of wounds; immune status not known	Hyperimmune human tetanus IG 250 iu in 1.0 ml with adsorbed Tet. Vac.[d]

[a] IG = Immunoglobulin ≡ ISG (US) immune serum globulin
[b] Dosage recommended by author (Dudgeon, 1974)
[c] ZIG = Zoster immune globulin
[d] IG and vaccine must be given in separate syringes and at separate sites
As the concentration of immunoglobulins may differ from one preparation to another depending on whether it is normal IG or a hyperimmune product, the dosages have been expressed in milligrams according to age, or millilitres per kilogram body weight

Measles

IG is extremely effective in preventing measles in susceptible contacts, but may have to be given repeatedly to children where there is a recognised contraindication to live measles vaccine. The use of smaller doses of IG as a method of attenuating a natural attack of measles is no longer advocated as live vaccine is more effective.

Rubella

Studies carried out by the Public Health Laboratory Service (1970) showed that IG was ineffective in preventing rubella in pregnant women after contact at home. Although it is correct to say that *routine* administration of IG to pregnant women contacts is contraindicated, there are circumstances when its use is justified, particularly where a pregnant woman wishes the pregnancy to go to term. In such circumstances it is important to know the immune status of the woman at the time of contact, or as soon as possible thereafter. Immunoglobulin should be administered in a sufficient dosage to achieve protection and laboratory tests for rubella antibody employed in order to determine whether seroconversion has or has not occurred in a patient initially found to be suceptible (Dudgeon, 1974).

Hepatitis type A

Normal IG is highly effective in preventing hepatitis A amongst contacts and in conferring protection for travellers (Krugman, 1963; Pollock, 1969).

Hepatitis type B

The effectiveness of the hyperimmune hepatitis B preparation in preventing congenital or perinatally acquired infection is currently under investigation. Its use, therefore, should be restricted to cases which qualify for inclusion in clinical trials currently being undertaken.

Zoster-immune globulin

Studies by Brunell et al (1969, 1972) have shown that hyperimmune zoster-immune globulin (ZIG) has a greater protective effect than normal IG. There are two situations in which the use of this preparation should be considered. First, to protect a neonate from perinatal infection and secondly, to protect children with leukaemia and other malignant disorders whilst on treatment. In the former, the main at-risk group are infants whose mothers develop varicella within four days of delivery and infants who developed the rash between the first five to ten days of life (Myers, 1974). This preparation is scarce and its use should be restricted to those groups at special risk.

Vaccine Production and Safety Testing

This important subject already referred to has been well reviewed by Perkins (1969, 1972 1973). As he says, three questions have to be asked before an immunological product can be considered for use in human beings. First, where was the vaccine made and by whom; secondly, what were the results of tests for hazardous extraneous agents, and thirdly, how effective will the prophylactic agent be in man?

Vaccine production in this country is carefully controlled at present by regulations laid down by the Licensing Authority under the Therapeutic

Substances Act. This control has been further extended by the Medicines Act of 1968 which requires that a comprehensive and detailed description of the method of production be submitted to the Licensing Authority and to seek advice when necessary from the Committee on Safety of Medicines. This advice includes consideration of very stringent testing of immunological products and if these tests are approved they are written into the licence. The regulations made under the Therapeutic Substances Act will be repealed shortly and their place will be taken by a Compendium which is being drawn up by the Licensing Authority with the advice of both industry and the Committee on Safety of Medicines, but will be more flexible as changes can be made more easily as compared with the old system.

Amongst the important general considerations are the design and inspection of the premises where vaccine is produced. Each product must be produced in a separate area physically separated from each other, or in the case of tetanus vaccine in an entirely separate area. Buildings can under certain circumstances, be used for sequential production provided that effective sterilisation and redecoration is carried out between the production of each vaccine (Perkins, 1969). Probably the most important aspect of vaccine production is consistency in production methods. More reliance can be placed upon a manufacturer who consistently produces a safe, potent vaccine which passes all the necessary requirements than on one where batches of vaccine periodically fail to pass the necessary tests.

The vaccine seed

Any vaccine, bacterial or viral, should be produced from a pure culture of the organism. It follows, therefore, that the seed, bacterium or virus, used to produce the vaccine must also be a pure culture. Reference has already been made to errors which have been made in the past where the seed strain has been found to be contaminated with some other organism (Wilson, 1967). Today, as much attention is paid to the development, production and safety testing of the seed pool as to the production of the final product. This is generally easier to achieve with bacterial vaccines than with viral vaccines where production of the seed virus system has to be rigidly applied so that each batch of vaccine originates from the approved seed.

Vaccine substrate

The production of bacterial vaccines on well-defined laboratory growth media is again comparatively simple compared with virus vaccines which require a living cell substrate. This is the fundamental point upon which the whole problem of safety depends. Tissues derived from animals may contain adventitious agents as, for example, the numerous simian viruses which have been detected in monkey kidney cell cultures used for the preparation of poliomyelitis vaccines. It is a general practice to test at least 25 per cent of tissues used for vaccine production to ensure, by appropriate tests, that they do not contain adventitious agents, bacteria or viruses (Perkins, 1973). In recent years there has been a move towards using human diploid cells for vaccine production maintained in a cell bank at low temperatures whose diploid karyotype and other characteristics are retained (Perkins, 1972). The widening of the powers of the TSA has allowed the manufacture of rubella and poliomyelitis vaccines to be made in human diploid cells.

Safety and potency testing

The safety of the product is tested at intervals during production and on the final product before and after it has been filled into the vials or ampoules. Clearly, the method of safety testing will depend on whether an inactivated or attenuated vaccine is being produced and, again, safety testing of viral vaccines is infinitely more complicated than with bacterial vaccines. The potency of the product is now usually related to the immunising capacity compared with a national or international reference standard product.

Efficacy of the product

The final question with which both manufacturers and the licensing authority are concerned as well as the health authorities who use the products, whether they be vaccines or immunoglobulin preparations, is do they work? Clinical trials on small groups of volunteers are an essential first step before a product licence is issued. Thereafter a system of surveillance is introduced which monitors the effectiveness of the product. The various bodies already referred to under 'Immunisation Strategy' have played an invaluable part in evaluating the effectiveness of pertussis, measles, poliomyelitis and BCG vaccines and more recently the National Rubella Surveillance Scheme was set up to study the effect of rubella immunisation on the incidence of congenital rubella defects (Dudgeon et al, 1973). Apart from studying the incidence of disease in the population after immunisation has been introduced, it is also important to sample a proportion of those immunised over a period of time for their immune status. In this way one can obtain additional information as to whether vaccine-induced immunity is being maintained. This can be of value in ascertaining the long-term effectiveness of poliomyelitis, measles and rubella vaccines.

THE PRESENT STATUS OF IMMUNISATION

Benefits and Problems

The penultimate problem concerned with immunisation is whether the vaccines employed afford protection and how their effectiveness can be assessed. This is where surveillance becomes so important. In the final analysis the efficacy of any vaccine can only be made by comparing the cost and risks of using it with the costs and risk of not doing so. The general trend of the effect of immunisation can be obtained by a comparison of statistical returns showing annual notifications and deaths for each disease for which immunisation is being used. It is also important to try to evaluate the economic consequences of immunisation in purely financial terms. The method of cost–benefit analysis takes into account the direct cost of implementing an immunisation programme compared with the direct and indirect benefits achieved by its use (Steinfeld, 1971). Dramatic changes have taken place in this country in the incidence of many of the severe forms of communicable disease since the early 1940s when immunisation against tetanus and diphtheria was first introduced. Although there was little change in morbidity before immunisation during this period, the mortality of many common infections such as scarlet fever, pertussis and measles was declining before any form of immunisation was introduced, due in all probability to the effects of improved hygiene, nutrition, chemotherapy and other environmental factors.

The data in Table 7.7 shows the notifications and deaths for the four principal communicable diseases, diphtheria, pertussis, poliomyelitis and measles from 1940 to 1974; the figures for 1974 being provisional. The deaths from tetanus are also included. From these figures can be calculated the fatality ratio (deaths per 100 notifications). The steady decline in the fatality ratio for pertussis and measles both before and after immunisation was introduced, did not occur either with diphtheria or poliomyelitis until immunisation was started. Despite the precipitous fall in notifications and deaths from diphtheria during the 1950s when notifications were still falling, the number of deaths, although small in number, were of no small significance in proportion to the number of cases notified. The fatality ratio was 4.5 in 1950 and 10.2 in 1960. This should be taken as a warning that if diphtheria reappeared as a result of a fall-off in immunisation the chances are that it would do so in a virulent form.

Another important aspect of immunisation is to study the acceptance rates of those eligible for vaccination. Figures of acceptance rates for the country as a whole in 1973 for diphtheria, pertussis, tetanus, poliomyelitis and measles vaccines were 81, 81, 81, 80 and 52 per cent respectively (DHSS, 1975). It remains to be seen whether the current concern over pertussis immunisation will be reflected in the 1974 figures for the use of triple vaccine, but otherwise the acceptance rates apart from measles vaccine are reasonably satisfactory, although there are almost certainly regional differences in acceptance rates. As far as rubella vaccines are concerned the numbers of girls aged 11 to 14 years being immunised is below 80 per cent, but of greater significance is the apparent delay in implementing the recommendation of immunising adult women known to be susceptible as a result of a serological test (CMO, 1974). Although rubella vaccination policy in the UK and US is different, as is the method of surveillance of congenital rubella defects, provisional figures from the US (Cooper, 1975) shows a marked decline compared with this country (Dudgeon, 1975). However it must be emphasised that continued surveillance

Table 7.7   Notifications and deaths from five infectious diseases 1940–1974

Year	Tetanus[c]	Diphtheria		Pertussis		Poliomyelitis			Measles	
						Non-para	Paralytic			
		N[a]	D[b]	N	D	N	N	D	N	D
1940		46281	2480	53607	678				409521	857
1941		50797	2641	173330	2383				409715	1145
1942		41404	1827	66016	799				286341	458
1943		34662	1317	96136	1114				376104	773
1944		23199	934	94044	1054				158479	243
1945		18596	722	62691	689		858	139	446796	729
1946		11986	472	92936	808		680	128	160402	204
1947		5609	244	92662	905		7776	707	393787	644
1948		3575	156	146383	748		1855	241	399606	327
1949		1881	84	102809	527		5982	657	385871	307
1950	71	962	49	157781	394	2195	5565	755	367724	221
1951	81	664	33	169441	437	1085	1529	219	616192	317
1952	63	376	32	114869	184	1163	2747	295	389502	141
1953	61	266	23	157842	243	1571	2076	338	545050	245
1954	61	173	8	105912	139	641	1319	134	146995	50
1955	48	155	12	79133	88	2619	3712	270	693803	176
1956	52	53	3	92410	95	1483	1717	137	160556	30
1957	46	37	4	85017	87	1667	3177	255	633678	94
1958	41	80	8	33400	27	575	1419	154	259308	49
1959	38	102	0	33252	25	289	739	87	539524	98
1960	32	49	5	58030	37	131	257	46	159364	31
1961	41	51	8	24469	27	169	707	79	763465	152
1962	29	16	2	8347	24	59	212	45	184895	39
1963	21	33	2	34736	36	12	39	3	601255	127
1964	28	20	0	31594	44	8	29	4	306801	73
1965	33	25	0	12945	21	36	55	3	502209	115
1966	27	20	5	19427	23	4	19	1	343642	80
1967	25	6	0	33531	17	3	16	0	440103	94
1968	22	15	1	17367	15	5	19	0	225789	47
1969	17	9	0	4866	5	1	9	0	131305	33
1970	21	22	3	16244	15	0	6	0	289893	40
1971	10	17	1	15933	23	1	5	1	126068	24
1972	13	4	0	1988	2	2	3	0	136147	29
1973	7	2	0	2437	2	1	4	0	152484	33
1974[d]	9	3	0	16225	13	0	5	0	109567	20

[a] Number of notified cases
[b] Number of deaths
[c] Deaths due to tetanus or fatal injuries complicated by tetanus
[d] 1974 figures are uncorrected

Dates when national immunisation campaigns were started:
Tetanus	1939	(the Armed Forces)
Diphtheria	1942	
Triple vaccine	1954	Programme started; fully implemented 1957
Poliomyelitis	1956	Salk-type inactivated poliovaccine (IPV)
	1961	Sabin-type oral poliovaccine (OPV)
Measles vaccine	1968	

The above figures apply in the main to England and Wales. Data extracted from the Annual Reports of the Chief Medical Officer, The Department of Health and Social Security is needed to determine efficacy of the rubella vaccines as not all defects are recognisable at birth, and a low reported incidence in the past year or so may underestimate the actual number of cases occurring.

It is important to achieve as high an acceptance rate as possible, approaching 90 per cent, in order to control pertussis, measles, rubella and poliomyelitis, whereas control of diphtheria can probably be achieved provided that at least two-thirds of the population are immunised. No immunisation campaign can be expected to succeed unless it is fully implemented and the current acceptance rates of measles and rubella vaccines fall far short of the objective. The same could apply to pertussis unless the present uncertainty about the use of triple vaccine in this country can be resolved. Doubts have been expressed as to the efficacy and safety of pertussis vaccines in use in this country which could have an adverse effect, not only on immunisation against pertussis, but against diphtheria and tetanus as well. Pertussis vaccines have been in use in the UK for the past 20 years and, except for a short period in the 1950s when some vaccines of marginal potency were used (MRC, 1959), because of a difference between the British and International standard vaccine, their use has been associated with a progressive fall in the annual notifications (Miller, Pollock and Clewes, 1974; Edsall, 1975). The principal cause of anxiety is related to the safety of triple vaccine containing the pertussis component which has been highlighted by reports by Dick (1974) and Kulenkamphh, Schwartzmann and Wilson (1974) on the incidence of neurological complications. Although it has been known for many years that symptoms which include sudden collapse, 'screaming attacks', convulsions and rarely encephalopathy may follow the use of pertussis and triple vaccine (Byers and Moll, 1948; Ström, 1967), the incidence of such complications is extremely difficult to assess and, moreover, the incidence varies from one country to another (Edsall, 1975). It has also been assumed, probably quite incorrectly, that the symptoms referred to under the general heading of 'cerebral' symptoms represent a spectrum of the same pathological process, whereas there may well be, as Cohen et al (1973) have suggested, a pharmacological reaction responsible for the cases of screaming or shock which could be totally different from the mechanisms responsible for encephalopathy. Recent studies from the Netherlands (Cohen and Hannik, 1973) have also revealed that four children with neurological symptoms following immunisation with combined DPT and inactivated poliovaccine were suffering from a primary infection with a neurotropic virus which could have caused the neurological symptoms. The essence of the problem is that the frequency of serious reactions to pertussis is not known, and it is important to obtain facts so as to establish how many children develop illnesses after vaccination *in excess of those which would otherwise have occurred*. Until this information is available the use of triple vaccine is recommended as a routine procedure for infants unless otherwise contraindicated, especially for children of large families in order to reduce the risk of cross-infection to young babies in such households.

The control of poliomyelitis is a major success story due to the effectiveness of modern poliovaccines. This is well illustrated in Figure 7.1 showing an intensive care unit for bulbar poliomyelitis cases during an epidemic in the US in 1949. A small outbreak in 1973 in the North of England from which wild strains of poliovirus were isolated, was well contained by efficient surveillance and vaccination of contacts (BMJ, 1974). Again this episode emphasises the need for maintaining a high vaccination rate throughout the country. A very slight risk still exists of developing paralysis from the vaccine or from contact with a recently vaccinated person, but the rate of 'recipient-associated' cases is of the order of 1.1 to 0.3 cases per million vaccine doses distributed

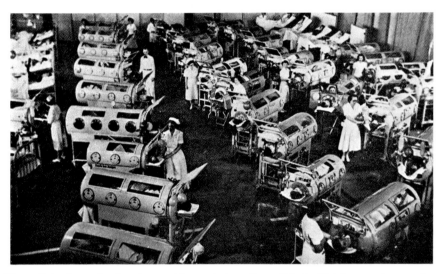

Figure 7.1 A ward of patients with paralytic poliomyelitis in Drinker respirators, Los Angeles, 1949, one of the first examples of an intensive care unit

during the period 1962 to 1972, and for 'contact-associated' cases, between 0.6 and 0.5 for the same period (Smith, 1975).

As stated earlier, the current policy in respect of BCG vaccination in this country is in need of reappraisal. Recent estimates indicate that vaccination could be responsible for the prevention of only one case per thousand vaccinated (Office of Health Economics, 1974), and this figure may fall to an even lower level. A comparison of the costs and the benefits would suggest that the finance used for vaccination could be diverted to other purposes. Sencer and Axnick (1973) have estimated that the costs associated with smallpox vaccination in the US in 1968 together with the costs of medical care for the complications of vaccination was $135 million. No cases of smallpox were reported in the US in that year. Major benefits have also accrued from the mass measles vaccination campaign in the US with savings estimated of up to $1.3 billion, over a 10-year period. The total direct and indirect costs for the treatment of thousands of multiple handicapped children as a result of the rubella pandemic in 1964 to 1965 in the US has been estimated at £1.4 billion, and this could well be a gross under-estimate. Rubella immunisation should prevent a repetition of such a disaster.

Future Prospects

The future prospects for the development of immunological products can be considered under two headings, both of which have already been referred to and listed in Table 7.1. First, there is the need for improvement in existing products and secondly the development of new vaccines against infections for which some form of prophylaxis is, or may be, required. Both aspects have been fully discussed at two international meetings on immunisation against infectious diseases (International Conference on Application of Vaccines, Washington, DC, 1971; International Symposium on Vaccination, Monaco, 1973). There clearly is a need to look more closely at methods of production of pertussis vaccines not only in respect of the protective antigen but to identify various factors which may be associated with toxicity such as the heat-labile endotoxin and histamine-sensitising factor (HSF) (Lehrer, Tau and Vaughan, 1974). Important advances have been made in the production of combined viral vaccines which can be administered in a single dose such as measles–rubella, measles–smallpox, measles–mumps–rubella vaccines (Hilleman et al, 1973a). The antibody response of the combined bivalent or trivalent products appears to be as satisfactory as with the monovalent vaccines. Advances have also been made in the development of improved adjuvants to increase the immunising capacity of killed vaccines. The development of a readily metabolisable peanut oil adjuvant with an emulsifier and stabiliser would seem to offer distinct advantages over mineral oil adjuvants (Hilleman et al, 1973b). Although immunisation against influenza is not required as a routine procedure for children, recent advances in vaccine production as a result of a major breakthrough in technology may have important applications with other vaccines. The purity of influenza vaccines has been improved by the use of zonal centrifugation and solvents to 'split' the virus, thus eliminating toxic properties. Another development of great potential is the use of the technique of recombination whereby new strains are produced in the laboratory by hybridisation of strains (Kilbourne, 1971). Genetic recombinant strains have been developed which have the high growth rate potential of an established laboratory strain and the antigenic properties of a recently isolated epidemic strain. Recombinant influenza A strains have also been developed by Beare and Hall (1971) for use as live attenuated influenza vaccines. Recombination appears to be a rapid and effective way of attentuation. However, as far as respiratory virus infections of children are concerned, a far more important problem is the amount of illness caused by the respiratory syncytial virus (RSV). Respiratory syncytial virus infection can cause a wide spectrum of respiratory illness from mild upper respiratory tract infection to severe bronchiolitis and pneumonia. It is undoubtedly a pathogen of the greatest importance in infancy with a mortality of about 4 per cent from bronchiolitis and pneumonia. Of greater importance, however, is the morbidity from this infection. Detailed studies by Gardner and his colleagues from Newcastle (Gardner et al, 1967; Gardner, 1975) have produced figures which, if applied to the whole country could mean that as many as 25 000 cases of RSV infection could be admitted to hospital in any one year. Initial attempts by Chanock et al (1971) to protect infants with an inactivated RSV vaccine led to the unexpected response of producing more severe disease in the vaccinated infants than in unvaccinated infants of the same age. This finding and other observations suggest that the pathogenesis of RSV infection is not due to a simple invasion of the respiratory tract but may well be caused by some immunopathological process. Until more is known about this the prospects for prevention by immunisation are not bright, although it may be possible to develop an attenuated RSV vaccine which, if given by the intra-nasal route, may stimulate local IgA and thus protect. Even if such a vaccine could be developed the question has to be asked, to whom it should be administered?

Rabies is not a problem in this country at present, but could be so before long, so that the question of postexposure treatment for children as well as adults has to be seriously considered. The duck-embryo vaccine at present in use although safe, is of questionable potency. The recent development of an inactivated vaccine in human diploid cells (Wiktor, 1971) has given encouraging results in experimental animals and may well prove to be a product of great value for treatment of human beings in the future.

Cytomegalovirus is the most common congenital virus and is a significant cause of mental retardation in children. Hanshaw et al (1973) has estimated that between 400 and 800 cases of children with mental retardation due to congenital CMV infection may be born in this country every year. Although many such cases are probably due to primary infection it is difficult to assess the role of reactivation infection which is known to occur in CMV infection. Here again a fundamental look at the epidemiology and natural history of CMV infection is required, but the obstacles to prevention by means of a vaccine are great indeed (Dudgeon, 1973).

The increasing prevalence of antibiotic resistant strains of *Neisseria meningitidis* and *Haemophilus influenzae* have led to studies for the development of protective vaccines. Progress has been made with polysaccharide vaccines against type C and A meningococcal infections (Artenstein, 1971; Artenstein et al, 1974; Goldschneider et al, 1973), but at present their use is restricted to epidemic situations. Similarly a vaccine has been prepared from the capsular antigen of the *Haemophilus influenzae* type B strains which also appear to be immunogenic (Smith et al, 1971).

Finally, some form of prevention of viral hepatitis is called for as both forms, infectious hepatitis type A and hepatitis type B, are infections of the greatest concern to health authorities at the present time. Krugman and Giles (1973) have recently reported that the serum from a known infective human serum from a case of hepatitis type B was immunogenic and conferred protection after inactivation by heat at 98°C. At a recent conference in Washington, two groups of investigators (Purcell et al, 1975; Hilleman et al, 1975) reported the development of an inactivated hepatitis B vaccine prepared from the non-infective surface antigen particle obtained from pooled human plasma. Preliminary tests for potency, safety and protection appear encouraging.

It is an intriguing thought that after so many years of progress in vaccine development, methods have turned full circle and once again human material is being considered as the source of a vaccine. Little progress can be reported with a vaccine against hepatitis A, which is a more important infection as far as children are concerned, but there is now fairly conclusive evidence that a third type of viral hepatitis exists which is unrelated to types A or B (Symposium on Viral Hepatitis, 1975).

In conclusion it would seem that the achievements of the past 50 years and the prospects for the future justify the validity of the opening sentence of this chapter.

REFERENCES

American Academy of Pediatrics (1974) *Report of the Committee on Infectious Diseases*, 17th edn. Evanston, Illinois, USA.

Artenstein, M. S. (1971) Polysaccharide vaccines against meningococcal infections. In *International Conference on the Application of Vaccines Against Viral, Rickettsial and Bacterial Diseases of Man*, pp. 350–352. Pan-American Health Organisation, Washington, DC: Scientific Publications no. 226.

Artenstein, M. S., Winter, P. C., Gold, R. & Smith, C. D. (1974) Immunoprophylaxis of meningococcal infection. *Military Medicine*, **139**, 91–95.

Ballard, E. (1868) On vaccination: its values and alleged dangers. A prize essay awarded by the Ladies Sanitary Bureau. London: Longmans and Green.

Beare, A. S. & Hall, T. H. (1971) Recombinant influenza A viruses as live vaccines for man. *Lancet*, **2**, 1271–1272.

Bowers, D. M. (1973) Smallpox: a historical survey. *Update*, **6**, 833–838.

British Medical Journal (1974) Poliomyelitis in England and Wales. *British Medical Journal*, **3**, 585.

Brunell, P. A., Ross, A., Miller, L. H. & Kuo, Betty (1969) Prevention of varicella by zoster immune globulin. *New England Journal of Medicine*, **280**, 1191–1194.

Brunell, P. A., Gershon, Anne A., Hughes, W. T., Riley, H. R. & Smith, J. D. (1972) Prevention of varicella in high risk children: a collaborative study. *Pediatrics*, **50**, 718–722.

Butler, N. R. (1972) Diphtheria, pertussis and tetanus vaccines. In *The Therapeutic Choice in Paediatrics*, Part IV, Immunisation. London: Churchill Livingstone.

Byers, R. K. & Moll, F. C. (1948) Encephalopathies following prophylactic pertussis vaccine. *Pediatrics*, **1**, 437–457.

Chanock, R. M., Kapikian, A. Z., Perkins, J. C. & Parrott, R. H. (1971) Vaccines in non-bacterial diseases other than influenza. In *International Conference on the Application of Vaccines Against Viral, Rickettsial and Bacterial Diseases of Man*, pp. 101–116. Pan-American Health Organisation, Washington, DC: Scientific Publications no. 226.

Chief Medical Officer (1974) Letter on vaccination procedures against rubella. (Circular letter to the Medical Profession).

Cohen, H. & Hannik, Charlotte, A. (1973) Pertussis immunisation. *Gelben Hefte*, **13**, 97.

Cohen, H., Hofman, B., Brouwer, R., van Wezel, A. L. & Hannik, Charlotte A. (1973) Combined inactivated vaccines. In *International Symposium on Vaccination against Communicable Diseases*, pp. 133–141. Symposium Series no. 22. Basel, London and New York: Karger.

Cooper, L. Z. (1975) Congenital rubella in the United States. In *Symposium on Infections of the Fetus and Newborn Infant*. March of Dimes, New York City (to be published).

Copeman, S. M. (1899) Vaccination: its natural history and pathology. Milroy Lectures for 1898. London: Macmillan.

Department of Health and Social Security (1972) *Immunisation Against Infectious Disease*, prepared by Health Departments of Great Britain and Central Office of Information. London: HMSO.

Department of Health and Social Security (1975) Personal communication.

Dick, G. (1974) Reactions to routine immunisation in childhood. *Proceedings of the Royal Society of Medicine*, **67**, 371–372.

Ducksbury, Christina, F. J., Elliott, A., Hutchinson, R., Lee, J. A., McCallum, D. I., McDonald, J. R., Parry, W. H., Periera, Marguerite S. & Pollock, T. M. (1972) Smallpox vaccination of normal and eczematous children with the attenuated CV1-78 strain of vaccinia virus. *Community Medicine*, **127**, 155–157.

Dudgeon, J. A. (1963) Development of smallpox vaccine in England in the 18th and 19th centuries. *British Medical Journal*, **1**, 1367–1372.

Dudgeon, J. A. (1973) Future developments in prophylaxis. In *Intrauterine Infections*, Ciba Foundation Symposium Series 10, ed. Katherine Elliott and Julie Knight, pp. 179–198. Amsterdam: North Holland, Elsevier, Excerpta Medica.

Dudgeon, J. A., Peckham, Catherine, S., Marshall, W. C., Smithells, R. W. & Sheppard Sheila (1973) National Congenital Rubella Surveillance Programme. *Health Trends*, **5**, 75–79.

Dudgeon, J. A. (1974) Gamma globulin and congenital rubella. *British Medical Journal*, **2**, 732.

Dudgeon, J. A. (1975) Congenital rubella in the United Kingdom. In *Symposium on Infections of the Fetus and the Newborn Infant*, March of Dimes, New York City (to be published).

Edsall, G. (1975) Present status of pertussis vaccination. *Practitioner*, **215**, 310–314.

Edsall, G., Elliott, M. W., Peebles, T. C., Levine, L. L. & Eldred, M. C. (1967) Excessive use of tetanus toxoid boosters. *Journal of American Medical Association*, **202**, 17–19.

Enders, J. F., Weller, T. H. & Robbins, F. C. (1949) Cultivation of the Lansing strain of poliomyelitis virus in cultures of various human embryonic tissues. *Science*, **109**, 85–87.

Gardner, P. S. (1975) Personal communication.

Gardner, P. S., Turk, D. C., Aperne, W. A., Bird, T., Holdway, M. D. & Court, S. D. M. (1967) Deaths associated with respiratory tract infection in childhood. *British Medical Journal*, **4**, 316–320.

Glenny, A. T. & Südmersen (1921) Notes on the production of immunity to diphtheria toxin. *Journal of Hygiene*, **20**, 177–220.

Goldschneider, I., Lepow, Martha L., Gotschlich, E. C., Mauck, F. T., Bachl, F. & Randolph, M. (1973) Immunogenicity of group A and C meningococcal polysaccharides in human infants. *Journal of Infectious Diseases*, **126**, 769–776.

Hansard (1808) 2nd June.

Hanshaw, J. B., Schultz, F. W., Mellish, M. M. & Dudgeon, J. A. (1973) In *Intrauterine Infections*, Ciba Foundation Symposium Series 10, ed. Katherine Elliott and Julie Knight, pp. 23–32. Amsterdam: North-Holland, Elsevier, Excerpta Medica.

Hilleman, M. R., Buynak, E. B., Roehm, R. R., Tytell, A. A., Bertland, A. U. & Lampson, G. P. (1975) Purified and inactivated human hepatitis B vaccine: progress report. In *Symposium on Viral Hepatitis*. National Academy of Sciences, Washington, DC, 17th–19th March 1975, pp. 401–404.

Hilleman, M. R., Buynaks, E. D., Weibel, R. E. & Villarejos, V. M. (1973a) Immunity responses and duration of immunity following combined live virus vaccines. In *International Symposium on Vaccination against Communicable Diseases*, Symposium Series no. 22, pp. 145–157. Basel, London and New York: Karger.

Hilleman, M. R., Woodhour, A. F., Friedman, A. & Weibel, R. E. (1973b) The safety and efficacy of emulsified peanut oil adjuvant 65 when applied to influenza virus vaccine. In *International Symposium on Vaccination against Communicable Diseases*, Symposium Series no. 22, pp. 107–121. Basel, London and New York: Karger.

Home, F. (1758) *Medical Facts and Experiments*. London: Millar.

International Conference on the Application of Vaccines Against Viral, Rickettsial and Bacterial Diseases of Man (1971) Pan-American Health Organisation, Washington, DC: Scientific Publication no. 226.

International Symposium on Vaccination Against Communicable Diseases, (1973) Symposium Series no. 22. Basel, New York and London: Karger.

Jenner, E. (1798) *An Enquiry into the Causes and Effects of the Variolae Vaccinae*. London: Sampson Low.

Jenner, E. (1799) *Further Observations on the Variolae Vaccinae in cowpox*. London: Sampson Low.

Kempe, C. H., Fulginiti, V., Minamitani, M. & Shinefield, H. (1968) Smallpox vaccination of eczema patients with a strain of attenuated live vaccinia (CV1-78). *Pediatrics*, **42**, 980–985.

Kilbourne, E. D. (1971) Influenza: the vaccines. *Hospital Practice*, **114**, 103–114.

King, M. (1966) *Medical Care in Developing Countries*. Nairobi: Oxford University Press.

Krugman, S. (1963) The clinical use of gammaglobulin. *New England Journal of Medicine*, **269**, 195–201.

Krugman, S. & Giles, J. P. (1973) Viral hepatitis type B (MS 2 strain): further observations on natural history and prevention. *New England Journal of Medicine*, **288**, 755–760.

Kulenkamphh, M., Schwartzmann, J. S. & Wilson, J. (1974) Neurological complications of pertussis inoculation. *Archives of Disease in Childhood*, **49**, 46–49.

Lehrer, S. B., Tan, E. M. & Vaughan, J. B. (1974) Extraction and partial purification of the new histamine-sensitising factor of *Bordetella pertussis*. *Journal of Immunology*, **113**, 18–26.

Medical Research Council (1959) Vaccination against whooping-cough: final report. *British Medical Journal*, **1**, 994–1000.

Memorandum on Immunological Procedures, Ministry of Defence (1971) London: HMSO.

Miller, C. E., Pollock, T. M. & Clewer, A. D. E. (1974) Whooping-cough vaccination: an assessment. *Lancet*, **2**, 510–512.

Morley, D. (1973) In *Paediatric Priorities in the Developing World*. London: Butterworth.

Myers, J. D. (1974) Congenital varicella in term infants: risks reconsidered. *Journal of Infectious Diseases*, **129**, 215–217.

Office of Health Economics (1974) *Vaccination*, no. 50, London.

Peebles, T. C., Levine, L. L., Eldred, M. C. & Edsall, G. (1969) Tetanus toxoid emergency boosters. *New England Journal of Medicine*, **280**, 575–580.

Perkins, F. T. (1969) Safety of vaccines. *British Medical Bulletin*, **25**, 208–212.

Perkins, F. T. (1972) The preparation and control of vaccines. In *The Therapeutic Choice in Paediatrics*, Part IV, Immunisation. Edinburgh and London: Churchill Livingstone.

Perkins, F. T. (1973) Safety testing of vaccines. In *International Symposium on Vaccination against Communicable Diseases*, Symposium Series no. 22, pp. 177–182. Basel, London and New York: Karger.

Pollock, T. M. (1969) Immunoglobulin in prophylaxis. *British Medical Bulletin*, **25**, 202–207.

Public Health Laboratory Service (1970) Report of working party on the effect of immunoglobulin in pregnancy. *British Medical Journal*, **2**, 497–500.

Purcell, R. H. & Gerin, L. G. (1975) Hepatitis B subunit vaccine: a preliminary report of safety and efficacy tests in chimpanzees. In *Symposium on Viral Hepatitis*. National Academy of Sciences, Washington, DC, 17th–19th March 1975, pp. 395–399.

Ramon, G. (1924) Sur La toxine et sur L'antoxine diphteriaques. *Annalles de L'Institut Pasteur*, **38**, 1–10.

Royal Commission on Vaccination (1889–97) A report on vaccination and its results, based on the evidence taken by the Royal Commission. *New Sydenham Society, London* (1898), Vol. 164.

Seminar on Immunisations in Africa, Kampala, 7th–10th December (1971) Paris: Centre Internationale de L'Enfance.

Sencer, D. J. & Axnick, N. W. (1973) Cost benefit analysis. In *International Symposium on Vaccination against Communicable Diseases*, Symposium Series no. 22, pp. 37–46. Basel, London and New York: Karger.

Smith, D. H., Johnson, R. B., Peter, G. & Anderson, P. (1971) Studies on a vaccine for *Haemophilus influenzae* B. In *International Conference on the Application of Vaccine Against Viral, Rickettsial and Bacterial Diseases of Man*, pp. 353–358. Pan-American Health Organisation, Washington, DC: Scientific Publications no. 226.

Smith, J. W. G. (1973) Immunisation schedules. In *International Symposium on Vaccination against Communicable Diseases*, Symposium Series no. 22, pp. 199–214. Basel, London and New York: Karger.

Smith, J. W. G. (1975) Personal communication.

Steinfeld, J. L. (1971) Cost-benefit analysis in the developed countries. In *International Conference on the Application of Vaccines Against Viral, Rickettsial and Bacterial Diseases of Man*, pp. 465–468. Pan-American Health Organisation, Washington, DC: Scientific Publications No. 226.

Ström, J. Further experience of reactions especially of a cerebral nature in conjunction with triple vaccination: a study based on vaccination in Sweden. *British Medical Journal*, **4,** 320–323.

Symposium on Viral Hepatitis (1975) National Academy of Sciences, Washington, DC, 17th–19th March (to be published).

Wiktor, T. J. (1971) New vaccines and the future of rabies prophylaxis. In *International Conference on the Application of Vaccine Against Viral, Rickettsial and Bacterial Diseases of Man*, pp. 66–72. Pan-American Health Organisation, Washington, DC: Scientific Publications no. 226.

Wilson, G. S. (1967) In *The Hazards of Immunisation*. London: The Athlone Press.

World Health Organisation (1974) *Weekly Epidemiological Records*, no. 47, 389–394.

World Health Organisation (1975) *Weekly Epidemiological Records*, no. 28, 28th July.

8

UNEXPECTED DEATH IN INFANCY

Early recognition of the 'at risk' situation

J. L. Emery

Unexpected and apparently inexplicable death in infants has been with us from at least biblical days and it is only in this century that the belief has developed that all normally formed children should be capable of surviving to adult life.

The natural right of all children to life and health entails assumptions whose implications have not yet been sufficiently explored. In the field of education the provision of free schools has not resulted in equal education for all. Parental influence and age at leaving school may decide whether a girl becomes a nurse or a doctor but does not limit her life expectancy or the emotional wealth of her life. The provision of a National Health Service does not ensure that all will receive equal benefit. If it is shown that non-utilisation of the health service can result in a baby's death, what then? If our practitioners and hospital services have developed so that they only function for the most highly motivated parents, what then? Whose is the responsibility? The recent exposure of the 'battered baby' situation has left us in a nice dilemma concerning the rights of the child and the rights of the parents, and the position of the social welfare workers in diagnosis and handling.

The Cause of Death?

Our studies of the backgrounds of cot deaths have brought us face to face with situations that are not the normal province of the traditional academic paediatrician. Before discussing possible ways of attempting to prevent 'unexpected' death in infants, it is necessary to set this large group of child deaths in perspective. Within hospital practice we clearly recognise that some children are at a greater risk of death than others. This is a component of 'prognosis' which is possibly the major art of clinical practice. But in hospital, except in rare circumstances, can we be exact? It is sometimes surprising how some children remain alive, particularly those with severe congenital deformities. Why does one child survive to perhaps the age of a year and pass as being almost normal when he or she has a gross hydranencephaly— probably due to infarction of almost the whole of the hemispheres around the time of birth—and yet in another child death is happily ascribed to a haemorrhage within a part of the brain without which another child appears to be able to survive for a considerable time. Within the hospital ward we have almost unconsciously accepted varying degrees of explanation of death. We see children whose death is expected continually and, at the same time, others in whom death comes quite inexplicably. It is not possible to explain why it occurred one day rather than a week earlier or a week later.

We have a very imperfect understanding of the onset and sequence of the series of what are vicious circles or terminal pathways leading to death. We know that at a certain ionic level irregularities in heart action occur but the serum level of an ion, while it is something we use as a monitor in treatment, is only a small part of the situation that determines whether or not a heart stops beating. There is a tendency to assume a knowledge of the cause of death of children in hospital when a known severe illness is also present. How many bronchopneumonias are really confirmed in children dying from chronic degenerative disease? But, when we are concerned with a child not under medical care and with no reliable history, our ignorance is exposed.

Where does out pattern of ignorance fit into the cot death situation? For the past 20 years all of the local cot deaths have been carried out by the Department of Pathology at the Children's Hospital and handled and treated as hospital deaths. Thus the records represent total child deaths. It was my practice to add to the index of lesions found at necropsy instances where the lesions found did not, of themselves, adequately explain death—a category of 'cause of death unknown'. This produced a graph shown in Figure 8.1. There is no increased incidence of unexplained death at the cot death age group. In immediate perinatal deaths the lesions found in the child do not explain death in almost half, although in almost all such cases death can often be explained in the sense that many hospital deaths are explained in conjunction with the obstetric and labour history.

The mortality rate from treatable disease such as meningitis and gastroenteritis in hospital is widely taught to relate largely upon the earliness of lateness of diagnosis and admission to hospital. The proliferation of emergency and resuscitation units in hospitals reflects the need to start treatment immediately in ill children. How much of this emergency work could have been prevented by a relatively simple alteration in regime a day or so earlier? In emergency treatment we treat the measurable aspects of abnormality, whether it be blood chemistry or an electric reaction and by so doing we have faith that we alter prognosis according to the system of medicine that we practice.

Approximately 30 years ago when I first started doing necropsies on infants referred to the coroner as being found unexpectedly dead, I was surprised to find often the same lesions in the cot deaths as I was finding in children who died after admission to hospital and who usually had the classical established symptoms of the disease found. Were there thus two groups of children with similar disorders, one with and the other without standard symptoms?

This stimulated my first planned study of 'cot deaths' 20 years ago (Emery and Cowley, 1956). Our then chief lady almoner visited the parents at home of a sequential series of 50 children, reported to the Coroner as being found dead, and who had been put to bed apparently fit. She visited them at home at about a week after the baby had been buried. She obtained a history of quite significant symptoms in all but one of these children, symptoms including convulsions, vomiting, diarrhoea lasting several days and, in over half, of

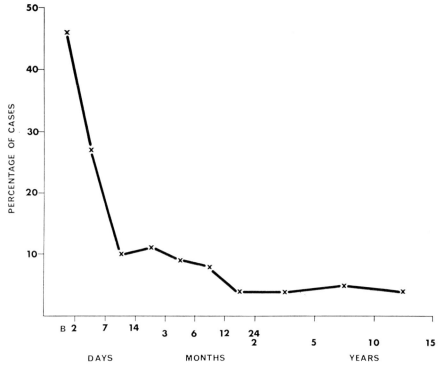

Figure 8.1 The proportions of children at different ages in which the necropsy alone failed to reveal an adequate cause of death. The cases include both hospital and cot deaths

at least a week's duration. The most dramatic case was one in whom I had found meningitis with a terminal sinus thrombosis. The history as given to the police and Coroner was completely negative. The real history was that this child had been convulsing periodically for several days but one of the parents was an incompletely controlled epileptic and convulsions were commonplace in that house. The infant's symptoms were thus unremarkable to the parents.

Since that time the problem of 'cot death', to me, has not been that of explaining the death of children with no symptoms but—

1. The recognition and evaluation of symptoms by parents, nurses and doctors and, in particular, against apparently similar symptoms in children who do not die.

2. The study of the mechanisms by which disease leads to death—this being equally applicable to hospital and 'cot deaths'.

The question arises as to what constitutes a 'cot death'. There has developed a belief that a large number of the children dying in the community do so 'completely out of the blue'—they are apparently completely healthy children who are simply found dead. We all have personal experience of relatives, or of professional and knowledgeable friends who have sustained such a child death. We all know good doctors who saw infants only a few hours before a baby died unexpectedly; many of us have had the same experience in hospital wards.

Sudden Infant Death Syndrome (SIDS)

Unexpected death at home, and occasionally in hospital, is a very real thing, but to the handful of experienced paediatric pathologists dealing with these child deaths in this country, the concept of the sudden infant death syndrome as a pathological entity is unconvincing.

The 'syndrome' concept of 'cot death' has arisen from a combination of factors:

1. The circumstance of death in these children leads to a police enquiry. The Coroner and forensic system in the past was concerned largely with the exclusion of unnatural death. This led to the examination of the children by forensic pathologists with grossly inadequate histories of the children and using non-specialist pathological investigations. Once there has been general acceptance that most of these deaths are due to natural causes, it has suited most Coroner's pathologists to put these children into a single category of natural though unexplained death. Indeed, if he wished to take the investigation further, he would be in difficulties. The statutory Coroner's fees would not provide a quarter of the laboratory cost of doing a full investigation.

2. The relatively recent 'discovery' of cot death in America was coupled with an extensive link up with parent groups. These groups facilitate the charitable counselling of parents and are also very active in obtaining funds for research purposes. In the counselling of such bereaved parents the raising of any grounds of even partial defect in service or responsibility raises in the parents an exaggeration of the often already unreasonable feelings of guilt. To mention contributory factors is unjustified and perhaps even harmful to the family unit. It is too late to do anything for the child and our responsibility lies with the parents and siblings. The use of a mystery disease thus helps the parents and counsellor. An extensive organisation now exists in the belief of the existence of a definite *sudden infant death syndrome* and this was the title of the book published in 1974 by the newly formed Canadian Foundation for the Study of Infant Deaths.

3. It suits the doctor or nurse or health authority to believe in 'SIDS' for if death was due to something outside medical knowledge, it is outside their responsibility. It suits the research worker to whom it gives the widest scope for speculation and experimentation.

Much of the confusion regarding unexpected death in infancy lies in the failure to realise that we are dealing here with a whole range of diseases and social situations and that any attempt to find 'a cause' for cot deaths or 'SIDS' is due for disappointment. Furthermore, it must be remembered that the final diseases causing death in different communities are likely to be different, particularly when we are dealing with widely differing mortality rates.

The definition of sudden infant death syndrome as generally accepted in the United States, was discussed by Beckwith (1970) at some length, at a symposium in 1970 which defined the conditions as 'the sudden death of an infant or young child which is unexpected by history, and in which a full postmortem examination fails to demonstrate an adequate cause of death'. He and others appreciated the inadequacy of this definition. The pathological entity turns on the absence of significant findings. Thus, the Seattle group insist on doing a blood culture at necropsy and if the blood culture is positive, then the child is not a case of SIDS. Does a positive blood culture provide an adequate cause of death? The same arises when one is concerned with the amount of pneumonia necessary in the lung to explain death. At that conference a group of pathologists worked out the minimal pathology work-up to enable a child to be included as a 'SIDS' for epidemiological purposes. They did not feel that blood or spleen cultures were essential but required histology of the brain, heart, liver, lungs and kidneys only. This leaves the histological and pathological definition of SIDS in a situation which even many general pathologists would consider inadequate. The interpretation of figures of causes of death of infants in different communities must be looked at against the background of the depth of study of the cases. This, obviously, varies very much from centre to centre, between university centres in this country, and even from hospital to hospital within a city. With postneonatal data for communities, total figures are the most reliably comparable ones and infant mortality in a community must be looked at as a whole.

Incidence

The increase in hospital clinical and laboratory paediatrics associated with the vast increase in number of paediatricians in this country has not been associated with a lowering of the mortality rate of children between the ages of two weeks and one year. At the same time, the mortality rates in countries such as Finland and Holland have fallen progressively (Figure 8.2). The figures for Sheffield follow the national trend and most of the subsequent observations will be based on our own work in Sheffield. Sheffield is an industrial city of approximately half a million persons situated almost exactly in the centre of England and having a fairly static population with long-standing socialist political control.

A breakdown of the site of death of children dying in Sheffield during the years 1968 to 1972 is shown in Figure 8.3. At this time the birth rate was static. It can be seen that approximately half of the postneonatal child deaths occurred in hospital and half occurred in the community presenting as unexpected child deaths, or 'cot deaths'. A small number of expected deaths (chiefly deaths of children with fatal diseases sent home to die) occurred at home.

There are many ways of analysing child mortality but one that we have found useful is to divide the deaths into four main groups related to the life-

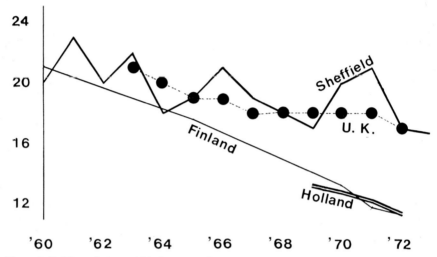

Figure 8.2   The relative total infant mortality rates (per 1000 live births) in 1960 to 1972 in the UK and Sheffield and in Finland and Holland

threatening situation as we see it today. The first group (group A) comprises children with gross congenital deformities such as hydrocephalus and spina bifida, gross congenital deformities of the heart or renal tract, children with chronic degenerative diseases of the central nervous system, leukaemias and other malignancies, i.e. children with very severe disease of long-standing in whom treatment tends to delay death rather than prevent it, or diseases for which no treatment is known. In many of these children continued life is difficult to explain! By far the greatest number of these are children with central nervous system and heart deformities. These are instances of, at present, probably inevitable death, no matter how early treatment be started.

The second group (group B) comprises potentially lethal conditions for which treatments are available. Conditions such as pneumonia, meningitis and gastroenteritis with hypernatraemia. In most of these conditions the prognosis depends upon how early a diagnosis is made and how soon adequate treatment commenced.

Group C comprises children who, at necropsy, reveal evidence of diseases liable to produce symptoms but not usually death. Such conditions are minor gastroenteritis without evidence of gross dehydration or uraemia, tracheitis, infection of the respiratory tract with otitis media, i.e. diagnosable disease but, with our present level of knowledge, with changes not severe enough to account for death. This group also contains children showing lesions such as necrosis of the vocal cord, i.e. at present non-assessable pathology.

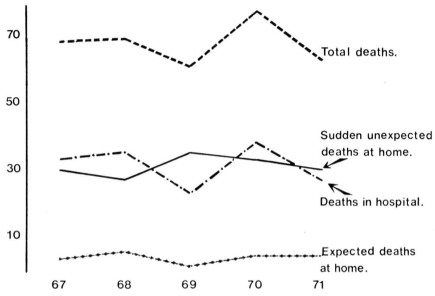

Figure 8.3 The numbers of deaths in children aged seven days to one year occurring in Sheffield during the years 1967 to 1971 and their location

Group D comprises children in whom no definite diagnosable disease is found. This group contains two subgroups—one (D1) in which histology reveals evidence that the child has been ill for some while, findings such as lack of growth in the rib, discharge of the thymus, fatty change in the liver indicating a metabolic response to some stimulus; and the other group (D2) in which no such changes are found, i.e. apparently completely disease-free children, using the tools available at our disposal.

Figure 8.4 shows a breakdown of all postneonatal child deaths in the city of Sheffield over a two-year period based on these criteria and also divided into whether death occurred in hospital or at home. In Sheffield no severely ill child is treated at home. All are referred to hospital so all home deaths, apart from a few group A deaths, are 'unexpected'.

It will be seen that the hospital deaths were largely of group A and the rest of the hospital cases are of group B. There are a small number of children with tumours (T). Of the children dying unexpectedly at home, a large number are in group B, a similar large number in group C and the number in the D1 and D2 groups is extremely small.

This figure was produced before we were fully utilising the vitreous humour in diagnosing hypernatraemia at necropsy. Since that time some of the children previously of the C group would reveal evidence of severe hypernatraemia and uraemia and thus have a treatable condition and thus, some of them belong to group B rather than group C. The dividing line between these

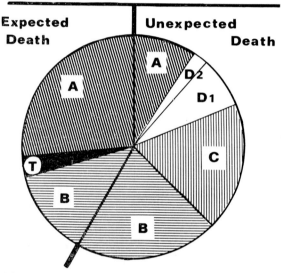

Figure 8.4 A 'pie' diagram showing a breakdown of the categories of death of all children dying in Sheffield between the ages of one week and one year in the years 1972 and 1973. The categories of death are broken down into the A, B, C, D groupings as mentioned in the text. T represents malignant tumours

groups cannot be clear cut. There are also a large number of children with non-lethal deformities who are not taken into consideration at all within this grouping, and these children are thus at least superficially normal from a life threatening point of view. There was not a single death in this age group from an accident or 'battering' in the city during this two years.

Two points are immediately obvious. First, that the majority of lethal diseases occurring in normally formed children occur outside the care of the hospital paediatrician. Indeed, it would seem that over half of the children who die in this age group do so without contact with a paediatrician after the perinatal period. Second, if we are to reduce mortality in children of this age group, our activities need to be centred in the community and not within the hospital.

Because a child's death is categorised in B group, it does not necessarily imply that if the child had been admitted to hospital a few hours before death it would necessarily have recovered. A large number of B deaths occurred in hospital but the conditions included in the B category are essentially those in which the prognosis is related to the duration of symptoms, and how early treatment had started. Indeed, much of the illness associated with gastroenteritis could have been prevented by the provision of adequate hydration. Most meningitic deaths could be prevented by earlier treatment. However we interpret the situation we cannot avoid the conclusions that something could have been done therapeutically for up to a third of the children dying and that therapy would have been likely to alter the course of the disease if applied early enough.

Regarding the C deaths, we are approaching the frontiers of our lack of skill and knowledge in paediatric pathology and it is in these deaths that much of the theoretical and experimental work concerned with child death lies. However, within this group, we have already found a group of children with severe hypernatraemia. This group of cases with hypernatraemia and uraemia that were diagnosed using the vitreous humour stimulated us to start an intensive local propaganda and educational scheme using the local press and radio and, subsequently, the numbers of children dying in the city of Sheffield with these changes in the vitreous humour has diminished remarkably and thus, the figures that Swift and I reported from Sheffield two years ago no longer apply, although they do still apply in some centres in the West Riding. Paediatric pathology colleagues who have adopted this use of vitreous humour assay at necropsy seem to find different results in different areas. Perhaps the most interesting came from Melbourne, Australia, where Alan Williams reports on the absence of hypernatraemia in his cot deaths, but the cot death rate there is considerably lower than in Sheffield and he finds the baby feeding patterns there also different from our own.

It is useful to look at general postperinatal mortality statistics related to the B, C and D deaths. The postneonatal mortality rate for England and Wales is reported as being around 6 per 1000 live births, as compared with that of 1.5 for Finland, and the details are well set out in the report on child care in Finland by Wynn and Wynn (1974). The incidence of unexpected death on the 'SIDS' definition is in the region of 2 per 1000 births in this country but the rate in Holland is probably in the region of 0.4 per 1000 (Baak and Huber, 1974) and that in Sweden is of the same order (Folin, 1974). If we look at the mortality 'pie' diagram for Sheffield (Fig. 8.4) it is apparent that if we were to eliminate the bulk of the group B deaths and some of the group C deaths, then our mortality statistics would be similar to those in Finland and Holland. It could well be that the 'cot deaths' in Sweden and Holland largely correspond only with some of our C and D groups here. A conclusion that we can draw is that our community contains a large number of infants in the postperinatal period who are not being diagnosed and treated clinically and who die with, if not from, conditions that are treatable, i.e. that there are a large number of theoretically preventable deaths and most of these are now presenting as 'cot deaths'.

A final point needs to be mentioned in conjunction with some of the C and D deaths. The situation of the non-accidental injury causing baby deaths is now well recognised. Such deaths are diagnosed by the evidence of gross degrees of physical violence to the baby. From our own evidence of post-mortem findings in children that have been truly accidentally smothered, it is, at the present time, not possible to distinguish clearly a baby, perhaps ill and crying with otitis media, that has its face held into a pillow until it stops crying, from one of our C deaths. We have evidence of the existence within our own postmortem material of a few instances of such deaths that we term the 'Gently Battered Baby' but we are not aware of any such case being upheld in court and it is unreasonable to expect any jury to accept medical evidence as significant of unnatural death that is widely accepted as being frequently found in a natural unexplained 'syndrome'. But the group must not be assumed to be absent because they are unprovable in court and are one good reason for maintaining our present system of handling all unexpected child deaths through the coroner's system.

In a study of 'cot deaths' one is always too late. Histories in retrospect are always liable to errors and after a baby death the situation becomes even more complicated as the complications of bereavement, guilt, frustration and rationalisation play different roles in different parents. Non-subjective data is only available in necropsy findings and in recorded health data before the child's death. Our necropsy material indicates that all but a very few children have been ill before death (Sinclair-Smith, Dinsdale and Emery, 1975); recorded health data is more difficult to obtain. In our early attempts to get at the background history and early history of children found unexpectedly dead, our first approach was through the local maternity and child welfare departments, to obtain the recorded details of the children. We found that there were no clinic records of at least half of these infants and we ran into a peculiar inability to trace even the health visitor's statutory first visit on many of the children. We had been aware from our interviews with many parents of cot deaths that many of them were certainly not in sympathy with their general practitioners, and frequently had not consulted them (Emery, 1972). It became obvious that it was not going to be possible to obtain adequate reliable data on such children through the present child health services, and some form of prospective study was necessary.

Physiopathological Mechanisms

As mentioned above, there are two separate aspects regarding unexpected death in infants—the sociological one concerned with the recognition of symptoms and the parental reaction that it stimulates, and the more physiopathological one of the mechanisms presponsible for death. Our present postmortem investigation tools are inadequate in both spheres but have been almost the only ones available to date. The epidemiology of cot deaths has been well worked out and discussed recently by Froggatt in Ulster (Froggatt, Lynas and MacKenzie, 1971) but has left us with only general factors. The study of 'missed' cot death—infants who would have been likely to have died unexpectedly but for some happy chance—are rare but we are uncertain of the effect of the collapse on the child and are aware of instances when a revived child has survived but with mental deficiency.

The question of 'cot deaths' has stimulated much needed research into mechanisms causing death and these have been greatly helped by recent researches in mechanisms of breathing and the physiology of sleep. The investigation into the sleep physiology related to 'SIDS' such as that described by McGinty and Harper (1974) indicates that if we are to get further into the aetiology of unexpected death during sleep, it will be necessary to identify the children at risk of abnormal periods of apnoea and hypoxia during sleep. This has been attempted by Steinschneider (1974) with the development of an apnoea monitor for detection of periods of apnoea in children who he considers susceptible to death by this means. The study by Wealthall, Whittaker and Greenwood (1974) of the breathing patterns of hydrocephalics, a group of infants very susceptible to unexpected death, perhaps indicates how this is a general problem and already applicable in some inpatient groups.

Other theories of cot death, such as that of anaphylaxic reaction to inhaled foreign material, such as propagated by Coombs (1965) require us to know, if we are to prevent the condition, the hypersensitivity of allergic state of infants prior to death. The same probably applies to the question of heart irregularities (Anderson et al, 1974), if indeed these are related in any way to unexpected death in infancy. In the instance of established epidemiological patterns between different viruses such as RS virus (Gardner, McQuillin and Court, 1970) and influenzae A virus (Nelson et al, 1975) and unexpected death, it is even more essential to identify infants at increased risk.

Whatever the mechanism that remains of either truly unexplained cot death, and even more of explained death, it is going to be essential to identify babies at risk of cot death, but we have to do this in such a way so as not to alarm parents.

Any attempts to study the physiological state of children prior to unexpected death with an incidence of about 1 in 500 in this country would require prospective clinical data on about 10000 children to anticipate 20 deaths, which is quite impractical (in Holland it would be 50000!).

Identification of Infants at Risk

It is essential to define a high risk group for study. Several epidemiological surveys on children dying as cot deaths have shown an almost unanimous finding that the factors that predispose to cot death are essentially the same as those predisposing to child death in general; the most locally relevant study was one recently carried out by Froggatt et al (1971) in Belfast.

Attempts at defining groups of children at risk have not been popular or effective, but this has probably been due to the inability to quantitate the relative numerical value of each factor. I was fortunate that the setting up of the Foundation for the Study of Infant Deaths brought me into contact with Robert Carpenter and, while discussing with him the need for a prospective study into children who come into the cot death category, he described a statistical tool that had been used with considerable success in identifying children who were likely to be repeated offenders after a period in Borstal. We decided to attempt this in the field of cot deaths.

To anticipate cot deaths it is necessary to determine the children at risk as near the time of birth as possible. The data must be available for all children and to give each factor a numerical rating we needed a statistically valid control group. The material used comprised the children who had died in Sheffield as unexpected deaths and whose necropsies had been carried out by the Department of Pathology of the Sheffield Children's Hospital. We confined our cases to children who had been born in the three principal maternity institutions in the city which were attached to the University of Sheffield, and where a reasonably competent uniform standard of antenatal and obstetric notes were available. The control for each case was the next normal child born within the same hospital who was not a twin and who had survived (Protestos et al, 1973). The information collected had to be confined to the information available in the case notes. The same applied to the postnatal state of the child. Several hundred features were tabulated and for the study, all cases of unexpected death, whether completely unexplained or partly unexplainted, or possibly explained, i.e. B, C and D groups, were treated as one group for discriminate analysis.

The whole data was first assessed comparing the cot deaths and the controls by a system of direct tabulation and 40 features were selected which gave evidence of there being statistical differences between the two groups. Following this stepwise discriminate analysis was carried out and an estimate made of the magnitude of the coefficient of difference (Carpenter and Emery, 1974). The discriminators that were finally used were: mother's age, birth order, blood group, attempt and intent to breast feed, the duration of the second stage of labour, presence of urinary infection during pregnancy, presence of polyhydramnios during pregnancy and prematurity based upon birth before 37 weeks and/or a birth weight of less than 2500 g (Table 8.1). The essential feature of the use of such coefficients is that each factor has different ratings on a mathematical scale. Thus, mother's age has a coefficient of minus 2.7 per year. Urinary infection during pregnancy has a score of 21.6 and thus, the scoring effect of urinary infection during pregnancy is completely obliterated by an increase of 10 years in the mother's age and similar effects of a slightly different order apply to blood groups and prematurity. For the purpose of this study an attempt was made to identify 50 per cent of the expected deaths within 12 per cent of the total child population.

The criteria such as blood groups which eventually came out as discriminators do not, superficially, make much sense. But the blood group difference may well have no direct relationship to actual blood groups but simply be an indication of ethnic grouping. Also, the importance of the intent to breast feed rather than actual breast feeding throughout infancy (which, of course, is not accessible at the time of birth) is probably an indicator of the mother's mental approach to the child and not any effect of the breast milk itself.

Table 8.2 Table of discrimination devised by R. G. Carpenter for the Sheffield prospective survey (Carpenter and Emery, 1974a)

Variable	Scale	Coefficient	s.e.
Mother's age	Years	−2.7	0.59
Birth order	Number	+5.9	1.82
Blood group:			
B or AB	Yes 1/No 0	+28.0	8.90
O	Yes 1/No 0	+14.5	5.87
Breast fed initially	Yes 1/No 0	−18.2	5.98
Duration second stage labour	Approx. log (time)	−7.5	3.17
Urinary infection in pregnancy	Yes 1/No 0	+21.6	9.46
Polyhydramnios in pregnancy	Yes 1/No 0	+40.9	18.23
'Premature', i.e. <37 weeks and/or <2500 g	Yes 1/No 0	+16.4	0.75

A similar attempt to construct a discriminate function for identifying high-risk babies was carried out by Kraus, Franti and Borhani for white Californian infants (Kraus, Franti and Borhani, 1972). They used the factors of mother's age, birth order, plural births, sex and birth weight but, as far as we are aware, they have not submitted these to a prospective trial and Winter and Lilos (1974) have suggested a similar system in Israel for scoring the risk of admission.

Our purpose in working out the discriminators was to follow up a group of children prospectively and a side issue of the analysis of the deaths gave an indication of how it would be necessary to carry this out. In the initial analysis of the data that we obtained from the hospital notes we found that the single most powerful criteria for identifying children at high risk of unexpected death was whether, when they had been given a clinical appointment on discharge from the maternity hospital, the appointment was kept or not. Only 44 per cent of the cases kept the appointment compared with 86 per cent of the controls. This has an important bearing upon the approach to babies at follow-up clinics. It indicated that it would be impractical to attempt a prospective survey of children at possible increased risk of cot death through any ordinary clinic system. It also indicated the extreme care that needs to be taken in

8

interpreting any data taken from infants attending the so-called normal follow-up clinics at maternity hospitals, as those attending the clinics are a self-selecting group of people who actively cooperate with the clinic holder. This poor hospital clinic attendance, together with the failure of our previous attempt to obtain data on babies later likely to be cot deaths through the services of health visitors and infant welfare clinics, indicated that our problem was not simply one of an abnormal physiology or pathology but one concerned with parental child health relations. It was obvious that a prospective study of cases at possible increased risk of cot death could not be carried out through routine services and a special organisation was needed to follow these children.

Details of the organisation of this system, which involved the active support of the community paediatrician and many others, has already been published (Emery and Carpenter, 1974). It involved a secretary who visited every maternity hospital in the area and abstracted data for the assessment protocol from every child on the day of its birth. Children with gross congenital deformities were identified and removed from the study. The residue were then assessed and graded 'at increased risk' or 'non-risk'. The 'increased risk' group were then divided randomly into two groups—a study group and a control. The study group were then subjected to a detailed follow-up by a special group of attached health visitors. At the same time, an also random group of non-risk children was taken so that the nursing and medical personnel dealing with the children did not know whether the children they were following were high risk or low risk. The health visitors worked as a team with my paediatric colleague, Dr Bruce Smith.

While we were concerned with the babies' deaths we were much more concerned with the identification of early pathological features and possible abnormal nervous reflexes, and abnormal sleeping patterns in children at increased risk. Thus the survey was truly represented to the parents as a study in child development. We initially had no definite evidence that any of the children may be at an increased risk of unexpected death.

Details have already been published for the first year of the study (Carpenter and Emery, 1974b) (see Fig. 8.5) and the second year produced almost exactly similar figures. The results of this prospective survey indicate that, taking every child born in the city over a period of two years, the discriminants produced an identification of 60 per cent of deaths within 15 per cent of the population (Carpenter and Emery, 1974a). What first surprised us was that in the group of normally formed increased risk infants that were handled and followed by our health visitors, there were no deaths that we felt were not preventable. One of these cases has been described elsewhere (Emery and Carpenter, 1974). This study from the point of view of discovering early symptoms of children later to present as unexplained cot deaths was thus a complete failure. Another unexpected finding of the division into children at possible increased risk of cot death and others was that the former group had a greater morbidity rate, as judged on the number of times the children required hospital admission for medical conditions. This ties in with the finding of Froggatt and others concerning the backgrounds of cot deaths which is common with other conditions in childhood, such as pneumonia. The morbidity aspect of this study may well in the end be more important than the mortality, in view of the much greater numbers involved and the effect of general disease on a child attaining his developmental potential.

Our health visitors on the other hand were working in quite different circumstances from others in the city. They were only concerned with children and they were working in direct contact with a consultant paediatrician, and

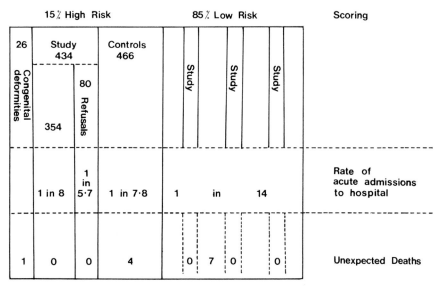

Figure 8.5   The results of the Sheffield prospective survey of all children born (6004 births) in the city in 1973, indicating the hospital admission rates and unexpected death rate in the different groups (Emery and Carpenter, 1974; Carpenter and Emery, 1974b)

they were based on the Children's Hospital (Owen and Portess, 1975). If they were in any way worried about a child, immediate paediatric advice was available and hospital admission in such cases was immediate, both for the care of the child and to facilitate detailed observation. The most important instances, however, were those where the health visitors found babies to be extremely ill but the parents were quite unaware of the child's state, and one child that required immediate transfusion on admission was brought to the hospital by the health visitor with the extreme reluctance of the parents. It is also apparent that some of the features described by Richards and McIntosh (1972) in Glasgow are equally active in Sheffield.

As judged from the publications of Margaret and Arthur Wynn (Wynn and Wynn, 1974) and our own observations in Holland, the intensity of nursing care that we introduced to the mother and child was less than the normal routine care given to every child in Finland and Holland, and the same probably applies in Sweden. To apply this intensity of health care to all infants in our local community would not be possible without at least doubling the number of health visitors in the area, and also redirecting much of their present activities. To utilise our present nurses to greater advantage it would thus seem that the identification of children at increased risk of death is essential, and if feasible, as our pilot study suggests, needs extending. The ideal time to recognise at-risk babies is not at birth but before birth. This is in the hands of the obstetricians. But the latter are unfortunately almost completely

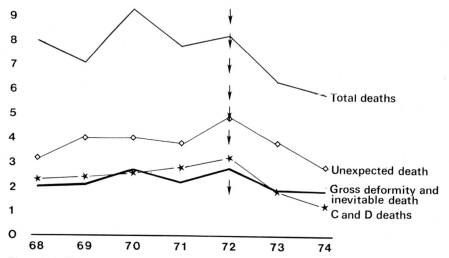

Figure 8.6   The death rates in Sheffield of children between the ages of one week and one year, per 1000 live births the previous year (i.e. population at risk of death). There appears to have been virtually no change in the inevitable (group A) deaths and an apparent fall in cot deaths due to a fall in the number of 'C' and 'D' deaths. The falling arrows indicate the commencement dates of our prospective study

concerned with perinatal mortality and usually completely divorced from later paediatric care. The situation in Holland is intriguing. In that country over 50 per cent of confinements occur at home but according to Visser (1975) the great fall in infant mortality in Holland is related to all mothers attending antenatal clinics and a careful selection of the risk and non-risk group. All the risk groups are brought into hospital for delivery.

The discriminate values that we used in our prospective study have not yet been published in detail and we have reason to believe that the discriminants are only valid for a particular community at a particular time. We are in the process of revising our local discriminants. During the period of our prospective study, the paediatric situation changed in Sheffield. The child births have fallen by about 1000 a year. But the local attitude to abortion has changed and it is now more easily obtainable. The cases of cot deaths associated with severe hypernatraemia also disappeared and following an intensive campaign on infant feeding and breast feeding, the rate of intent to breast feed of women in the major lying-in hospitals has changed over a year from 40 to 60 per cent. At the same time the number of cot deaths has also fallen (Fig. 8.6).

The recognition tools that we are using to date were only designed to cover 60 per cent of the children at risk of unexpected death, and we are now attempting to obtain data on all children at the age of four weeks in an attempt to throw in a second screen to raise the proportion to at least 90 per cent, but this will take much time. Meanwhile, we would like to see discriminants set up in other parts of the country for two reasons—apart from attempting to confirm our results. While our present child nursing services are so inadequate it is essential to direct our available resources to where there is greatest need. Second, we are unlikely to get much further in our understanding of the causes of the truly unexplained child death until our other partly explained and probably preventable deaths have been eliminated.

REFERENCES

Anderson, R. H., Bouton, J., Burrow, C. T. & Smith, A. (1974) Sudden death in infancy— a study of cardiac specialised tissue. *British Medical Journal*, **2**, 135.

Baak, J. P. A. & Huber, J. (1974) The incidence of S.I.D.S. in the Netherlands. In *S.I.D.S. 1974*, pp. 157–168.

Beckwith, J. B. (1970) *Sudden Infant Death Syndrome*, ed. Bergmann, Beckwith & Ray, p. 17. Seattle: University of Washington.

Carpenter, R. G. & Emery, J. L. (1974a) The identification and follow-up of high risk infants. In *S.I.D.S. 1974*, pp. 91–96.

Carpenter, R. G. & Emery, J. L. (1974b) Identification and follow-up of infants at risk of sudden death in infancy. *Nature*, **250**, 729.

Coombs, R. (1965) An experimental model for cot-deaths. In *Sudden Death in Infants*, ed. Wedgewood, R. J. & Benditt, E. P., pp. 55–74. US Department of Health Education and Welfare.

Emery, J. L. (1972) Welfare of families of children found unexpectedly dead (cot deaths). *British Medical Journal*, **1**, 612.

Emery, J. L. & Carpenter, R. G. (1974) Clinical aspects of the Sheffield prospective study of children at possible increased risk. In *S.I.D.S. 1974*, pp. 97–106.

Emery, J. L. & Cowley, E. M. (1956) Clinical histories of infants reported to Coroner as cases of sudden unexpected deaths. *British Medical Journal*, **2**, 1578–1579.

Folin, L. (1974) S.I.D.S. occurrence in Stockholm 1968–72. In *S.I.D.S. 1974* (2).

Froggatt, P., Lynas, M. A. & MacKenzie, G. (1971) Epidemiology of sudden unexpected death in infancy (cot death) in Northern Ireland. *British Journal of Preventative Medicine*, **25**, 119.

Gardner, P. S., McQuillin, J. & Court, S. D. M. (1970) Speculation on pathogenesis in deaths from respiratory syncytial virus infections. *British Medical Journal*, **1**, 327–330.

Kraus, J. F., Franti, C. E. & Borhani, N. V. (1972) Discriminatory risk factors in post-neonatal sudden unexpected deaths. *American Journal of Epidemiology*, **96**, 328–333.

McGinty, D. J. & Harper, R. M. (1974) Sleep physiology and S.I.D.S. In *S.I.D.S. 1974*, pp. 201–230.

Nelson, K. E., Greenberg, M. A., Mufson, M. A. & Moses, V. K. (1975) The sudden infant death syndrome and epidemic viral disease. *American Journal of Epidemiology*, **101**, 423–430.

Owen, B. & Portess, M. (1975) Prospective investigations into cot death—health visitors experience. *The Health Visitor* **48,** 379–381.

Protestos, C. D., Carpenter, R. G., McWeeny, P. M. & Emery, J. L. (1973) Obstetric and perinatal histories of children who died unexpectedly (cot death). *Archives of Diseases in Childhood*, **48,** 835–841.

Richards, I. D. S. & McIntosh, H. T. (1972) Confidential enquiry with 226 consecutive infant deaths. *Archives of Diseases in Childhood*, **47,** 697.

Sinclair-Smith, C., Dinsdale, F. & Emery, J. (1976) Evidence of duration and type of illness in children found unexpectedly dead. *Archives of Diseases in Childhood* (in press).

Steinschneider, A. (1974) The concept of sleep apnoea as related to S.I.D.S. In *S.I.D.S. 1974,* pp. 117–190.

Sudden Infant Death Syndrome (1974) Proceedings of the Francis Camps International Symposium on Sudden and Unexpected Death in Infancy, ed. Robinson, R. R. Published by The Canadian Foundation for the Study of Infant Deaths.

Visser, H. K. A. (1975) *Paediatrics and the Environment.* Fellowship of Postgraduate Medicine, London.

Wealthall, S. R., Whittaker, G. E. & Greenwood, N. (1974) The relationship of apnoea and stridor in spina bifida and other unexplained infant deaths. *Developmental Medicine and Child Neurology*, **32,** 107.

Winter, S. T. & Lilos, P. (1974) Prediction of hospitalisation during infancy—scoring the risk of admission. *Paediatrics*, **53,** 716–772.

Wynn, M. & Wynn, A. (1974) *The Protection of Maternity and Infancy: A Note on Services in Finland and Britain.* Council for Children's Welfare, London.

Wynn, M. & Wynn, A. (1974) *The Right of Every Child to Health Care: A Study of Protection of the Young Child in France.* Council for Children's Welfare, London.

9
THE EPIDEMIOLOGY OF RESPIRATORY DISEASE IN CHILDHOOD

J. R. T. Colley

In childhood, respiratory diseases are still an important cause of illness, and sometimes of death. If management is to improve further knowledge is needed of the precise aetiology, of the underlying and contributory causes, and of the long-term consequences. The aetiology may be viral, bacterial or allergic. Adverse environmental factors may change the illness from a relatively minor disorder into one that produces permanent structural damage in the respiratory tract. Among such factors are the social and domestic circumstances under which children live, their exposure to air pollution, and later their smoking habits. Both the age at which children have respiratory illness and the form and intensity of adverse environmental factors can determine the extent of permanent structural damage and subsequent susceptibility to other environment factors. Knowledge on the role of these external factors in the provocation of chest disease in children and on their long-term effects is a necessary preliminary to limiting, or hopefully preventing, their effects.

A large part of the epidemiological effort expended on investigating respiratory disease in childhood has concentrated on the common upper and lower respiratory illnesses including asthma. Many of the epidemiological studies have been conducted in the United Kingdom. This is as much a reflection of an awareness that respiratory disease may be a particular problem in the United Kingdom as the presence in this country of epidemiologists with an interest in this subject.

SOURCES OF DATA

The United Kingdom, with other developed countries, routinely collects data on mortality. By linking deaths with the populations out of which they arose, death rates may be calculated for specific causes of death by age, sex, area and also for some other categories. These data form a readily available and important source of information for those diseases where death occurs in a significant proportion of those affected. Respiratory diseases, particularly those involving the lower respiratory tract, continue to have an appreciable mortality in children.

In contrast to these mortality statistics, data on illness is seldom available to the same extent. In England and Wales the major source of routinely collected morbidity data is that obtained from a 10 per cent sample of hospital discharges, and this constitutes the material published annually as the Hospital Inpatient Enquiry. Apart from notifications of selected infectious diseases, such as influenza and pertussis, there are no other routinely collected national morbidity data for children that are published centrally on an annual basis in England and Wales.

One major source of information is the morbidity data derived from ad hoc studies. Among these have been two studies in England and Wales, in 1955–1956 and 1970–1971, on morbidity in general practice. These provide useful information on the patterns of illness as seen by the primary care physician. Also there are many epidemiological field studies on various aspects of respiratory disease in children, many of which attempted to answer specific questions, particularly on the aetiology, underlying causes, and long-term consequences of respiratory disease in children.

Vital Statistical Data

Mortality—international comparisons

As countries improve their registration of deaths, and enumeration of their populations, so more data have become available to allow comparisons to be made between countries. For example in 1973, the data on mortality for the year 1969 had been published for 25 out of the 32 member countries of the European Region of the World Health Organisation. These data are compiled by the United Nations and published in World Health Statistics Annual, using a uniform format in respect of age groups, diagnostic groups and time periods. A comparison has been performed for countries in the European region who provided data for the year 1969, using the eighth revision of the International Classification of Diseases.

MORTALITY WITHIN COUNTRIES

In Figures 9.1 and 9.2 the age and sex specific mortality rates from pneumonia and bronchitis (ICD 480–486, 490–493) are given for two countries—the Netherlands and Romania. Both these countries show the typical age pattern for mortality from these diseases; mortality is high in infancy, drops to a minimum in childhood and early adult life and then rises progressively throughout middle and old age. However, although the age patterns are not too dissimilar the absolute levels of mortality in the two countries are not the same. In Romania, at each age, mortality exceeds that found in the Netherlands. This is most striking for ages under one year, and between one and four years. In addition, in Romania mortality rates in infancy are similar to those seen in middle and old age. The Netherlands, in contrast, show a quite different pattern; rates in infancy being lower than those in middle and old age. These contrasting patterns of mortality serve to emphasise

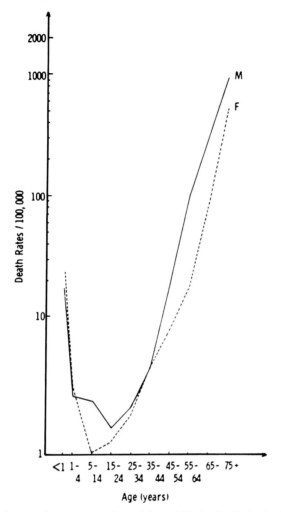

Figure 9.1 Death rates from pneumonia and bronchitis in the Netherlands, 1969 (WHO, 1974)

the continuing wide differences in mortality that exist between countries within the same continent.

The precise reasons for the lower mortality rates in middle and late childhood in comparison with the high rates in infancy are not known. It is probable that this mainly reflects the increasing immunity that follows repeated exposure to respiratory infections as children grow up. The high initial mortality would also remove those who are most susceptible, leaving the more resistant.

In both countries, there is a sex difference in mortality in middle and late

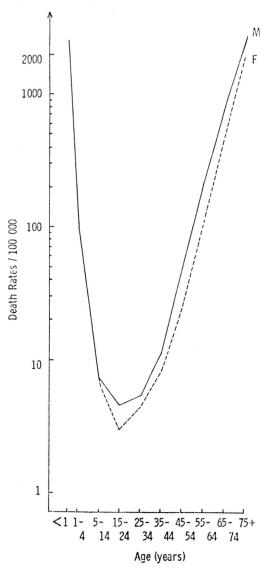

Figure 9.2   Death rates from pneumonia and bronchitis in Romania, 1969 (WHO, 1974)

childhood, where male rates exceed those of females; a pattern that is accentuated in adult life.

MORTALITY BETWEEN COUNTRIES

Further comparison of mortality between countries, at specific ages, emphasises the different mortality rates current in these countries. In Figures 9.3, 9.4 and 9.5 mortality from pneumonia and bronchitis is given by rank

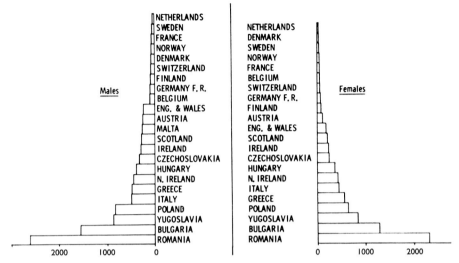

Figure 9.3 Mortality from pneumonia and bronchitis for European countries, 1969 (rate per 100000): aged under one year (WHO, 1974)

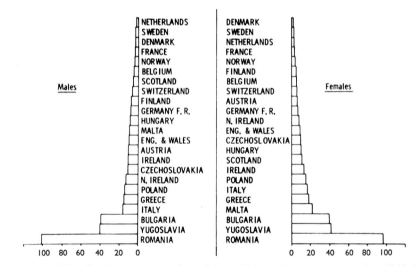

Figure 9.4 Mortality from pneumonia and bronchitis for European countries, 1969 (rate per 100000): ages one to four (WHO, 1974)

for 23 countries in the European region at three ages; under one year, one to four, and 15 to 24 years. The major contrast between these countries is in their mortality in children under one year old. Here the Netherlands has the lowest rates, and Romania the highest (Fig. 9.3). A male mortality excess is present at this age although this is not large or wholly consistent. The rankings, by country, for mortality at this age are almost the same for males and females.

This raises the possibility that the differences in mortality between the sexes are primarily a result of innate differences in susceptibility and not due, for example, to differential exposure either to environmental factors or contact with infections.

In the one to four year olds (Fig. 9.4), mortality rates are considerably lower than in the under one year olds. The contrasts between countries in their levels of mortality are also smaller, and there is now no consistent sex difference. Turning to the 15 to 24 year olds (Fig. 9.5) mortality from pneumonia and bronchitis is now very low. At this age the ranking of countries seen at younger ages tends to break up, and a male mortality excess reappears.

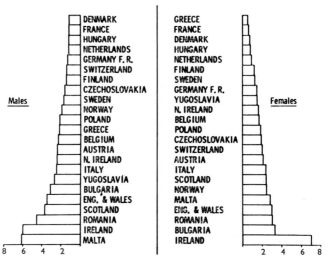

Figure 9.5 Mortality from pneumonia and bronchitis for European countries, 1969 (rate per 100 000): ages 15 to 24 (WHO, 1974)

The reasons for these wide differences in mortality, particularly for children under one year old, are not obvious. There are a number of possible explanations. The first to consider is that these differences may be artefacts. This may arise due to the different death certification habits of physicians in the various countries, as may happen when physicians do not employ uniform diagnostic standards. In addition, differences may also arise if uniform criteria for coding of the diagnoses are not used. Often, where such doubts arise it is customary to study the patterns of mortality using wide diagnostic groupings. For example, to take mortality from all respiratory diseases, instead of a narrow group of conditions as pneumonia and bronchitis. In this way any differences of classification such as may arise between individual categories of respiratory disease, would not influence comparisons between countries and thus lead to spurious differences in mortality. When the patterns of mortality for all respiratory diseases were examined for these 23 countries, only minor changes were found in comparison with the patterns for pneumonia and bronchitis. This suggested that differences in certifying and coding practices were unlikely to explain more than a small part of the mortality differences between countries, and strengthens the view that these mortality rates reflect the true patterns of disease. However, there is clearly a need to investigate current certifying and coding practices before we can be sure of this point.

These remarks apply less forcefully to comparisons within a country, whether between different age-groups, or between males and females. Here most physicians who certify causes of death in children are likely to have a broadly similar medical training and thus would tend to employ similar diagnostic labels. Likewise, the coding rules for death certificates are unlikely to differ within a country.

Time trends in mortality

ALL RESPIRATORY DISEASES

In England and Wales mortality from all respiratory diseases has declined sharply since the early 1940s. This can be seen in Figures 9.6A and B. Here mortality for the period 1968 to 1972 is plotted on an annual basis, and year to year fluctuations can be seen in the rates. In the earlier periods, mortality rates are based on four or five years data and this has the effect of smoothing any large year to year variations. In infants under one year old, mortality declined at a high rate to the mid 1950s and then levelled out. In the remaining age groups mortality continued to decline throughout the period, although there are fluctuations in the annual rates from 1968. There are a number of possible reasons for the overall fall in mortality. At first sight, in the earlier years, this might seem to be primarily the result of the continuing introduction of new antibiotics. This is unlikely to be the whole explanation as mortality from respiratory disease has been falling steadily since the early 1900s well before the introduction of chemotherapy. Improvements in the social and economic circumstances of the population may well have contributed substantially to this fall in mortality. Studies in the 1920s and 1930s, reviewed by Collins, Kasap and Holland (1971), demonstrated the close association between, for example, overcrowding and respiratory mortality. It is thus reasonable to infer that improvements in these and other social and economic factors, have contributed to the decline in mortality.

The small change in mortality since the mid-1950s in infants under one year old, in comparison with the trend in older children, suggests that factors influencing mortality may differ at these ages. In the neonatal period respiratory infections are infrequent and the main causes of mortality are either the consequences of immaturity or of problems associated with delivery, where environmental factors play little part. In contrast, in the postneonatal period respiratory infections are a major cause of mortality and here social and

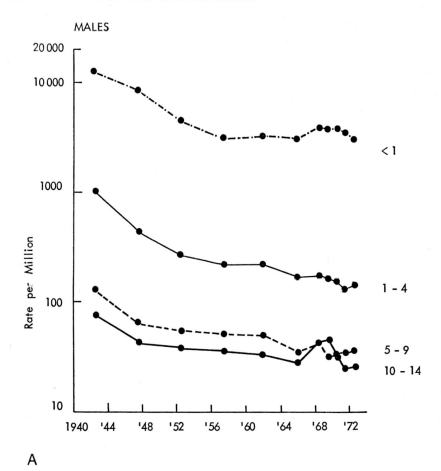

A

Figure 9.6A and *B*   Mortality for all diseases of the respiratory system (rate per million), 1940 to 1972 for England and Wales. Data for 1940 to 1967 adapted from Collins, J. J., Kasap, H. S. and Holland, W. W. (1971) *American Journal of Epidemiology*, **93**, 10–22. Data for 1968 to 1972 from *Registrar General's Annual Reports for England and Wales*

environmental factors have important influences (Heady and Heasman, 1959). Thus while improvements in social and environmental factors have influenced mortality at older ages, this has happened to a lesser extent in infants under one year of age. The experience of other countries, notable the Scandinavian and Northern European group (Fig. 9.3), suggests that considerable potential exists for further reducing mortality at this age in England and Wales.

A further way of examining the potential benefits of improved social, environmental and therapeutic agents is by cohort analysis. In this form of analysis the mortality rate is examined at successive ages in a single generation

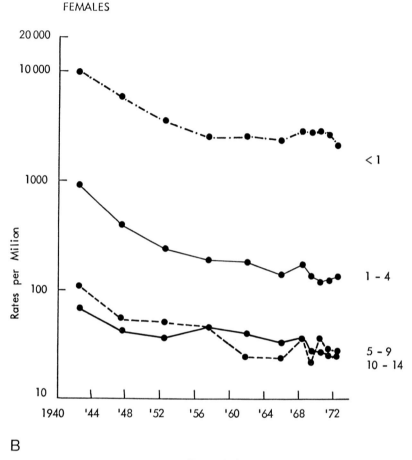

Figure 9.6B

followed from birth. The mortality rates for bronchitis in succeeding generations of children born in 1921, 1931, 1941 and 1951 are given in Figure 9.7
which has been prepared from data of Case and Harley (1958), Case, Coghill
and Harley (1968), and from the Registrar General's Annual Reports.
Successive cohorts can be seen to have a reduction in bronchitis mortality.
Thus generations who experience high mortality in infancy continue to show
this high mortality throughout life. This suggests that circumstances in early
childhood determine subsequent mortality from bronchitis. Colley (1971)
further analyses the cohort data by also plotting the mortality ascribed to
bronchopneumonia, and lobar and undefined pneumonias. He noted that
deaths due to lobar and undefined pneumonias showed the most obvious and
continuing reductions, particularly in the cohort born around 1936 to 1940.
This was thought to be a consequence of the introduction of the sulphona-

mides in the late 1930s and of penicillin in the 1940s. That such large changes did not occur in mortality ascribed to bronchitis and bronchopneumonia suggests that these deaths may have been mainly a result of viral infections, whereas deaths ascribed to lobar and undefined pneumonia were mainly bacterial in origin.

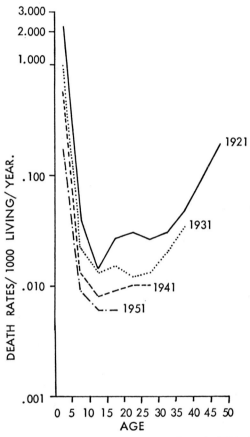

Figure 9.7   Bronchitis death rates in male generations born in 1921, 1931, 1941 and 1951

ASTHMA

Asthma mortality in childhood appears to vary between countries. For example, Gordis (1973) noted that asthma mortality in the United States in persons under the age of 20 years had remained steady between 1958 and 1967, at three deaths per million population. In contrast Japan over the same period had higher asthma mortality rates, and these rates varied between 9 and 11 deaths per million population. How far these differences between Japan and the United States represent differences in certification and coding practices, or reflect a true difference in incidence or case fatality, is not clear.

One major feature of the epidemiology of asthma has been the changes in asthma mortality during the 1960s in some countries. This was particularly marked in England and Wales where mortality from asthma rose between 1959 and 1966, and thereafter fell. This can be seen in Figure 9.8. The data for 1968 to 1973, which were classified under the eighth revision of the ICD, have been adjusted to correspond to the seventh revision classification used

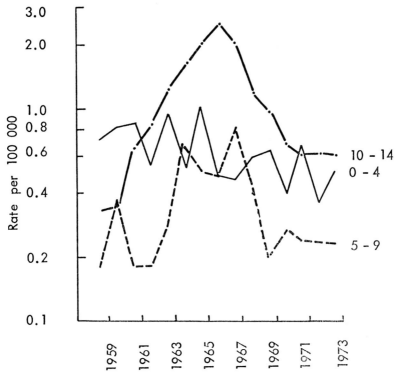

Figure 9.8   Mortality from asthma in England and Wales, 1959 to 1973 (rate per 100000). Deaths 1959 to 1967 and 1968 to 1973 classified by seventh revision ICD to rubric 241. Data supplied by the General Register Office

before 1968. Little change in mortality occurred in children under five between 1959 and 1973. The other two age groups show an upward trend, with a peak in 1966 for the 10 to 14 year olds, and 1967 for the five to nine year olds. Thereafter the rates fall to steady levels in 1971 to 1973.

The largest rise in mortality was in the 10 to 14 year olds, where a sevenfold increase occurred. Although mortality subsequently dropped, this has now stabilised at a higher level than that before the rise started in 1961. This pattern can be demonstrated in another way by calculating the proportional mortality rates. Among the 10 to 14 year olds in 1959 to 1960, asthma accounted for about 1 per cent of all deaths, and in 1966 for 7.2 per cent, where it became the fourth most common cause of death (Inman and Adelstein, 1969). By 1973 asthma mortality had dropped, accounting for 2.2 per cent of all deaths. Mortality in the five to nine year olds, in contrast, only showed a fourfold rise and has now returned to initial levels. There has been considerable debate about the cause of this rise in mortality and its subsequent fall. The most satisfactory explanation, and the one that best fits the available data, is that this rise was caused by the excessive use of pressurised aerosol bronchodilators. The publicity that followed this suggestion led to a fall in their use, and this was accompanied by a fall in asthma mortality. Inman and Adelstein (1969) were able to examine the changes in use of pressurised aerosol bronchodilators, both in their type and the delivered dose, in relation to asthma mortality and hospital admissions for this disease. In the absence of any other satisfactory explanation they concluded that excessive use of these aerosols was the major factor in the rise of asthma mortality. While this may be an adequate explanation for the situation in England and Wales, in other countries where aerosol bronchodilators were also used, for example in Canada and the United States, no change in asthma mortality seems to have occurred.

Hospital Admissions and Discharges

Hospital admission is often determined by a number of factors other than the severity of the disease or the strict necessity for inpatient care. Among these factors are the adequacy of home conditions for management of an ill child, availability of hospital beds, distance from hospital, and preparedness of the general practitioner to manage the child at home. These factors will tend to vary from area to area within a country; for children, in addition, their age may influence whether or not admission is thought necessary. For example, it may be more likely for a child under the age of one year with a lower respiratory infection to require admission to hospital than would be the case with an older child.

These preliminary remarks are intended to draw attention to the possible limitations of such data when used to indicate the presumptive effects of environmental and other factors on the incidence of disease. These data do, however, provide information on the use being made of hospital inpatient facilities. This can be seen in Table 9.1 where estimated total discharges among boys for diseases of the respiratory system from hospital in England and Wales are given for the year 1972. Some 11 per cent of all discharges in 13 and 14 year old boys, and 31 per cent of all discharges in boys aged five to nine years old are due to respiratory causes. Thus as a group, respiratory diseases comprise an important cause of hospital inpatient care in childhood. Discharge rates (per 10 000 home population) for major subcategories of respiratory disease are given in Table 9.2. Admission rates are highest in the first year of life where acute respiratory infections, including influenza, pneumonia, and bronchitis are major causes of respiratory admissions. In the one to four year age group the rates are lower, both for all causes, and for respiratory causes. At this age admissions for hypertrophy of tonsils and adenoids, which will include children admitted for tonsillitis as well as children having tonsillectomy and/or adenoidectomy, exceed those for

Table 9.1 Estimated number of hospital discharges for selected diagnoses in England and Wales, 1972, males

Diagnostic group (ICD A list)	Age group (years)				
	Under 1	1–4	5–9	10–12	13–14
All causes (A 1–150)	110270	138060	160850	60400	33370
Diseases of respiratory system (A 89–96)	14680	32000	49760	9160	3700
Discharges for respiratory diseases as a percentage of all discharges	13	23	31	15	11

Source: *Report on Hospital Inpatient Enquiry for Year 1972*, Part 1. HMSO, London, 1974

Table 9.2 Estimated hospital discharge rates for selected diagnoses per 10000 home population for England and Wales, 1972, males

Diagnostic group (ICD A list)	Age group (years)				
	Under 1	1–4	5–9	10–12	13–14
All causes (A 1–150)	2922	868	767	509	445
Diseases of respiratory system (A 89–96)	389	201	237	77	49
Acute respiratory infections including influenza (A 89, 90)	234	89	38	14	7
Pneumonia and bronchitis (A 91, 92, 93a)	110	28	8	4	2
Asthma (A 936b)	5	17	12	10	6
Hypertrophy of tonsils and adenoids (A 94)	2	51	156	34	18

Source: *Report on Hospital Inpatient Enquiry for Year, 1972*, Part 1. HMSO, London, 1974

pneumonia and bronchitis. In the next age group, five to nine year olds, these differences widen. Here 65 per cent of admissions for respiratory diseases are for hypertrophy of tonsils and adenoids, and these account for 20 per cent of all admissions in boys. At ages over nine, while all causes admission rates continue to drop, those for respiratory causes show much larger reductions, comprising 15 and 11 per cent of all admissions in the 10 to 12, and 13 to 14 year groups respectively. At these ages, although admission rates for hypertrophy of tonsils and adenoids drop, they still remain a major cause of respiratory admissions. The data for females has not been tabulated to save space but the pattern is broadly similar to that for boys except that the rates are lower.

Epidemiological Field Methods in Childhood Respiratory Disease

Routinely collected data on mortality and morbidity, while providing useful indications to broader aspects of the influence of environmental factors, often cannot provide the more detailed assessment needed. Recourse has then to be made to field studies, where clinical and other measurements are made on every individual within a defined population. The basis of the epidemiological approach in the investigation of aetiological factors involves comparisons between the disease experience of groups who have different exposure to the factor under investigation. Thus in the case of an aetiological factor, such as air pollution, the respiratory disease experience of children exposed to high levels of air pollution could be compared with a group of children exposed to lower levels. It is implicit in such comparisons that not only should the populations be similar, for example, in their age distribution, but that the methods used to assess disease experience should also be identical. If this is not the case it may prove difficult, if not impossible, to evaluate any differences, or lack of differences in disease experience between the populations. This problem has already been referred to earlier when attempts were made to evaluate differences between countries in their mortality from respiratory disease. To facilitate comparisons between groups having dissimilar exposures to environmental factors, epidemiologists have expended considerable effort in developing measurement techniques that are not only valid but can be readily standardised for use in field studies. Many epidemiological field studies into childhood respiratory disease have used standardised questionnaires, a limited clinical examination and simple tests of ventilatory function. The use of a standardised questionnaire ensures that each subject is asked exactly the same set of questions. In most studies on children these questions are completed by the parents. Two techniques are used; the first involves trained interviewers asking the questions of the parents, while in the second the parents fill in the questionnaire themselves. The latter method has been extensively used. It has major advantages in its low cost and ready application, simultaneously, to large populations. The information recorded by questionnaires, apart from the usual demographic data, often consists of past history of episodes of respiratory tract illness. Uncertainty may surround such information as the diagnostic labels attached to such illness may not be uniform. In practice, certainly in the United Kingdom, this has not proved an impediment to its use. To circumvent this type of problem, and in addition to record evidence of minor respiratory disability, questions on respiratory symptoms have been developed; for example, questions to elicit the presence of cough and wheeze. Sets of such questions received extensive development for studies in adults, and have subsequently been adapted and widely used since for studies on children.

Clinical examination is of limited value in field studies. In particular, assessment of clinical signs in the chest may be virtually worthless due to the unacceptably large variation found between observers in their assessment of these signs (Armitage, Blendis and Smyllie, 1966). Clinical examination may be more acceptable where a single observer makes the assessment on all subjects, provided he does not alter his criteria for such assessment during the course of the study. The clinical measurements most often used in field studies include examination for evidence of ear pathology, such as perforated or scarred ear drums, sinus opacities, and presence or absence of tonsils.

The clinician has available a wide range of tests of lung function. For field studies the epidemiologist primarily needs tests that need inexpensive and portable equipment, and are both simple in operation and acceptable to the population being examined. In practice such tests, for example the measurement of peak expiratory flow rates, tend to be less precise than some of the techniques in current use in pulmonary laboratories. On the other hand, as comparisons in field studies are often made between the mean ventilatory function of groups of children, some loss in precision is acceptable in order to gain the other advantages.

ENVIRONMENTAL AND OTHER FACTORS

In this section specific environmental factors, such as air pollution, as well as social and familial factors, are reviewed for evidence of their effects upon respiratory disease in children. The evidence presented is drawn from studies of mortality and to a greater extent from epidemiological field survey.

Air Pollution

In 1970 a Committee of the Royal College of Physicians of London published a review of the evidence on the health effects of air pollution. The report covered the role of air pollution in the aetiology of chronic respiratory infections in children as well as in adults. A distinction was drawn between the effects of short-term exposure to high levels of air pollution and those following long-term chronic exposure to lower levels.

Acute effects

The acute, and exceptionally severe, air pollution episode in December 1952 in London resulted in some 4000 'excess' deaths. These deaths occurred mainly in adults in the older age groups, many of whom already had chronic illnesses. However, children under the age of one year also showed a mortality excess, although this was not seen in children over this age (Logan, 1953). This whole episode served to emphasise the potentially lethal effects of short-term exposure to high levels of air pollution. The conclusion drawn was that infants, along with those older adults who have existing chronic diseases, are a particularly susceptible group to the effects of high levels of air pollution.

While mortality is an important index of the severe effects of air pollution it does not furnish a measure of the overall effect on health, as could be provided by measurement of morbidity. Unfortunately the morbidity resulting from this air pollution episode could not be measured very precisely. Recently, however, an attempt has been made to see whether infants exposed to this air pollution episode showed any adverse effects on the respiratory tract in early adult life. This study involved a comparison between those born in London in the weeks before, and after, the 1952 fog episode and was conducted in two stages (Waller, Brooks and Adler, 1975). In the first, 800 18-year-olds who were exposed in infancy to the 1952 fog were examined. In the second stage a further group of 800 were examined also at the age of 18, but who were all born after the fog episode. When the results from a standard questionnaire on respiratory symptoms and tests of ventilatory function were compared, no differences between these two groups were found that could be attributed to exposure to the fog. The reasons for the lack of any difference between these two groups was discussed. One possibility was that infants at the time of the fog would have been kept indoors and thus protected, in small part, from exposure to the higher levels of air pollution out of doors. The two groups would, however, have been exposed throughout their childhood to the high levels of air pollution that prevailed in London in the 1950s and early 1960s, and this might have tended to obscure any differences caused by the fog. Doubt must therefore still remain on whether or not exposure of young children to very high air pollution leads, in those who survive, to any long-term effects upon the respiratory tract.

Chronic exposure

Reid (1969), when he reviewed the conditions that appear to favour the onset of bronchitic disease in children, remarked upon the higher mortality from bronchitis among preschool children living in urban areas in England and Wales. In Table 9.3 mortality rates from bronchitis and pneumonia for the years 1959 to 1963 in England and Wales are given for three age groups in childhood. In both boys and girls under one year, mortality is lowest in rural areas and there is a trend for mortality to rise with increase in size of urban area, although in the boys this is not consistent in the conurbations and urban areas of 100 000 and over. In the one to four year age group the pattern breaks up and the rural mortality advantage lessens in boys and disappears in the girls. At the 5 to 14 year age group also, there is no consistent pattern, although at this age the rates may be unreliable as they are based on a small number of deaths. This pattern of mortality in the under one year olds is at least suggestive of urban residence, and at that time, i.e. 1959 to 1963, exposure to air pollution, as explaining in part the urban–rural gradients. Various suggestions have been made for the lack of a gradient in the older children. This could be a result of greater exposure of children in rural areas to vegetable or other allergens, or more likely to their encountering infections rather later than children in the towns. Thus the susceptible town child might well suffer greater exposure to respiratory infections in the first year of life, and therefore show higher mortality then, while the country child has this exposure, and mortality, postponed to later years. Interpretation of these data is further complicated by the different urban–rural distribution of the social classes.

Table 9.3 Death rates per 1 000 000 per annum from bronchitis (ICD 500–502) and pneumonia (ICD 490–493, 763) in England and Wales 1959–1963

	Age group in years		
	Under 1	1–4	5–14
Death rates in males			
England and Wales (overall rate)	4015	194	30
Conurbations	4390	193	23
Urban areas of:			
100 000 and over	4672	204	33
50 000–100 000	4095	174	28
under 50 000	3689	210	33
Rural districts	3201	180	33
Death rates in females			
England and Wales (overall rate)	3065	165	24
Conurbations	3414	159	18
Urban areas of:			
100 000 and over	3384	173	24
50 000–100 000	2988	131	18
under 50 000	2831	176	28
Rural districts	2492	177	34

Source: Registrar General's Decennial Supplement, England and Wales, 1961, Area Mortality. HMSO, London, 1967

Semiskilled and unskilled workers and their families suffer higher respiratory mortality than families of skilled and non-manual workers. In addition they tend to live more often in the large industrial cities. The higher respiratory mortality rates in the large urban areas may thus be more a reflection of the social class composition of their populations rather than of exposure to higher levels of air pollution.

Collins et al (1971), in their investigation of environmental factors and mortality in childhood, demonstrated that various social and environmental factors, including air pollution, were so closely correlated that their individual effects could not be separated. The evidence for an increased risk of mortality following chronic exposure to lower levels is thus not as firm as the evidence for the immediate effects of exposure to very high levels of air pollution. From such mortality studies it is necessary to turn to field surveys of morbidity to investigate the role of air pollution further.

Much of the earlier work in the United Kingdom on the relationship between air pollution and respiratory disease had been on adults, and specifically on working populations. Various problems in interpretation arose with these studies. For example, cigarette smoking and occupational exposure, both of which can influence the incidence and severity of respiratory disease, could mask or exaggerate possible effects of air pollution. Studies of children seemed one way to circumvent these problems. Few children and particularly those of primary school age, i.e. less than 11 years old, would not yet smoke sufficiently for this to be an important complication in interpreting possible air pollution effects. In the same way, as children do not go out to work, they would not yet have suffered exposure to occupational factors.

Some of the earlier studies involved young men undergoing medical examination prior to induction into the armed forces. Lee (1957) investigated chronic otitis media and noted high prevalence rates in young men coming from the predominantly industrial areas of Clydeside and south-east Lancashire, which contrasted with the lower rates in those from the London area. As he had also found chronic otitis media more frequently reported in young men coming from low social class families he could not be sure how much of the excess prevalence in chronic otitis media in young men from the industrial areas could be explained by the differences in social class distribution. Rosenbaum (1961) also studied a sample of young men who were called up into the armed forces. He followed them for any subsequent admissions for respiratory illness, to army medical units, and found that those who had been called up from industrial areas had higher rates of admission for respiratory illness, than men from country districts. This pattern was independent of where they were stationed while in the army. These findings demonstrate the continuing adverse effects of urban residence, but like Lee (1957) cannot satisfactorily separate possible social class from air pollution effects.

Since these earlier studies a number of field surveys of young children in the United Kingdom, notably those by Wahdan (1963), Douglas and Waller (1966), Lunn, Knowelden and Handyside (1967) and Colley and Reid (1970), have shown associations between air pollution and lower respiratory disorders. In the national sample of 3866 children studied by Douglas and Waller, the incidence and severity of lower respiratory tract illnesses was found to increase with the level of air pollution. This trend was also found in children from the same social group, but exposed to different levels of air pollution. Similar findings were reported in schoolchildren by Wahdan (1963) and Lunn et al (1967). The latter group reported a further study of their Sheffield schoolchildren which suggested that the reduction in air pollution in the city since the first study, had been followed by a fall in respiratory morbidity (Lunn, Knowelden and Roe, 1970). In England, Colley and Reid (1970) found a gradient for past history of bronchitis and current cough; the lowest rates were observed in rural areas, where air pollution was at a minimum, and the highest rates among children living in the most heavily air-polluted towns. These differences were most striking among children of semiskilled and unskilled workers. In the children studied in South Wales, where smoke pollution is relatively low, the respiratory morbidity rates were far in excess of those found in English areas with comparable levels of air pollution. No very satisfactory explanation was found for these differences and it is likely that there are some special circumstances, unrelated to air pollution or social class, affecting respiratory morbidity among children in South Wales.

In contrast to the general agreement between the findings of these studies on the association between air pollution and lower respiratory tract illness, no such agreement was found in relation to upper respiratory tract disease. Thus Wahdan (1963) and Lunn et al (1967) found such an association, whereas Douglas and Waller (1966) and Colley and Reid (1970) did not. There is no ready explanation for these conflicting findings.

The studies by Wahdan (1967), Lunn et al (1967), Holland et al (1969) and Colley and Reid (1970) were unable to show any unequivocal association between chronic exposure to air pollution and a reduction in ventilatory function. So the effects of chronic exposure to air pollution on ventilatory function are uncertain. In contrast, evidence from Japan suggests that exposure to very high levels of air pollution can be associated with reduction in ventilatory function. Toyama (1964), working in Tokyo, reported that during the winter months, when air pollution was at its highest, mean peak expiratory flow-rates were lower in exposed children than in non-exposed children living nearby. When air pollution dropped the peak-flow rates in the exposed children returned to normal levels. These findings appear to indicate that in children exposure to high air pollution over a few weeks can cause a reduction in ventilatory function which returns to normal levels when air pollution drops.

The long-term effects of childhood exposure to air pollution are more difficult to measure. However, the follow-up of the cohort of children born in 1946 (Douglas and Blomfield, 1958), and investigated in childhood for the effects of air pollution exposure (Douglas and Waller, 1966), have permitted examination of this aspect when these children reached the age of 20. At this age, when due allowance had been made for other factors, there was little residual effect of air pollution upon the prevalence of chronic cough (Colley, Douglas and Reid, 1973). However, since then, when this group were resurveyed at the age of 25, the effects on chronic cough of childhood exposure to air pollution were more obvious. It is thus possible that as the cohort ages, the effects of childhood exposure may become more apparent.

The evidence thus far points to children in early childhood, and particularly in the first year of life, being most susceptible to the effects of air pollution. In comparison with the effects of other factors, air pollution probably exerts only a small effect on respiratory morbidity. Nevertheless it is a factor, in contrast to others to be discussed later, that is amenable to change.

Social Factors

Social factors have been recognised to powerfully influence the patterns of respiratory mortality and morbidity in childhood. Probably nowhere has this been such a feature of respiratory disease in childhood than in the United Kingdom. Social class gradients in respiratory disease have been a prominent finding in the past (Payling Wright and Payling Wright, 1945; Grundy and Lewis-Faning, 1957; Douglas and Blomfield, 1958; Logan, 1960; Miller et al,

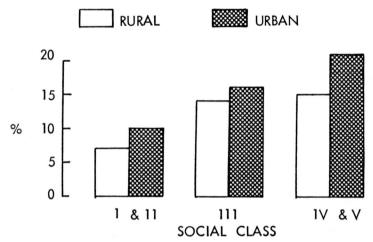

Figure 9.9 Prevalence (percentage) of chronic cough in 6 to 10 year old schoolchildren by social class and area

1960). The trend has always been for mortality and morbidity to be low in the children of parents in the professional and managerial group (social class I and II in the Office of Population Censuses and Surveys, Classification of Occupations, 1970), and to be highest among children of labourers and semi-skilled workers (social class IV and V). These gradients were found not only for the lower respiratory tract illnesses, but also for those of the upper respiratory tract.

With the changes in social, economic and other circumstances of life that have occurred over the last quarter century in the United Kingdom, it might be expected that these gradients would tend to diminish or even disappear. However, this has not happened; gradients in respiratory morbidity remain a striking feature of this group of illnesses (Holland et al, 1969; Colley and Reid, 1970). This can be seen in Figure 9.9, when the prevalence of cough in 6 to 10 year olds is given for social class and also urban and rural area of residence (data from study by Colley and Reid, 1970). Prevalence of cough rises from social class I and II to a maximum in social class IV and V. In addition, within social class, prevalence is higher in the urban than rural children. Social class is a rather vague concept that is based, in the Office of Population Censuses and Surveys classification, primarily upon the occupation of the head of the family. It is not at all easy to establish what are the precise features of social class that contribute to these gradients. A number of factors, such as parental education, family size, income, housing standards, are linked with social class and themselves influence the incidence of respiratory infections. These and other factors are so closely interrelated that it has proved difficult to separate their individual effects and thus assess the contribution they make to the social class gradients.

There is ample evidence that domestic and economic circumstances do have large effects upon respiratory disease in children. Respiratory mortality has been found to be higher among children living under the least satisfactory conditions (Payling Wright and Payling Wright, 1945; Grundy and Lewis-Faning, 1957). Domestic overcrowding, in particular, has been shown to be closely related to respiratory mortality in infancy and childhood. A study of the epidemiology of respiratory infections in working class families found that overcrowding increased the risk of transfer of respiratory infections within the family (Brimblecombe et al, 1958). In addition those children with inadequate clothing suffered more respiratory illnesses than children who were better clothed. Low standards of maternal care given to children under one year old (Grundy and Lewis-Faning, 1957) and under five years old (Miller et al, 1960) has also been found to be associated with high respiratory morbidity rates.

As noted earlier, social, domestic and economic factors tend to be interrelated. There is a need for further studies with the major aim of separating the individual effects of these important factors. This is a necessary preliminary to influencing the incidence, severity and longer term consequences of these illnesses.

There is reason to believe that the marked social class gradients seen in the United Kingdom may not be present to the same extent in other countries. If this is so, then it is suggestive of the effects on respiratory disease of some general factors present in the circumstances of life in these islands.

Familial Factors

Reference has already been made to the importance of overcrowding in the transfer of respiratory infections within the family (Brimblecombe et al, 1958). Recently, interest has been shown in the relationships between respiratory disease in parents and children. The use, in the parents, of the now widely accepted and well-validated questionnaire developed by the Medical Research Council's Committee on the Aetiology of Chronic Bronchitis (1960), allows a standardised assessment of the parents' respiratory symptoms. Two reports have shown that a close relationship exists between parents' and children's respiratory disease. One study demonstrated this association between parents and their school-age children (Colley, 1974), while the other between parents and preschool children (Colley, Holland and Corkhill, 1974). In the first of these studies the prevalence of chronic cough in the children was at a minimum of 13.5 per cent when both mother and father did not have winter morning phlegm, and at a maximum of 44.2 per cent when both parents reported phlegm. These associations persisted after due allowance was made for parental smoking habits, social class and family size. Several explanations for this association suggest themselves. Sharing of a similar, genetically determined susceptibility between parents and child could be one reason, as could the greater opportunity for transmission of respiratory infections from parents with respiratory disease to their children. Twin studies, involving assessment of the concordance in respiratory symptoms between monozygotic and dizygotic adult twin pairs is suggestive of a genetic influence (Cederlöf et al, 1967). However, there has as yet been no study of the influence of genetic factors in the relationship between parents' and children's respiratory experience.

A further aspect of these relationships has been the influence of parents' smoking habits. Adults who smoke have a higher prevalence of respiratory symptoms than those who are non-smokers; thus at least a part of the association between parents with respiratory symptoms and their children's respiratory experience will be this effect of parents' smoking. There remains, however, the possibility that children may inhale tobacco smoke generated when their parents smoke at home and thus suffer ill effects as a result. This potential effect was examined in children of school age and after allowing for the effects of parental phlegm, social class, and family size, no residual effect of such 'passive smoking' could be found (Colley, 1974). On the other hand in preschool children a quite definite effect upon the incidence of pneumonia and bronchitis was found (Colley et al, 1974). In this study infants with parents who did not have winter morning phlegm, and who were both non-smokers, had an incidence of pneumonia and bronchitis of 7.6 per cent in the first year of life, in contrast to an incidence of 15.2 per cent among infants when both parents smoked between them 25 or more cigarettes per day. No such effect was observed in the children over the age of one.

Harlap and Davies (1974), in a study of admissions to hospital for pneumonia and bronchitis in the first year of life, came to the same conclusions on the effects of passive smoking. They however only included the mother's smoking habits, and did not take account of parental respiratory symptoms and father's smoking habits. Thus the evidence points to the passive inhalation of tobacco smoke being associated with an increased risk of lower respiratory tract illness in the first year of life. In this context it is worth recalling that in children, only those under the age of one year appeared to show excess mortality during the 1952 London fog. The mechanism by which passive smoking effects the incidence of pneumonia and bronchitis is not known. It is possible that the infant's susceptibility to respiratory pathogens is in some way increased following exposure to tobacco smoke.

Smoking

The reports prepared by the Royal College of Physicians (1962) and the Surgeon General of the Public Health Service of the United States (1964) reviewed among other items the evidence linking smoking in the aetiology of chronic bronchitis in adults. The more recent report from the Royal College of Physicians (1970) further emphasised the role of smoking in this disease.

Smoking is not a habit that is confined to adults only, as Bewley, Day and Ide (1973) show in their review of the literature on smoking in children in Great Britain. A study of 10000 school children in Kent, by Holland and his co-workers, found children of secondary school age who were already regular smokers (Holland and Elliott, 1968). In addition, those who smoked had higher prevalence rates for cough and phlegm than children who did not smoke. In the following years some children gave up the habit and their prevalence of respiratory symptoms diminished. At the children's initial examination ventilatory function was measured and no differences were found in these measures between smokers, and non-smokers. Children who smoke usually do so at relatively low intensity, and will only have done so for a few years at the most. It is unlikely therefore that changes would have been produced in the respiratory tract sufficiently to cause more than very minor changes in ventilatory function.

Most of the earlier studies of children's smoking habits had been done on secondary school children. Bewley, Halil and Snaith (1973) reported a study of smoking habits and respiratory symptoms in 8682 10 and 11 year olds in Derbyshire. They found that 6.9 per cent of the boys and 2.6 per cent of the girls were regular smokers. As in studies on older children, those 10 and 11 year olds who smoked had a higher prevalence of respiratory symptoms than those who did not. For example 48 per cent of the boy smokers reported cough during the day or night in the winter, in comparison with 20 per cent in the non-smokers. These findings emphasise that even at primary school smoking can be a problem, and that effects upon the respiratory tract, as indicated by the presence of symptoms, may already be apparent.

It has been a consistent finding in the studies of secondary school children that boys have a higher prevalence of smoking than girls, and that they start earlier. The prevalence of smoking rises with age in both sexes, and up to 50 per cent of boys and 36 per cent of girls may be smoking by the age of 17. The pattern of smoking varies from school to school, but in general this seems to reflect more the background of the child, for example whether or not the parents smoke, than the features of the school.

Bewley et al (1973) concluded that antismoking campaigns directed at children had not been successful in deterring them from smoking. They also emphasised the complicated nature of the relationship between social environment and the psychological and social characteristics of the child smoker. It seems unlikely that any single action will have the desired effect in either persuading children not to start the habit or in those who already smoke to give up. The prevention or control of smoking are areas of research into which further resources need to be placed as the potential long-term benefits to health from not taking up the habit will be large.

LATE EFFECTS OF EARLY CHILDHOOD CHEST ILLNESS

It is often difficult to be sure that recovery from a chest illness has been complete. This is particularly the situation where young children have suffered such illnesses. This aspect can be investigated by comparing the prevalence of chest symptoms and ventilatory function in late childhood in those who did, and did not, suffer chest illnesses in early childhood. Where this has been studied, the child who suffered an early childhood chest illness is more likely to have chest symptoms and lower ventilatory function in later childhood than children who escape such illnesses. For example Colley and Reid (1970) found that primary school children who had a history of pneumonia or bronchitis in early childhood had a significantly higher chance of having winter cough than children who had not suffered such illnesses. Ventilatory function also differed. A combination of a history of bronchitis or pneumonia in early childhood and the presence of a current winter cough was associated with a mean peak expiratory flow rate of 213 litres/min. On the other hand children who neither had a history of bronchitis or pneumonia, nor a current winter cough, had a mean peak flow rate of 228 litres/min; these peak flow rates are significantly different $(0.02 > P > 0.01)$. Other studies in the United Kingdom, notably by Wahdan (1963), Lunn et al (1967), Holland et al (1969) and Bland, Holland and Elliott (1974), also found that children with a history of early childhood chest illness had significantly lower ventilatory function than children without such history. These studies indicate that the child with a history of lower respiratory tract illness is more likely to have lower ventilatory function and more respiratory symptoms than the child who escapes such illnesses.

DISEASE IN CHILDHOOD AND ADULT LIFE

There has been speculation for a number of years about the influence of events in childhood upon the later development of chronic respiratory disease in adult life (Reid, 1969). It is a common observation that, as chesty children grow up, many lose their proneness to chest illness. These observations match the patterns of mortality at different ages described earlier, where mortality is high in the first year of life and drops to a minimum in late childhood (Figs. 9.1 and 9.2). Also the age pattern of the prevalence of respiratory symptoms suggests that it is at its lowest in the older children. This trend might suggest that no excess risk would be present for these chesty children when they reach adult life for the development of chronic non-specific lung disease, i.e. chronic bronchitis.

The paediatrician's view of any link between childhood and adult disease may well be influenced both by being unable to continue observation of these children after they reach adolescence, and by selective referral of the more severe cases for his advice and treatment. In adult life, the chest physicians will tend to see those persons who already have moderately severe or even disabling respiratory disease, often already 40 to 50 years old. At this age there will be considerable uncertainty in obtaining reliable histories about events in childhood, such as whether or not attacks of pneumonia and bronchitis occurred, and at what age. Even where such histories can be obtained it may prove impossible to decide whether or not this reported early experience is any different from those persons of the same age who do not have chronic bronchitis. Due to the limitations inherent in both the paediatrician's and the chest physician's view, a purely clinical approach cannot resolve this issue. There is, however, epidemiological evidence that does suggest such a link between childhood and adult respiratory disease. It is worth spending time on this evidence, as the finding of such a link has implications for the general view we take of the importance of childhood chest disease.

The epidemiological evidence can be divided into that which is indirect, i.e. which stems from finding similar patterns of respiratory disease in children and adults, and direct, which involves following children's respiratory experience as they grow up and become adults.

The indirect evidence involves searching for similarities between the levels of respiratory disease in children and adults who live in similar social and environmental conditions. For example, in England and Wales in adults, there is a social class gradient for mortality from pneumonia and bronchitis. Mortality is lowest in social class I and rises steadily to a maximum in social class V. This pattern is similar to that found for mortality and morbidity from respiratory disease in children.

A similar match can be found, as Reid (1969) pointed out, between high mortality in infancy and middle age in urban areas, and lower mortality at these ages in rural areas. Colley and Reid (1970) compared the prevalence of cough in schoolchildren in five contrasting areas, with male adult bronchitis incapacity for work, and male and female bronchitis and pneumonia mortality rates in the same areas. They likewise found a consistent relationship between these measures of respiratory disease in children and adults.

The mortality in successive generations, noted earlier, also suggests that experience in infancy and early childhood determines the subsequent pattern of mortality. If mortality is high early in life, then this will also be the case in later life. Similarly, the associations between parents and children in their respiratory experience provide additional evidence of similarities between adults and children.

The evidence, thus far, is quite consistent with the hypothesis that children with a poor respiratory history grow up to be those with chronic respiratory disease in later life. However, this evidence only demonstrates associations between groups, whereas direct evidence is needed of individual children with respiratory disability growing up and developing chronic respiratory disease. There has been no study where this was done with a large enough population, or where follow-up extended long enough into adult life.

The study by Rosenbaum (1961) of young men who were called up for military service suggested that they take with them, when posted elsewhere in the country, the adverse effects of childhood environmental exposure. Those young men from industrial areas continued to show high rates of respiratory disease, even when removed from these areas.

Harnett and Mair (1963) chose to study adults who they had identified as attending in childhood the Mackenzie Institute of Clinical Research at St Andrews, Scotland, between 1920 and 1927. Examination of the case notes, which had been stored intact since that time, resulted in a group of 114 children being identified as having attended the Institute for recurrent bronchitis and repeated upper respiratory tract infections—and called catarrhal children. At the same time a matched control group was obtained by drawing case notes for those children who did not have such histories, and a total of 181 children was so identified. Harnett and Mair then attempted, in 1961 and 1962, to contact these individuals, some 30 to 40 years after their original attendance. Out of the original group they were able to contact and interview 47 per cent. The interview involved administration of the MRC questionnaire on respiratory symptoms (1960) and measurement of ventilatory function. The findings were suggestive that the catarrhal group had a higher prevalence of respiratory symptoms as adults than the controls, although there were no differences in ventilatory function. However, the catarrhal group had a higher proportion of males, and smokers. The small size of the study did not permit an adequate investigation of these and other factors which can influence respiratory symptoms in adult life. In addition the majority of those seen were under the age of 40 at the time, and this may have been too early for gross differences between the catarrhal and control groups to be apparent.

The thousand families study in Newcastle upon Tyne, where 1000 infants born in 1946 have been followed up, provides evidence for a link between early and middle childhood experience and that at the age of 15 years (Miller et al, 1974). These workers identified a group of 205 children who suffered a large number of respiratory illnesses in the first 10 years of life, and a group of 95 who had an average number of such illnesses. At the age of 15 some 13 per cent of the control children had chronic respiratory symptoms compared with 52 per cent in those with the poor respiratory experience under the age at 10. These findings strongly suggest that respiratory disability can persist into later childhood in a substantial proportion of chesty children.

The final source of data is provided by the follow-up of the 1946 national birth cohort. These individuals as already noted in an earlier section were contacted when they were aged 20 and enquiry was made about the presence of respiratory symptoms and smoking habits, using the MRC symptom questionnaire (1960). By linking the previously documented history of chest illness under the age of two years with chest symptoms and smoking habits at age 20, the influence of the early chest illnesses could be assessed (Colley et al, 1973). Among non-smokers at 20, a history of one or more chest illnesses under the age of two was associated with a prevalence of cough of 9.1 per cent, in non-smokers who escaped such illnesses the prevalence of 5.2 per cent. The corresponding prevalence rates for those smoking at age 20 were 16.5 per cent and 13.7 per cent. It proved possible to analyse these data in more detail, and the major influence at age 20 on respiratory symptoms was found to be the smoking habits, and to a smaller extent early childhood chest illness, both having a statistically significant effect. Social class and past exposure to air pollution had only a small and statistically non-significant effect. These 20 year olds have been followed to age 25 and the questionnaire reapplied (Kiernan et al, 1975). The findings at age 25 are substantially the same except that the effects seen at age 20 are accentuated and the influence of father's occupation now reaches statistical significance.

The findings from this study, taken with the other evidence, seem to have established the link between early childhood respiratory experience and respiratory disability in early adult life. The apparent increase in the effect of these early illnesses upon chest symptoms between the age of 20 and 25 makes it more likely that, as the cohort ages, these effects will be further accentuated. If this is the case, then we may reasonably expect that those with chest symptoms in their early 20s will be most likely to develop chronic lung disease in middle adult life. The social background in childhood, as was emphasised earlier, is a dominant factor in determining the experience of respiratory disease during the childhood years. It is of some interest to find that there are residual effects of such childhood social class background at the age of 25.

ASTHMA

This remains one of the major chronic respiratory tract disorders in childhood. Although the incidence of asthma is not high in comparison with other lower respiratory tract illnesses it nevertheless has an appreciable mortality and may cause considerable disability and permanent respiratory impairment.

9

Definitions

Investigation of the epidemiology of this condition in children, as in adults, has been bedevilled by problems of definition. This remains an impediment to epidemiological studies of this condition. In the investigation of respiratory diseases in general epidemiologists, as already noted, have usually attempted to develop methods that employ recognition of symptoms and abnormalities of function rather than use diagnostic labels, for it often proves impossible to obtain agreement on these. The Ciba Guest Symposium (1959) in discussing the definition of chronic non-specific lung diseases concluded that 'Asthma refers to the condition of subjects with widespread narrowing of the bronchial airways, which changes its severity over short periods of time either spon- taneously or under treatment . . .'. This functional definition was not wholly acceptable and a recently convened Ciba Foundation Study Group (1971) attempted to resolve this problem. However, the group failed to agree on a definition of asthma. These continuing problems of definition are a hinderance to the adequate comparisons of the findings of different epidemiological studies of asthma.

The problems in defining asthma are further complicated by the consider- able group of children who have had one or more episodes of wheezing, yet do not develop frank asthma. There appears to be a spectrum of illness consisting of children who may have only a single episode of wheezing, to children who have several attacks of wheezing which may or may not be labelled asthma, and finally, a group of children with undoubted severe and disabling asthma. It is within the intermediate group that most disagreements about whether or not a child has asthma are likely to arise. As will be seen later the lack of agreement on the definition of asthma may contribute to the apparent differences in prevalence of asthma found in some of the studies of this condition.

Prevalence of Asthma

International comparisons

It may be no surprise to find differences between studies in their prevalence of asthma. Logan and Cushion (1958), in their study of morbidity in general practices in England and Wales, report 1.23 per cent of boys and 0.6 per cent of girls under 15 years with asthma. These rates may underestimate the population prevalence as they were based entirely upon children who attended the general practitioner. Studies on schoolchildren, as they are usually accessible and representative of children of this age, have been the main source of information on asthma prevalence. In Birmingham in the United Kingdom, Morrison Smith (1961) obtained a prevalence of asthma in 5 to 15 year olds of 2.3 per cent among boys and 1.8 per cent in girls. A study in the Isle of Wight (Graham et al, 1967) of 9 to 11 year olds yielded an overall prevalence rate of 2.0 per cent. In Aberdeen, Scotland (Dawson et al, 1969), an overall prevalence rate of 4.8 per cent was found in 10 to 15 year olds, and a ratio of 2.2 boys to each girl. These three studies employed different methods for the primary identification of cases, and this may in part account for any lack of agreement in their findings.

Two studies in Scandinavia reported rather lower rates. In Sweden, Kraepelien (1954) found a prevalence of 1.4 per cent in 7 to 14 year olds in Stockholm, while in Finland, Peltonen, Kasanen and Peltonen (1955) found a prevalence of 0.85 per cent in children. Williams and McNicol (1969) report that among 10 year olds in Melbourne, Australia, 3.7 per cent had unequivocal asthma. However, they also identified a further group, 7.7 per cent of their population, who at some time had asthma or asthmatic bronchitis diagnosed by their doctor, giving an overall prevalence of 11.4 per cent. A rather similar finding was reported from Tecumseh, Michigan, by Broder, Barlow and Horton (1962), where cumulative overall prevalence (which included children who at any time in their life had definite asthma and also those in whom the diagnosis was less certain) was 14.4 per cent in six to nine year olds, and 12.1 per cent in 10 to 14 year olds.

Unfortunately there are no simple ways to establish whether these international differences in prevalence of asthma are, as seems likely, mainly due to differences in definitions and methods, or whether the disease truly varies in prevalence from place to place. If such true variations are found they may provide important clues to aetiological factors, in particular to environmental effects.

Age and sex

The prevalence of asthma is higher in younger children (Morrison Smith, 1961), and this is consistent with the clinical observation that the onset of asthma is more often in the preschool age group and that a large proportion lose their symptoms before puberty. Gordis (1973) reviews the evidence on age of onset and concludes that well over half of those who develop asthma in childhood do so before the age of five years.

A puzzling finding in asthma has been the unequal sex ratio. Those studies that report prevalence rates for the sexes separately show a male predominance (Gordis, 1973). It is unlikely that differential reporting or ascertainment of asthma in these field studies can adequately explain the sex differences. There is no reason to suppose that girls with asthma are less often referred to doctors than boys, or that doctors are more reluctant to make the diagnosis in girls. The conclusion must therefore be that the condition affects boys more than girls. There is also evidence that boys tend to suffer a more severe form of asthma than girls. The reasons for the sex difference in asthma are obscure.

Social class

There is a widespread clinical impression that asthma affects children from higher social classes more than those from low social class. As already discussed in relation to other respiratory diseases, social class gradients have been a prominent feature of childhood morbidity and mortality in the United Kingdom. In the study by Graham et al (1967) a higher prevalence of asthma was found in children in social classes I and II, than in IV and V; a gradient in the opposite direction to that for other respiratory diseases. They considered various sources of bias that might produce this finding, but concluded that these were unlikely to have resulted in these social class gradients. However, the information on asthma that they used came substantially from school medical records, and as working class mothers seem to attend school medical examinations less frequently than do middle class mothers, under-reporting of asthma in lower social classes may have occurred.

General practice consultation rates for asthma show a similar social class gradient to that observed by Graham et al (1967). Logan (1960) reports consultation rates for asthma in children under 14 years old, at 9.4 per 1000 for social class I, and 5.6 per 1000 for social class V.

In contrast Dawson et al (1969) in their study in Aberdeen found quite the opposite pattern. There was an excess of asthmatic children in families of manual workers in comparison with families of non-manual workers, although these differences were not statistically significant. A study in Vancouver, Canada, found no relationship between socio-economic group and asthma (Robinson et al, 1967).

In view of the uncertainties about whether or not true differences in asthma prevalence exist in the population between the social classes, it would be wise to refrain at present from speculation on probable reasons for any such differences. This is one aspect of the epidemiology of asthma that needs further study.

Area

Contrasts between the prevalence in urban and rural areas, as noted earlier, may provide clues to the influence of urban factors, such as air pollution. This is an aspect of the epidemiology of asthma in childhood that has so far been largely ignored. There is an absence of mortality data on asthma in urban and rural areas, although general practice consultation rates (Logan and Cushion, 1958) in urban and rural areas suggest that these are lowest in rural areas. Such differences are not easy to interpret, as they may reflect, for example, poor rural transport facilities, rather than the disease being less common. As with social class, possible area differences in the prevalence of asthma await further epidemiological investigation.

Natural history

In several studies asthmatic children have been followed up to see what eventually happens to their asthma. As Gordis (1973) points out in his review, due to differences in the composition of these groups of children in respect of age, treatment and length of follow-up, some clear statement on the natural history of childhood asthma is not possible, although it does seem that the majority eventually lose their asthma. A further problem is that for many of these studies the asthmatic children were identified after attendance at hospital clinics. As it is probable that those with more severe asthma will attend such clinics, overall outcome may appear worse than it really is. The only wholly satisfactory method to study the natural history of asthma, and of those factors that influence prognosis is by means of longitudinal studies on asthmatics derived from well-defined populations.

Treatment

As with other respiratory illnesses, doubts have been expressed on the adequacy of treatment of asthma in children. The rise in mortality from asthma in some countries, possibly as a result of misuse of bronchodilators, serves to underline this point. As well as inappropriate there is evidence that some asthmatic children may not receive sufficient treatment. McNicol and Williams (1973), in particular, considered that some of the most severely affected children had been given totally inadequate treatment. They thought that this resulted from doctors and parents often not appreciating the severity of the illness. It is difficult to escape the conclusion that such deficiencies primarily arise due to lack of adequate instruction, at undergraduate and postgraduate level, in what is after all a fairly common chronic respiratory disorder in children.

The house-dust mite, *Dermatophagoides pteronyssinus*, has now been implicated as probably the single most important cause of the allergenicity of house dust (*Lancet*, 1974). This assumes importance when it is realised that house-dust sensitivity is thought to be the commonest cause of allergic asthma. Recently interest has been growing in the feasibility of assisting allergic subjects to avoid contact with the mite and its products. The bedroom and especially the mattress, appear to be the major breeding area and source of mites. The apparent improvements seen in asthmatics after antimite measures suggest that this may be a useful line of treatment. For example, Sarsfield et al (1974), observed the effects on mite-sensitive asthmatic children, among other procedures, of covering the mattress with a plastic jacket as a means of limiting contact with mites. They report improvements in symptoms as a result of these measures. However encouraging these results may appear some caution is needed in their interpretation. In this study no controls were available to assess the relevance of treatment to the improvements in symptoms. Also the number of asthmatics studied was small and follow-up limited. There does seem to be a need for a more rigorous evaluation of this form of mite avoidance in the management of asthma.

Relationship Between Asthma and Bronchitis

Comments are often made that the bronchitic and pneumonic episodes recorded by parents in epidemiological field surveys may in reality be episodes of asthma or asthma-like illnesses. There is a certain amount of evidence to suggest that this is not the case. These two groups of disorders do not have a similar frequency, in that cumulative prevalence rates for asthma, which vary from as low as 0.6 per cent to as high as 11 to 14 per cent, are substantially less than those rates reported for past bronchitis. For example Colley and Reid (1970) found 18 to 25 per cent of primary schoolchildren with a history of past bronchitis. The social class pattern, as already noted, is not the same in these two disorders. While a consistent excess of bronchitis and other indices of respiratory disease are found in the lower social classes, asthma has no social class gradient or the gradient is in the opposite direction.

Bronchitis has a higher prevalence in urban than rural areas, after due allowance has been made for differences in social class (Colley and Reid, 1970). As noted earlier there is little firm evidence on the distribution of asthma in urban and rural children. The evidence, such as it is, suggests that asthma may be more prevalent in rural than urban children.

The seasonal distribution of asthmatic attacks suggests a peak in the late summer and early autumn (Gordis, 1973), and this matches the peaks in asthma mortality reported by Inman and Adelstein (1969). In contrast, as Inman and Adelstein (1969) noted, other respiratory diseases show a rise in mortality during the last quarter of the year and reach a peak in the first quarter of the following year.

The evidence therefore, as far as it goes, does suggest that all or a major proportion of those illnesses reported in epidemiological studies as being bronchitis, are not, as some think, asthmatic episodes.

PREVENTION AND CONTROL

Environmental and Social Factors

As things stand at present it is necessary that children be exposed to common respiratory infections so that general and specific immunity to such infections can be acquired. Apart from immunisation against pertussis and to a lesser extent influenza, there are no other common respiratory pathogens for which protection can be readily provided by immunisation. Thus prevention of respiratory infections is not usually possible. In these circumstances attempts to limit a child's exposure to pathogens, to ensure that massive and frequent exposure does not occur, would seem a sensible objective.

Some of the studies already cited suggested that exposure to respiratory infections is substantially determined by environmental circumstances, for example, by overcrowding. Here it may be possible to effect a change in crowding by moving the family to a larger dwelling. However, such a move could not be guaranteed to change the subsequent respiratory experience of the children. It is one thing to identify factors that are associated with a higher prevalence, or incidence, of respiratory disease, and another to assume that by changing exposure to such factors the levels of respiratory disease will also change. This might or might not happen and will depend in part on whether the associations indicate a causal relationship between the factor and respiratory disease. Where such associations are thought to be causal, changes in the factor might reasonably be expected to result in a change in respiratory disease.

There is more than an impression that as the general, social and economic circumstances of life improve, so the severity and possible incidence of respiratory infections fall. For these reasons it might be worth considering the active manipulation of one or two of the environmental factors that appear to have powerful associations with respiratory disease, to see if reductions in respiratory disease incidence and severity of illness follow. It is essential, as with the introduction of new drugs or treatments, to test in a rigorous manner whether or not such active environmental changes do in fact alter the subsequent pattern of illness. The only wholly satisfactory way of doing this is to conduct randomised controlled trials. For example improved house heating by installing central heating might be considered a reasonable step to reduce the impact of respiratory disease. In conducting such a trial, families, all of whom would be living in non-centrally heated houses, would be randomly allocated either to having central heating installed or keeping their existing heating. The randomisation would ensure, as far as possible, that the two groups are comparable at the start of the study in all important respects; both groups would then be observed for an appropriate period of time and respiratory illnesses documented. At the end of the observation period the number of illnesses in the two groups would be compared and on the basis of any differences observed conclusions could be drawn on the effect, or lack of effect as the case may be, of the change in house heating.

There have been no adequate controlled trials on any aspect of domestic environmental changes, and it might be worth considering what could be done, and whether this would be sensible. There is little doubt from the studies already reviewed that poor social conditions have a major effect on the respiratory experience of children. Domestic overcrowding, large families, low social class, living in urban areas, have all been shown to have independent effects on respiratory disease. Improvements in the domestic environment could reasonably be expected to confer benefit not limited only to respiratory diseases, but maybe also, for example, to behaviour problems. It could be argued that adequate housing is a fundamental right and thus an adequate reason, quite apart from any medical indications, for improving the housing of those living in poor domestic circumstances. For this reason it may be doubted whether there it is worth the effort to rigorously test the effects on health of improvement in the physical aspects of the domestic environment, as these changes will hopefully occur in the absence of evidence of their necessity for better health.

There remains a considerable lack of information on the relation of domestic microenvironment to the spread and severity of respiratory illnesses. This has recently become, as already noted, of particular importance in relation to the role of mites in the natural history of asthma.

Investigations need to be conducted into the precise role in respiratory disease of different methods of domestic heating in relation to, for example, temperature levels, changes in temperature, humidity and indoor air pollution. Such studies have greater priority within the United Kingdom as, in comparison with other Western European countries, domestic heating is often inadequate. As noted earlier, the apparent excess of respiratory mortality in the United Kingdom is unexplained, and it may in part be a result of these inadequacies in domestic heating in comparison with other countries of similar socio-economic level.

Air pollution, both acute exposure to very high levels and long-term exposure to low levels, has been shown to influence chest illness in children. The feasibility and acceptability on economic grounds of reducing air pollution has been amply demonstrated in the United Kingdom. There can be little excuse for failing to take action when air pollution levels are still unacceptably high, and continuing efforts at national and local level will be needed to ensure reduction in air pollution is achieved, and maintained.

Parental Chest Illness and Smoking

Turning to other areas for preventive action, that related to parental chest symptoms and smoking stands out as not only important in the size of their effects on children's respiratory experience, but also as being potentially amenable to change. The effects of passive smoking by infants in their first year of life on incidence of chest illness suggests that parents who smoke should at least not do this in the presence of their infant, and at best should not smoke at all. The evidence implicating cigarette smoking in the aetiology of lung cancer and chronic non-specific lung disease in adults is so overwhelming that for this reason alone parents could be advised to give up smoking. It is likely that those smokers who have respiratory symptoms, such as cough and phlegm, will, if they give up the habit, notice a lessening in symptoms. If the major reason for the association between parents' chest symptoms and their children's respiratory experience is the ready transfer of respiratory infections from parent to child, then ceasing to smoke could reasonably be expected to result in fewer infections being transmitted from parent to child. A further and longer term benefit of parents ceasing permanently to smoke, is the possible lesser chance of the child taking up the habit. It is doubtful whether we need to test whether when parents give up smoking, this reduces the risk of chest illness in their children. Such a study would not be easy to conduct and resources might be more usefully employed in investigating ways of persuading parents and older children not to smoke. Taking a long-term view, such efforts to persuade children not to smoke, if successful, will have substantial benefits in lessening the chance of development of chronic nonspecific lung disease when they reach adult life and may, in addition, result in their children in turn having fewer chest illnesses. Smoking stands out as one of the major factors in the evolution of chronic respiratory disease and as such merits considerable efforts on the part of clinicians, and paediatricians in particular, to persuade the general public, as well as parents, not to smoke.

Use of Health Services

Data on hospital admissions and discharges, and general practice consultations, provide measures of the use being made of these services. They cannot, however, provide information on children who require medical care, yet are not taken either to their general practitioner or to hospital. The 1000 families' study (Miller et al, 1974) indicated that a large proportion of illnesses in the preschool years received no medical help. They found, for example, that 42 per cent of all recorded episodes of illness did not receive medical help or supervision, and these illnesses included one in five attacks of bronchitis and pneumonia occurring in children under one year old. That parents sometimes do not seek help for potentially serious chest illnesses indicates a need for education in this aspect of child care.

Management of Respiratory Illnesses

There is a widespread suspicion that these illnesses are not always adequately treated by doctors involved in primary medical care. In view of the link between respiratory disease in childhood and early adult life, the effective management of these illnesses takes on a further importance, as adequate and early treatment may minimise the degree of pulmonary damage these illnesses cause. This is one aspect of childhood respiratory disease that has not yet been adequately studied. As a start, the interval between onset of chest illness and the first contact with a doctor could be investigated to discover if delay in seeking treatment is widespread, and what the characteristics of such families are, and the reasons for such delay. A further aspect involves the adequacy of treatment given by the doctor. It is said, and again evidence to support this opinion is incomplete, that due to deficiencies in undergraduate and postgraduate training in child health, doctors may not always correctly diagnose respiratory illness in young children and thus give inappropriate or no treatment. There is an impression that antibiotics are often used in these illnesses at incorrect dosages and for a duration either too short or too long. Miller et al (1974) comment that they suspected many children were receiving chemotherapy at too small a dose for too short a time. In addition they found that in children with otorrhoea, many received no chemotherapy at all.

For those illnesses with an allergic component, treatments such as hyposensitisation often tend to be overprescribed, follow inadequate investigation, and use unsatisfactorily refined allergens. In this context, the recent epidemic of deaths in asthmatic children is an example of the need for the continuous monitoring of vital statistics to detect changes in mortality at an early stage, so that appropriate action may be taken quickly.

REFERENCES

Armitage, P., Blendis, L. M. & Smyllie, H. C. (1966) The measurement of observer disagreement in the recording of signs. *Journal of the Royal Statistical Society, Series A,* **129,** 98–109.

Bewley, B. R., Day, I. & Ide, L. (1973) *Smoking by Children in Great Britain. A Review of the Literature.* London: Social Science Research Council and Medical Research Council.

Bewley, B. R., Halil, T. & Snaith, A. H. (1973) Smoking by primary schoolchildren: prevalence and associated respiratory symptoms. *British Journal of Preventive and Social Medicine,* **27,** 150–153.

Bland, J. M., Holland, W. W. & Elliott, A. (1974) The development of respiratory symptoms in a cohort of Kent schoolchildren. *Bulletin Physio-pathologie Respiratoire,* **10,** 699–716.

Brimblecombe, F. S. W., Cruickshank, R., Masters, P. L., Reid, D. D., Stewart, G. T. & Sanderson, D. (1958) Family studies of respiratory infections. *British Medical Journal,* **1,** 119–128.

Broder, I., Barlow, P. P. & Horton, R. J. M. (1962) The epidemiology of asthma and hayfever in a total community, Tecumseh, Michigan. I. Description of study and general findings. *Joutnal of Allergy,* **33,** 513–523.

Case, R. A. M., Coghill, C. & Harley, J. L. (1968) *Death rates for 1956–1960 and 1961–1965. Supplement to death rates by age and sex for tuberculosis and selected respiratory diseases, England and Wales, 1911–1955,* by R. A. M. Case, & Joyce L. Harley (1958). The Chester Beatty Research Institute, London.

Case, R. A. M. & Harley, J. L. (1958) *Death rates by age and sex for tuberculosis and selected respiratory diseases, England and Wales,* 1911–1955. The Chester Beatty Research Institute, London.

Cederlöf, R., Edfers, M. L., Friberg, L. & Jonsson, E. (1967) Hereditary factors, 'spontaneous cough' and 'smoker's cough'. A study on 7800 twin-pairs with the aid of mailed questionnaires. *Archives of Environmental Health,* **14,** 401–406.

Ciba Guest Sympsoium (1959) Terminology definitions and classification of chronic pulmonary Emphysema and related conditions. *Thorax,* **14,** 286–299.

Ciba Foundation Study Group No. 38 (1971) *Identification of Asthma,* ed. Porter, R. & Birch, J. Edinbrugh: Churchill Livingstone.

Colley, J. R. T. (1971) Respiratory disease in childhood. *British Medical Bulletin,* **27,** 9–14.

Colley, J. R. T. (1974) Respiratory symptoms in children and parental smoking and phlegm production. *British Medical Journal,* **2,** 201–204.

Colley, J. R. T. & Reid, D. D. (1970) Urban and social origins of childhood bronchitis in England and Wales. *British Medical Journal,* **2,** 213–217.

Colley, J. R. T., Douglas, J. W. B. & Reid, D. D. (1973) Respiratory disease in young adults: influence of early childhood lower respiratory tract illness, social class, air pollution and smoking. *British Medical Journal,* **3,** 195–198.

Colley, J. R. T., Holland, W. W. & Corkhill, R. T. (1974) Influence of passive smoking and parental phlegm on pneumonia and bronchitis in early childhood. *Lancet,* **2,** 1031–1034.

Collins, J. J., Kasap, H. S. & Holland, W. W. (1971) Environmental factors in child mortality in England and Wales. *American Journal of Epidemiology,* **93,** 10–22.

Dawson, B., Horobin, G., Illsley, R. & Mitchell, R. (1969) A survey of childhood asthma in Aberdeen. *Lancet,* **1,** 827–830.

Douglas, J. W. B. & Blomfield, J. M. (1958) *Children Under Five*. London: Allen and Unwin.

Douglas, J. W. B. & Waller, R. E. (1966) Air pollution and respiratory infection in children. *British Journal of Preventive and Social Medicine*, **20**, 1–8.

Gordis, L. (1973) *Epidemiology of Chronic Lung Diseases in Children*, Ch. 2. Baltimore and London: The Johns Hopkins University Press.

Graham, P. J., Rutter, M. L., Yule, W. & Pless, I. B. (1967) Childhood asthma: a psycho-somatic disorder? Some epidemiological considerations. *British Journal of Preventive and Social Medicine*, **2**, 78–85.

Grundy, F. & Lewis-Faning, E. ed. (1957) *Morbidity and Mortality in the First Year of Life: a Field Enquiry in Fifteen Areas of England and Wales*. London: The Eugenics Society.

Harlap, S. & Davies, A. M. (1974) Infant admissions to hospital and maternal smoking. *Lancet*, **1**, 529–532.

Harnett, R. W. F. & Mair, A. (1963) Chronic bronchitis and the catarrhal child. *Scottish Medical Journal*, **8**, 175–184.

Heady, J. A. & Heasman, M. A. (1959) *Social and Biological Factors in Infant Mortality*. Studies on Medical and Population Subjects, No. 15. London: HMSO.

Holland, W. W. & Elliott, A. (1968) Cigarette smoking, respiratory symptoms, and anti-smoking propaganda: an experiment. *Lancet*, **1**, 41–43.

Holland, W. W., Halil, T., Bennett, A. E. & Elliott, A. (1969) Factors influencing the onset of chronic respiratory disease. *British Medical Journal*, **2**, 205–208.

Inman, W. H. W. & Adelstein, A. M. (1969) Rise and fall of asthma mortality in England and Wales in relation to use of pressurised aerosols. *Lancet*, **2**, 279–285.

Kiernan, K., Colley, J. R. T., Douglas, J. W. B. & Reid, D. D. (1975) Chronic cough in young adults in relation to smoking habits, childhood environment and chest illness. *Respiration* (in press).

Kraepelian, S. (1954) The frequency of bronchial asthma in Swedish school children. *Acta pediatrica*, Suppl., **100**, 149–153.

Lee, J. A. H. (1957) Chronic otitis media among a sample of young men. *Journal of Laryngology and Otology*, **71**, 398–404.

Logan, W. P. D. (1953) Mortality in the London fog incident, 1952. *Lancet*, **1**, 336–338.

Logan, W. P. D. (1960) *Morbidity Statistics from General Practice*, Vol. 2. Studies on Medical and Population Subjects, No. 14. London: HMSO.

Logan, W. P. D. & Cushion, A. A. (1958) *Morbidity Statistics from General Practice*, Vol. 1. Studies on Medical and Population Subjects, No. 14. London: HMSO.

Lunn, J. E., Knowelden, J. & Handyside, A. J. (1967) Patterns of respiratory illness in Sheffield infant schoolchildren. *British Journal of Preventive and Social Medicine*, **21**, 7–16.

Lunn, J. E., Knowelden, J. & Roe, J. W. (1970) Patterns of respiratory illness in Sheffield junior schoolchildren. A follow-up study. *British Journal of Preventive and Social Medicine*, **24**, 223–228.

McNichol, K. N. & Williams, H. B. (1973) Spectrum of asthma in children. 1. Clinical and physiological components. *British Medical Journal*, **4**, 7–11.

Medical Research Council. Committee on the Aetiology of Chronic Bronchitis (1960) Standardised questionnaires on respiratory symptoms. *British Medical Journal*, **2**, 1665.

Miller, F. J. W., Court, S. D. M., Walton, W. S. & Knox, E. G. (1960) *Growing Up in Newcastle upon Tyne: a Continuing Study of Health and Illness in Young Children Within Their Families*. London: Oxford University Press.

Miller, F. J. W., Court, S. D. M., Knox, E. G. & Brandon, S. (1974) *The School Years in Newcastle upon Tyne*. London: Oxford University Press.

Morrison Smith, J. (1961) Prevalence and natural history of asthma in schoolchildren. *British Medical Journal*, **1**, 711–713.

Office of Population Censuses and Surveys (1970) *Classification of Occupations, 1970*. London: HMSO.

Payling Wright, G. & Payling Wright, H. (1945) Etiological factors in bronchopneumonia amongst infants in London. *Journal of Hygiene, Cambridge*, **44**, 15–30.

Peltonen, M.-L., Kasanen, A. & Peltonen, T. E. (1955) Occurrence of allergic conditions in schoolchildren. *Annales Paediatriae Fenniae*, **1**, 119–129.

Reid, D. D. (1969) The beginnings of bronchitis. *Proceedings of the Royal Society of Medicine*, **26**, 1–6.

Robinson, G. C., Anderson, D. O., Moghadam, H. K., Cambon, K. G. & Murray, A. B. (1967) A survey of hearing loss in Vancouver school children: Part 1. Methodology and prevalence. *Canadian Medical Association Journal*, **97,** 1199–1207.

Rosenbaum, S. (1961) Home localities of national servicemen with respiratory disease. *British Journal of Preventive and Social Medicine*, **15,** 61–67.

Royal College of Physicians of London (1962) *Smoking and Health*. London: Pitman Medical.

Royal College of Physicians of London (1970) *Air Pollution and Health*. London: Pitman Medical.

Sarsfield, J. K., Gowland, G., Toy, R. & Norman, A. L. E. (1974) Mite-sensitive asthma of childhood. Trial of avoidance measures. *Archives of Disease in Childhood*, **49,** 716–721.

Toyama, T. (1964) Air pollution and its health effects in Japan. *Archives of Environmental Health*, **8,** 153–173.

United States Public Health Service (1964) *Smoking and Health*. Report of the Advisory Committee to the Surgeon General of the Public Health Service. Public Health Service Publication No. 1103.

Wahdan, M. H. M. E. H. (1963) *Atmospheric pollution and other environmental factors in respiratory disease of children*. Thesis for Ph.D. degree, University of London.

Waller, R. E., Brooks, A. G. F. & Adler, M. W. (1975) Respiratory symptoms and ventilatory capacity in a cohort of Londoners from 1952–53. In *Proceedings of an International Symposium on Recent Advances in the Assessment of the Health Effects of Environmental Pollution*. Paris (in press).

Williams, H. & McNicol, K. N. (1969) Prevalence, natural history, and relationship of wheezy bronchitis and asthma in children. Epidemiological study. *British Medical Journal*, **4,** 321–325.

World Health Organisation, Regional Office for Europe (1974) *Respiratory Disease in Europe. Report on a Study*. Copenhagen: WHO.

10
MANAGEMENT AND PROGNOSIS OF RENAL DISEASE IN CHILDHOOD
Glomerulonephritis

C. Chantler

It is hoped that this chapter will help the paediatrician to decide the safest and most economical way to investigate the child with renal disease and to determine treatment. The intention has been to cover a wide field and therefore only the necessary discussion of pathogenesis, classification and fundamental research is included. Some selection has been necessary and only those conditions which are usually managed in a general paediatric service rather than a nephrology unit are included. Prognosis is always important in the communication with the family and such information, wherever possible, is included. The technology available to diagnose and treat the child with renal disease has increased considerably over the last few years and it is expensive. Electron microscopy and immunofluorescent studies of renal biopsy material, dynamic renal scintillography using the gamma camera, ultrasonography and haemodialysis are examples. The management of a child may require his transfer to a unit where these facilities are available. The decision to effect this transfer must take account of other factors which only the paediatrician can evaluate, and it is hoped that the knowledge of what is available and might be achieved will help him to decide. The establishment of centres specialising in paediatric nephrology means a change in patterns of care. Good communication between the centre and the area it serves is essential. Every attempt must be made to ameliorate the financial burden sustained by families whose children are transferred to regional centres for treatment.

GLOMERULONEPHRITIS

The child with glomerular disease is likely to present in one of the following seven ways: acute nephritic syndrome, nephrotic syndrome, haematuria and proteinuria, haematuria, proteinuria, acute renal failure or chronic renal failure. Unfortunately knowledge of presentation does not enable the renal pathology to be predicted (Table 10.1) and the prognosis appears to be more related to the histological classification (White, 1970) than to the clinical syndrome. Much experimental work concerning the pathogenic mechanisms of glomerulonephritis has been done over the last decade (Dixon and Wilson, 1972) but the specific aetiology of these conditions is usually not known and therefore a clinical classification is useful; it implies no assumptions about aetiology.

Table 10.1   Clinical and pathological correlations in children with glomerulonephritis

	Acute nephritic syndrome	Nephrotic syndrome	Haematuria	Proteinuria	Haematuria proteinuria
Minimal change	−	+ + +	+ +	+ + +	±
Proliferative:					
Mesangial	+ +	+ +	+ +	+ +	+ +
Mesangiocapillary	+ +	+ +	−	−	+ +
Extracapillary	+ +	+ +	−	−	+
Acute exudative	+ + +	+	−	−	+ +
Endo-extra capillary					
sclerosing	+ +	+ +	−	−	+
Membranous	−	+ +	−	+	+
Focal proliferative	+	+	+ +	+	+
Focal sclerosis	−	+ +	−	+ +	+

Acute Nephritic Syndrome (AGNS)

The typical syndrome comprises the sudden onset of oliguria, haematuria, proteinuria, reduced glomerular filtration rate (GFR), oedema and hypertension. However, the disease may be mild and be manifest by the presence of haematuria only. In poststreptococcal AGNS only a minority of affected children have symptoms (Dodge, Spargo and Travis, 1967). Evidence of a previous streptococcal infection should be sought, for the prognosis is good in poststreptococcal disease, whereas this is not necessarily so in other cases. Various serotypes of group A beta-haemolytic streptococci have been implicated (Travis et al, 1973) and some strains do not stimulate an immediate antibody response to streptolysin, so that other antibodies, such as anti-hydaluronidase, and antideoxyribonuclease B should be looked for if the antistreptolysin titre is normal. Serum C3 complement activity is depressed in nearly all children with poststreptococcal nephritis but usually returns to normal within 12 weeks. Some children with poststreptococcal AGNS continue to have low C3 levels for up to four years after the illness (Popovic-Rolovic, 1973), although this is unusual and suggests the possibility of mesangiocapillary or lupus nephritis. Final confirmation of poststreptococcal aetiology may depend on finding the typical histological appearances at renal biopsy (Travis et al, 1973). Where strict criteria for accepting a streptococcal aetiology are adopted poststreptococcal AGNS accounts for about 60 per cent of all cases of sporadic AGNS in Texas (Travis et al, 1973) and about

32 per cent in Illinois, USA (Lewy et al, 1971). Recently Meadow (1975) found that the streptococcus was implicated in a third of the patients with AGNS in Leeds. It may well be that the pattern of the disease is changing for AGNS may be seen with other infections (Table 10.2). Many of these non-streptococcal infections produce an acute exudative inflammation and presumably the prognosis is similar to streptococcal AGNS though this is not certain. Table 10.1 shows the other histological appearances associated with AGNS; various appearances may be found apart from the acute exudative lesion characteristic of poststreptococcal AGNS. These renal lesions of unknown aetiology have differing prognoses.

Table 10.2   Causes of acute nephritic syndrome

Beta-haemolytic streptococcus	
Other bacteria	Pneumococcus, staphylococcus, non-haemolytic streptococcus, secondary syphilis
Viruses	Mumps, ECHO, EB, influenza, varicella, hepatitis, virus B (Australia antigen)
Glomerulonephritis of unknown aetiology	Rapidly progressive, mesangiocapillary, mesangial proliferative, focal proliferative, IgA mesangial disease, interstitial nephritis
Multisystem disease	Henoch–Schonlein, systemic lupus polyarteritis, Wegener's granuloma, Goodpasture's syndrome, subacute bacterial endocarditis
Drugs	Phenylindanedione, phenylbutazone (vasculitis) penicillin (interstitial nephritis)

Management

When the only manifestation is haematuria other causes of bleeding must be excluded. A 10-day course of a suitable antibiotic, usually penicillin, is given to eradicate streptococcal infection. If there is evidence of fluid overload or a raised blood pressure or if there is oliguria, the child should be admitted to hospital. The plasma creatinine should be measured as an index of glomerular filtration rate (GFR) at the start of the illness and checked sequentially to monitor progress. There is no specific treatment which is effective in AGNS and steroids and immunosuppressive drugs are not indicated. Steroids by increasing salt retention are dangerous. Bed rest is reasonable during the acute stage of the illness until the fluid overload has subsided. Long-term bed rest is not useful and does not effect the eventual outcome (Joseph and Polani, 1958). Some exacerbation of haematuria after exercise or during an upper respiratory infection is sometimes noted in the healing phase and can be disregarded as long as it is not associated with a deterioration in the GFR.

Salt and water overload. Salt and water retention is a consequence of the low GFR and increased proportional reabsorption of glomerular filtrate in the proximal tubule; it is responsible for the hypertension which can be life threatening and associated with pulmonary oedema, hypertensive encephalopathy and cerebral haemorrhage. Plasma renin activity is usually low in AGNS with fluid overload (Powell et al, 1974). The dietary sodium should be restricted to 1 mEq/kg body weight/day in the young child and not more than 40 mEq/day in the adolescent. If oliguria is present the fluid intake should be restricted to the insensible loss (about 25 ml/kg/day in the infant and 10 ml/kg/day in the adult) plus the urinary output. Intravenous frusemide will remove sodium; 1 to 2 mg/kg is the usual dose but doses as large as 5 to 8 mg/kg have been used in the presence of severe oliguria.

Hypertension. Restriction of salt and water intake and where necessary the use of intravenous frusemide is often sufficient to control the raised blood pressure. If in spite of these measures the diastolic pressure exceeds the normal for a child of that age then it should be reduced. Intravenous or intramuscular hydrallazine 0.5 to 1 mg/kg 6 hourly or intramuscular reserpine 0.05 to 0.1 mg/kg 4 hourly are usually effective. When these drugs fail then intravenous diazoxide 3 to 5 mg/kg given as a rapid injection is effective.

Oliguria and renal failure. The oliguria of AGNS is usually associated with a high urine osmolality (> 500 mosmol/kg) and a low sodium concentration (< 20 mEq/litre) and this is useful in distinguishing from other causes of acute renal failure such as tubular necrosis. When anuria supervenes peritoneal dialysis may be required; other indications for dialysis are hyperkalaemia, fluid overload unresponsive to the treatment already discussed and severe electrolyte disturbance with acidosis. Such treatment is probably best undertaken in specialised units and arrangements for transfer should be made before such complications become a threat to life. Hyperkalaemia can often be temporarily corrected for the journey by giving calcium/potassium exchange resin 1 g/kg orally and rectally, by correcting an acidosis, or rarely by giving glucose and insulin though this may be hazardous and should only be used if a doctor is accompanying the patient.

Renal biopsy

There is no doubt that the ability to study the pathology of glomerular disease whilst it is still evolving has contributed much to the understanding of the pathogenic mechanisms involved, to the delineation of different types of inflammation with differing prognoses, and to the rational assessment of therapy. The procedure is relatively safe and causes only minor discomfort if properly performed. Most of the fatal complications reported in the past have been attributed to general anaesthesia. In babies under six months and over five years of age we generally use sedation and local anaesthesia. The main risk to the biopsied kidney is damage to a large artery causing persistent haemorrhage necessitating nephrectomy. Careful selection of cases excluding those with small kidneys, control of hypertension, the use of fluoroscopic screening to visualise the kidney after injection of contrast media should reduce the potential hazard. In over 1800 needle biopsies in adults and children over the last 10 years, we have not seen persistent haemorrhage necessitating nephrectomy.

The child with acute nephritic syndrome secondary to a streptococcal infection whose clinical course is following the expected course to recovery will not need a renal biopsy. Biopsy is indicated when there is severe oliguria necessitating dialysis as some of these children will have severe extra-capillary proliferation and a poor prognosis. Similarly a deterioration in GFR (rising plasma creatinine) from 10 to 14 days after the onset of the disease may be due to a more severe lesion than the acute exudative proliferation of poststrepto-coccal nephritis. Two recent patients demonstrated this. A 10 year old girl was admitted with acute renal failure and no history of haematuria. The renal biopsy showed an acute exudative lesion with only minor epithelial cell proliferation and after 10 days of peritoneal dialysis a diuresis occurred. No other treatment was given and six months later she had normal renal function.

Table 10.3   Renal biopsy was performed on 66 of 174 children under 15 years who presented with AGNS but without systemic vasculitis (Guy's Hospital, 1964–74)

Biopsy findings	No. of patients	Percentage
Endothelial, exudative or mesangial proliferative only	49	74
Mesangiocapillary nephritis	11	17
Extracapillary nephritis with extensive crescents	3	4.5
Focal and segmental glomerular sclerosis	0	0
Minimal glomerular changes	0	0
Membranous nephropathy	3	4.5
Total	66	100

In contrast the renal biopsy of a seven year old West Indian girl with AGNS following a streptococcal throat infection showed an acute exudative lesion but she was still oliguric and the plasma creatinine was raised after two weeks. A second renal biopsy showed the picture of rapidly progressive nephritis with semicircumferential epithelial crescents in 70 per cent of the glomeruli. Immunosuppression and anticoagulation (Brown et al, 1974b) was associated with a steady improvement and GFR is now normal (Fig. 10.1).

The indications for biopsy are severe oliguria or anuria, progressive disease, persistent hypocomplementaemia and failure of normal course of resolution. It is important that the child with rapidly progressive nephritis should be diagnosed early before renal failure supervenes. After the initial illness the haematuria and proteinuria should steadily diminish and renal biopsy should be considered if there is persistent microscopic haematuria at one year or significant proteinuria at six months after the onset. Our own experience of renal biopsy in AGNS over the last 10 years is shown in Table 10.3.

Prognosis

The prognosis of AGNS will depend on the renal lesion (Fig. 10.2). Poststreptococcal disease is associated with virtually complete resolution (Perlman et al, 1965). In an extended prospective study of sporadic disease in Texas the probability of complete resolution has been estimated at 92 to

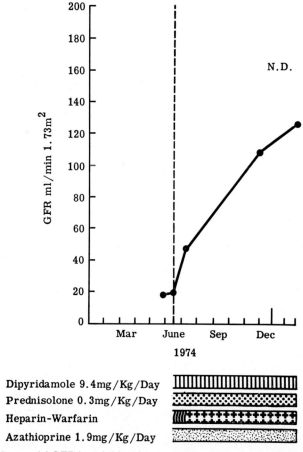

Figure 10.1 Sequential GFR in a child with acute poststreptococcal nephritis who developed severe epithelial proliferation. GFR was measured with ^{51}Cr-EDTA (Chantler and Barratt, 1972). Therapy with immunosuppression and anticoagulation is shown

98 per cent excluding cases of rapidly progressive disease (Travis et al., 1973) Whether the long-term (20–30 years) prognosis will be equally good is unknown. It has been suggested that over a third of patients will eventually manifest renal damage sustained during poststreptococcal AGNS (Baldwin et al, 1974). The prognosis in cases other than poststreptoccal AGNS depend on the nature of the underlying disease.

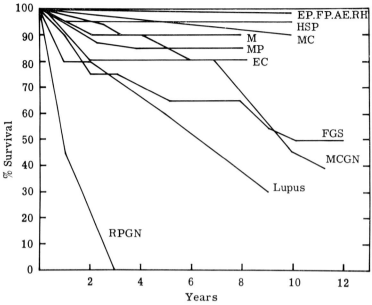

Figure 10.2 Actuarial survival for children with various histological and clinical variants of glomerulonephritis (modified from Cameron, 1972). EP, endothelial proliferation; FP, focal proliferation; AE, acute exudative (acute poststreptococcal AGNS); RH, recurrent haematuria; HSP, Henoch–Schonlein purpura; MC, minimal change; M, membranous; MP, mesangial proliferation; EC, extracapillary (with less than 50 per cent crescents); FGS, focal glomerulosclerosis; MCGN, mesangiocapillary; RPGN, rapidly progressive nephritis (extracapillary with 70 per cent crescents)

Primary (Recurrent) Haematuria

The syndrome of recurrent macroscopic haematuria sometimes with persistent microscopic haematuria but without proteinuria and with normal renal function can be regarded as a subgroup of AGNS. Other causes of haematuria as shown in Table 10.4 need to be excluded. Some children with

Table 10.4 Causes of haematuria in children

Infections including tuberculosis
Trauma
Acute nephritic syndrome
Chronic nephritis
Benign recurrent haematuria
Familial nephritis
Tumours
Meatal ulcers
Renal calculi
Henoch–Schonlein purpura
Haematological disorders including sickle cell disease
Systemic disorders (SBE, SLE, etc.)
Urological malformations
Drugs

resolving poststreptococcal AGNS not infrequently suffer exacerbations of haematuria following exercise or an upper respiratory infection.

Primary recurrent haematuria affects males more commonly than females; the onset is abrupt and often associated with an upper respiratory infection or follows exercise. Symptoms are mild except when renal colic occurs though dysuria or loin pain may be experienced. Proteinuria is usually absent or only slight and renal function is normal. It is important to confirm the presence of blood by microscopy of a fresh urine sample. Casts are rarely seen. The presence of casts suggests severe glomerulonephritis such as AGNS, mesangiocapillary nephritis, extensive epithelial proliferation or focal sclerotic lesions (Gill, Visy and Chantler, 1975). It is important to exclude Alport's syndrome or hereditary nephritis by a careful history and examination for deafness.

Management

Other causes of haematuria should be excluded (Table 10.4) and the renal function should be checked by measuring GFR and 24-h urine protein excretion (Barratt and Chantler, 1975). Cystoscopy is usually not indicated unless the blood is not mixed with the urine and the haematuria is more marked at the beginning or end of micturition. Suprapubic tenderness or a pelvic mass or urinary retention would also suggest the possibility of bladder pathology. Renal biopsy is not necessary unless there is evidence of renal dysfunction or proteinuria, for the histology is usually normal on light microscopy or shows a mild focal segmental proliferation or mesangial proliferation (Table 10.1). All these lesions carry a generally good prognosis. An association has been found between primary haematuria and deposits of IgA in the mesangium (Berger, 1969) and this may be useful in confirming the kidney as the site of the haematuria in children with otherwise normal renal biopsies. The presence of significant proteinuria (>200 mg/24 h) is an indication for biopsy to detect more serious renal lesions such as focal sclerosis or mesangiocapillary glomerulonephritis (Hendler, Kashgarian and Hayslett, 1972). Sites of infection should be located and the infection eradicated otherwise no specific treatment is required. Full activity can be allowed and the family reassured about the diagnosis and prognosis.

In the neonate haematuria is always an important sign which should be fully investigated. A primary cause such as renal venous thrombosis or obstructive uropathy is found in about two-thirds of the infants (Emanuel and Aronson, 1974).

Prognosis

The recurrent episodes of bleeding subside in about half the patients over a five year period and even where bleeding continues renal function is usually well maintained (Johnston and Shuler, 1969; Singer et al, 1968). Thus a good prognosis can be given and the episodes of haematuria largely disregarded

There are two qualifications to this statement, firstly the diagnosis should be reviewed if the symptomatology changes or is prolonged and secondly, two out of 98 patients admitted to our renal failure programme at Guy's Hospital had a classical recurrent haematuria from childhood until their final illness at ages 23 and 34 years; it is also apparent that the occasional patient with mesangial IgA deposition may develop progressive disease (Sissons and Woodrow, 1975). It seems wise to keep the children under surveillance until the haematuria has subsided.

Nephrotic Syndrome

Nephrotic syndrome (NS) affects about 18 children per million per year under the age of 14 years. The maximum incidence is from one to five years of age and 95 per cent of these children have minimal change lesions on biopsy. Haematuria, and hypertension are uncommon, serum C3 complement is invariably normal and the differential protein clearances usually show a highly selective pattern (Cameron, 1968). About 80 per cent of all children with NS will respond to steroids (prednisolone 60 mg/m^2 per day) within eight weeks after the start of treatment and only about 5 per cent of children with minimal change lesions fail to respond (Abramowicz et al, 1970). A response is defined as the complete loss of proteinuria. Thus about 15 per cent of children with NS will have a more serious lesion such as focal sclerosis or mesangiocapillary disease. About half the children who fail to respond to an initial eight week course of steroids will do so during or after cyclophosphamide therapy, and a slightly smaller proportion will do so with prolonged intermittent prednisolone treatment (International Study, 1974), or perhaps with no specific treatment at all. The vast majority of these late responders have minimal change disease and probably only about 1 per cent of all minimal change cases fail to respond to either steroids or cyclophosphamide.

A proportion of children who respond to steroids will relapse at some time after steroids are withdrawn or when the dose is reduced. Estimates of the number who behave in this way vary from 30 to 90 per cent (Cameron, 1972). The International Study found 25 per cent of an unselected group became frequent relapsers (Abramowicz et al, 1970).

About a quarter of the children with a frequent relapsing course enter a permanent remission in the first year after onset of the disease but after 10 years of follow-up about 80 per cent appear to be permanently better (Siegel et al, 1972). Some continue to relapse, one patient did so for 49 years (Niall, 1965).

Cyclophosphamide has proved effective in a number of children with a frequent relapsing course (Barratt and Soothill, 1970). The percentage remaining in remission after a single course is shown in Figure 10.3. About 35 to 40 per cent of these children can expect a permanent remission (Cameron et al, 1974). If relapse occurs these children are sometimes more responsive to steroids than before cyclophosphamide (Bergstrand et al, 1973). A second course of cyclophosphamide is usually as effective as the first treatment. It is now well recognised that cyclophosphamide can cause gonadal damage leading to sterility (Fairley, Barrie and Johnson, 1972). Whilst it is still too soon to be completely sure it appears that an eight week course of 3 mg/kg/day given prepubertally usually is safe but gonadal damage has been reported after a 12 week course (Pennisi, Grushkin and Liebermann, 1975).

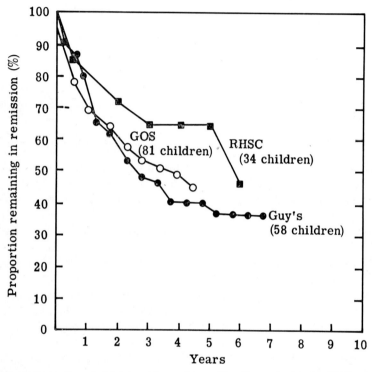

Figure 10.3   Proportion of children with steroid sensitive frequent relapsing NS in remission after a single course of cyclophosphamide. Guy's (Guy's Hospital, London; Cameron et al, 1974); GOS (The Hospital for Sick Children, Great Ormond Street, London; Barratt et al, 1975); RHSC (Royal Hospital for Sick Children, Glasgow; MacDonald, Murphy and Arneil, 1974)

Management

The diagnosis is usually straightforward. The presence of haematuria a low C3 complement level, hypertension, a moderate or poorly selective proteinuria or an older child make the possibility of a lesion other than minimal change more likely and may indicate the need for an early renal biopsy. Urinary infection which appears to be more frequent in these children should be excluded. The most important and potentially fatal complication of

NS in childhood is hypovolaemic shock caused by the sudden transfer of salt and water from the plasma to the extracellular fluid compartment (Egan et al, 1967). This occurs within a few days of the onset of the relapse whilst the oedema is accumulating; clinical evidence of hypovolaemia can be lacking with a normal pulse and blood pressure. One child recently seen at Guy's Hospital had a marked hypokalaemic alkalosis with a high plasma aldosterone level secondary to hyperreninaemia caused by the fall in renal perfusion following hypovolaemia. Plasma volume as judged by the rise in haematocrit had fallen by a quarter but pulse and blood pressure were normal. Another child collapsed with a haematocrit twice normal after an episode of vomiting; her pulse and blood pressure over the previous 12 h had shown no systematic alteration. Abdominal pain is a frequent complaint in children with hypovolaemia. Frequent assessment of haematocrit is an easy way to exclude hypovolaemia. A rising blood urea and falling urine output with highly concentrated urine is often noted.

Hyponatraemia is found if water is ingested in excess of salt for these children are usually thirsty. Treatment consists of intravenous plasma infusions. Diuretics should not be used to control oedema during the early stages of a relapse because of the danger of exacerbating hypovolaemia. An increased susceptibility to infection, classically cellulitis or pneumococcal peritonitis is a well-recognised feature of the nephrotic state. Penicillin prophylaxis during this time seems reasonable but can be discontinued after remission. Pancreatitis especially in patients on steroids has been reported. Oedema can sometimes become uncomfortable and prevent activity or accumulate around the eyes; infusion of double strength plasma with intravenous frusemide is generally effective. Care must be taken not to precipitate circulatory overload when the odema fluid is mobilised into the plasma space. Salt-free albumin is best avoided because it may lead to hyponatraemia. Bed rest is discouraged in relapse unless there is circulatory instability or the child feels unwell.

It is obviously impractical and inadvisable to admit all children in relapse to hospital. Our practice is to ask the parents to report the relapse so that steroid policy can be decided. They are told *to bring the child to hospital* if he is unwell, has abdominal pain, vomits or has diarrhoea or is feverish.

Prednisolone 2 mg/kg ideal weight for height/day up to a maximum of 60 mg/day is given orally. The mode time for remission is in the second week. Failure to respond to steroids in four to eight weeks is an indication for biopsy. If a minimal change lesion is found steroids may be continued or a course of cyclophosphamide (3 mg/kg ideal weight for height/day) is given. After a remission has been induced the steroids are reduced over an eight week period. A further relapse is treated with prednisolone as before. After two relapses the child is left on a long term course of alternate day steroids in a dose of 10 to 20 mg on alternate days. If he relapses on a dose of steroids sufficient to cause steroid toxicity (including growth retardation) then treatment with cyclophosphamide is considered. During cyclophosphamide therapy the WBC is monitored weekly; a fall in total polymorphonuclear leucocyte count to below $1000/\mu l$ is an indication for stopping therapy and restarting at half the dose after the blood count has returned to normal. Alopecia is usually mild but cystitis with haematuria may lead to bladder fibrosis and is an indication for stopping therapy altogether. Relapse after cyclophosphamide is treated with steroids as before. Persistent relapses in spite of steroid prophylaxis in children who have received cyclophosphamide is a difficult problem; we try where ever possible to avoid a second course of cyclophosphamide. Azothioprine appears ineffective in maintaining remission (Abramowicz et al, 1970) though occasionally it may enable a smaller dose of prednisolone to maintain remission. The judicious and careful use of diuretics may enable the nephrotic state to be tolerated and if oedema is only mild no specific treatment need be given.

If steroid resistance is encountered in a child previously steroid sensitive, renal biopsy should be considered for such a child may have a focal sclerotic lesion rather than minimal change. Occasionally a child with a focal sclerosis will respond to steroids (International Study, 1974). The aetiology of minimal change disease is obscure but occasionally a relation to reaginic hypersensitivity has been noted. Desensitisation in such cases has proved effective (Hardwicke et al, 1959).

Congenital Nephrotic Syndrome

This condition is exceedingly rare and generally fatal (Kaplan, Bureau and Drummond, 1974). It should be suspected in any child with NS under the age of one year. Knowledge of placental weight is invaluable in confirming that the NS was present at birth for the placental weight is usually increased due to oedema. Congenital nephrotic syndrome may be primary and of unknown aetiology or secondary to a congenital infection such as syphilis (Wiggelin-Khuizen et al, 1973), cytomegalovirus or toxoplasmosis. Treatment of the underlying infection usually leads to resolution of the nephrosis. Primary congenital nephrotic syndrome is of two types and both appear to be inherited as an autosomal recessive. In the type described mainly but not exclusively in children of Finnish ancestry there is cyst-like dilatation of the proximal tubules. This appearance has been poorly termed infantile microcystic disease. In the other type the glomerular lesion is that of a focal and global sclerosis (Habib and Kleinecht, 1971).

Management

Congenital infection should be excluded and a renal biopsy should be carried out to confirm the diagnosis and to enable a prognosis to be given. In the primary type little can be done and no specific therapy is of value; steroids and immunosuppressives are ineffective. In a child presenting after the neonatal period it is important to exclude a very early minimal change lesion which may be responsive to steroids; we have seen one such case presenting at six months of age. Management is largely supportive and consists of preventing and treating infection for these children are particularly prone to Gram-negative sepsis. Growth is usually poor but occasionally oedema can be controlled with diuretics and food intake, and growth may improve. If the child survives long enough then renal transplant can be considered and has been performed successfully at aged two years (Hoyer et al, 1973). Such treatment is not generally available and the uncertainty of the long-term results may not commend it in children so young. In a disease so rapidly fatal it is usually possible for a family to have at least one normal child if they are prepared to undertake the 1:4 risk associated with the inheritance. However, we have one family with all three children affected; two have died but the eldest aged nine years has just had a successful transplant.

Prognosis

In the Finnish type death usually occurs from septicaemia or renal failure within the first year. In the focal sclerotic type deterioration is slower but renal failure usually occurs before the end of the first decade. Prenatal diagnosis is now possible.

Symptomless Proteinuria

Persistent proteinuria in the absence of haematuria or other urinary abnormalities and when there is no structural renal tract abnormality is relatively benign (Antoine, Symrouldis and Dardenne, 1969). Orthostatic proteinuria has an excellent prognosis (Cameron, 1971).

Management

If persistent proteinuria is confirmed the urine should be cultured and tested for blood. Plasma creatinine should be measured. Postural orthostatic proteinuria can be excluded by testing the first urine passed before rising in the morning. An intravenous urethrogram (IVU) will exclude structural anomalies. If the GFR is normal, no other abnormalities are discovered and the urine protein excretion is less than $1 \text{ g}/1.73 \text{ m}^2/\text{day}$ then no further action is required except for occasional outpatient review. In some children the proteinuria disappears. If the proteinuria is moderate or heavy enough to alter the plasma protein concentration then a renal biopsy should be considered (Table 10.1).

Prognosis

The prognosis is excellent unless there is some underlying urological disease, infection or nephritis.

Haematuria and Proteinuria

The combination of haematuria and proteinuria suggest the possibility of some serious form of glomerulonephritis (Table 10.1). The histological appearances which may be found are as follows.

Minimal change

This implies that the renal histology is normal to light microscopy although on electron microscopy there is fusion of the foot processes of the epithelial cells which are applied to the outer surface of the glomerular basement membrane. Immunofluorescent studies reveal no deposition of immunoglobulins, complement or fibrinogen in the glomeruli. The prognosis of this lesion has been discussed and is shown in Figure 10.2.

Focal glomerulosclerosis

This condition is easily mistaken for a minimal change lesion; the presentation is usually with heavy proteinuria and microscopic haematuria. The lesion is focal in that in its earliest stages it affects only a proportion of the glomeruli especially in the juxtamedullary region (Habib, 1970) and segmental, only affecting part of the glomerular tuft. Focal tubular atrophy may be seen, and electron microscopy or immunofluorescent studies may aid in distinguishing the condition from minimal change disease. No lasting response to therapy has been noted (Cameron, 1972) although proteinuria may occasionally diminish during treatment with steroids or immunosuppression. The prognosis is poor.

Membranous nephropathy

Membranous nephropathy is unusual in children; it may be primary or secondary to lupus, malignant disease, etc. (Row et al, 1975). It is characterised by diffuse thickening of basement membrane with deposits of IgG and complement components on the epithelial surface of the membrane. The prognosis over the mid-term (10 years) in children is quite good although the long-term outlook is unknown. Treatment is generally ineffective but an occasional response coincident with therapy has been noted in some patients (Row et al, 1975).

Proliferative nephritis

Various types of proliferative glomerulonephritis can be distinguished on renal biopsy; prognosis differs accordingly. The common feature is the increase in glomerular cells.

Acute exudative glomerulonephritis. This appearance is typical of acute poststreptococcal nephritis and has been discussed above. Prognosis is good.

Mesangial proliferation. Mesangial cells and mesangial matrix material are increased but the capillary walls are normal. Immunofluorescence may show deposition of immunoglobulins and sometimes complement in the mesangium. These appearances may be seen with any glomerular syndrome (Table 10.1) or in resolving AGNS. The prognosis is good (Fig. 10.2) and treatment is usually not necessary and generally ineffective. Oedema when present as part of a nephrotic syndrome should be controlled with careful use of diuretics until the proteinuria subsides. Occasionally difficulty is experienced in distinguishing this lesion from minimal change with mesangial prominence and in such cases a trial of steroids or cyclophosphamide may be justified.

Focal proliferative glomerulonephritis. Only some glomeruli and then only one segment of the glomerular tuft is involved. The condition may be seen as part of a generalised vasculitis when the prognosis is not necessarily good but in isolation healing usually occurs spontaneously. Differentiation from focal sclerosis can be difficult, but the presence of IgA deposits in the mesangium may be helpful.

Mesangiocapillary nephritis (Habib et al, 1973)

The lesion is characterised by mesangial and endothelial hypercellularity, increased mesangial matrix and irregular thickening of the basement membrane either with subendothelial or intramembranous deposits. Electron microscopy and immunofluorescence where the deposition of C3 complement and IgG is marked, aid in establishing the correct diagnosis. Presentation may be with nephrotic syndrome, acute nephritic syndrome, haematuria and proteinuria or with acute renal failure. Partial lipodystrophy is occasionally associated (Peters et al, 1973). Plasma C3 complement is often reduced. A rapidly progressive picture is sometimes superimposed with marked epithelial cell proliferation. Prognosis is poor with a 50 per cent 10-year survival (Fig. 10.2). although the clinical course is variable and prolonged spontaneous clinical remissions are seen. The evaluation of therapy is difficult and no controlled data is available although response to steroids (McAdams, McEnery and West, 1975) and to anticoagulation and immunosuppression in both rapidly and slowly progressive disease (Gill et al, 1975) has been reported.

Extracapillary glomerulonephritis

The characteristic feature is proliferation of epithelial cells producing crescentic formations of cells pushing the capillary tuft to one side; the crescents also contain fibrin-like material. This lesion may be seen in a variety of acute clinical situations such as acute poststreptococcal nephritis, mesangiocapillary nephritis, and Goodpasture's syndrome where there is a circulating antibody to glomerular basement membrane. The prognosis appears to depend on the severity of the lesion (Sisson et al, 1974; Habib, 1970) with an 80 per cent 10-year survival for those with less than 50 per cent of glomeruli involved. When 70 to 80 per cent of glomeruli are involved with large occluding crescents the prognosis is poor with a 50 per cent mortality in one year and a 90 per cent mortality over two to three years. This condition has been termed *rapidly progressive nephritis.* Treatment with anticoagulants and immunosuppression has recently been demonstrated to be effective in a non-controlled study of adults and children (Brown et al, 1974) but only if applied early in the evolution of the disease. The importance of suspecting this lesion and arranging renal biopsy in any child with AGNS or nephrotic syndrome whose clinical course is unusual is obvious.

Endothelial (endocapillary) proliferative nephritis

This is the largest and least well-defined type of proliferative nephritis. Endothelial and mesangial cells are increased in number with patchy scarring and obliteration of glomeruli. Clinical presentation is with nephrotic syndrome with haematuria, or with haematuria and proteinuria. Chronic renal failure may be manifest at the time of diagnosis. Prognosis is uncertain, estimates vary from less than 10 to 30 per cent mortality over four years (Cameron, 1972). No effective treatment is available at the present time.

Interstitial Nephritis

Diffuse interstitial inflammatory cell infiltration with lymphocytes, plasma cells, and occasional eosinophils and neutrophils is an unexpected finding on renal biopsy of an infant or child presenting with acute renal failure, or haematuria and proteinuria with diminished renal function. The glomeruli are more or less normal but the condition is considered here because of the similarity of presentation to some varieties of glomerulonephritis. Interstitial nephritis may be confused with chronic bacterial infection. The possible relationship between interstitial nephritis and abacterial pyelonephritis caused by the persistence of *Escherichia coli* antigen in the interstitium which leads to an immunologically mediated inflammation (Aoki et al, 1969) needs further clarification.

The aetiology is often obscure (Simenhoff, Guild and Dammin, 1968); hypersensitivity to drugs such as analgesics, penicillin, sulphonamides and diuretics and phenindione, an unusual response to streptococcal infection, radiation, hyperuricaemia and transplant rejection will all cause an interstitial reaction, but the majority of cases are idiopathic. An association with iridocyclitis has been noted. Prognosis is good and spontaneous recovery or improvement with steroids usually occurs. We have seen three children with this condition in the last two years and all have recovered; two after steroid therapy. Apart from an associated iritis in one child, no definite aetiology was established and attempts to implicate virus infection were unsuccessful.

Systemic Disorders and Glomerulonephritis

Viral hepatitis type B with deposition of antigen/antibody complexes in the kidney has been found in association with endocapillary proliferative disease, mesangiocapillary, membranous, and extracapillary proliferative nephritis (Brzosko et al, 1974).

The association of haematuria, proteinuria and renal damage with subacute infective endocarditis has been recognised for many years. The histological lesion in the kidney appears to be diffuse or focal segmental proliferation and many cases show deposition of antigen/antibody complexes in the affected glomeruli (Boulton-Jones et al, 1974).

A severe proliferative glomerulonephritis may follow a chronically infected ventriculoatrial shunt in children with hydrocephalus. Antibody/antigen complexes with the infecting bacteria are deposited in the kidney (Kaufman and McIntosh, 1971); plasma and C3 component of complement may be decreased. Considerable improvement in renal function with resolution of epithelial crescents is possible after removal of the shunt (Wegmann and Leumann, 1973).

Henoch-Schonlein Purpura

About 30 per cent of children with Henoch–Schonlein purpura develop a nephritis; the clinical manifestations vary from haematuria with proteinuria, to acute nephritic syndrome, nephrotic syndrome or a rapidly progressive nephritis leading to renal failure. Renal biopsy is equally variable ranging from a mild focal segmental proliferation to severe extracapillary proliferation. Fibrin related material and immunoglobulins especially IgA may be demonstrated by immunofluorescent studies.

Only a small proportion of affected children (about 20 per cent) develop chronic glomerulonephritis and perhaps 5 per cent of those affected may reach terminal renal failure in one to two years after the onset of the purpura (Meadow et al, 1972). In the remainder the haematuria and proteinuria slowly disappears though this may take several years and exacerbation of haematuria during intermittent infections is common and need not cause concern. The overall prognosis is uncertain but a 10 year survival of about 95 per cent for affected children has been calculated (Cameron, 1972). It is likely that a few children with chronic glomerulonephritis will slowly deteriorate and enter renal failure perhaps after many years. Results of therapy are difficult to evaluate for in a disease with a high spontaneous remission rate it is not surprising that apparent improvement with steroids and immunosuppression is sometimes seen; in other children therapy has had no effect on the progression to renal failure (Meadow et al, 1972). Recently we have noted a dramatic response to anticoagulation and immunosuppression in a three year old boy with a rapidly progressive picture and 80 per cent epithelial crescents on biopsy; GFR rose from 20 ml/min/1.73 m^2 to normal levels after nine months treatment (Brown et al, 1974b). Our policy at present is to measure GFR in children with renal involvement and then consider biopsy and treatment if renal function is below normal or deteriorates. Follow-up continues until all renal abnormalities have disappeared. Care must be taken not to miss the child with severe renal involvement and rapidly deteriorating function early on in the disease. The children in whom the general Henoch–Schonlein manifestations persist or recur after three months seem particularly at risk and the prognosis of those with acute nephritis or nephrotic syndrome is worse than those whose renal involvement is manifest by haematuria and proteinuria alone.

Systemic Lupus Erythematosus and Other Vascular Diseases

This condition is fortunately rare amongst children in the United Kingdom though the incidence is higher in non-Caucasian immigrants especially those of African or Chinese descent. Renal involvement occurs in about half the patients with the deposition of soluble DNA antibody complexes in the kidney. Renal biopsy shows diffuse proliferation or focal segmental proliferation, minimal change or pure membranous nephropathy. The diffuse proliferative lesion has a much worse prognosis in general and untreated five year survival may be as low as 10 per cent; treatment with high dose corticosteroid or lower dose prednisolone and azathioprine improves the outlook with a five year survival of about 50 per cent (Cameron, 1972). Intensive treatment reduces the mortality of renal lupus but increases the danger of fatal infection or severe steroid complications. Some clinicians favour using drugs to keep the various immunological manifestations of the disease such as the low serum complement, antibody to DNA, abnormal urine light chain protein excretion, etc., within normal limits (Epstein, 1973) though this will inevitably lead to complications of treatment. Our own policy is to rely on the measurement of renal function particularly accurate assessment of GFR, using ^{51}Cr-EDTA single injection clearances (Chantler and Barratt, 1972), to determine the intensity of treatment. Considerable increases in GFR have been seen during treatment with prednisolone and azathioprine.

Polyarthritis nodosa, Wegener's granulomatosis (Raitt, 1972) and Goodpasture's syndrome (Sissons et al, 1974) are frequently associated with severe glomerulonephritis. The presentation is usually an acute nephritic syndrome. Biopsy is useful for diagnosis and to determine prognosis for extensive epithelial crescent formation and a rapidly progressive picture are common.

Haemolytic Uraemic Syndrome

The acute onset of haemolytic anaemia, thrombocytopenia and renal failure either in association with septicaemia or occurring without obvious cause is now well recognised by all paediatricians (Liebermann, 1972). The majority of affected children are under one year of age, though the condition appears later in childhood and has been reported in adults. Gastrointestinal symptoms of vomiting and diarrhoea which is often bloody and may be mistaken for ulcerative colitis or Crohn's disease is usually the initial event in the illness. The main pathological feature is the consumption of platelets and a microangiopathic haemolytic anaemia with distortion and fragmentation of red cells. Consumption of other clotting factors is not a prominent feature and recent reports suggest no constant decrease in fibrinogen survival (George et al, 1974). The importance of fibrin deposition in the pathogenesis of the renal damage has also been questioned recently for it is not always found in renal biopsy material though it may be marked in the presence of renal cortical necrosis.

The main current controversy concerns treatment. There is no doubt that survival has improved dramatically over the last 10 years and current estimates of mortality are less than 10 per cent (Liebermann, 1972). This is probably due to the improved management of acute renal failure. The use of heparin to stop intravascular coagulation remains unsubstantiated by controlled studies, and whilst some units ascribe the falling mortality to heparin therapy (Liebermann, 1972) other centres have noted similar improvements without heparin (Tune, Leavitt and Gribble, 1973). More recently the use of fibrinolytic agents such as streptokinase or urokinase have been advocated to reduce the mortality from renal failure and the incidence of later renal hypertension (Monnens et al, 1972).

Fatal haemorrhage is a complication of both heparin and fibrinolytic therapy (Stuart et al, 1974). The recent doubt over the importance of fibrin deposition in the pathogenesis is an extra reason for caution. Our own experience is difficult to evaluate; one patient died of a cerebral haemorrhage whilst receiving heparin, in one thrombocytopaenia continued for three weeks after admission but disappeared with improvement in red cell morphology within three days of starting heparin and in a third renal function rapidly deteriorated with recurrence of haemolytic anaemia when the heparin was withdrawn after 28 days treatment; in spite of restarting heparin renal failure occurred and was irreversible.

Our current management is based on the undoubted facts that most children will recover spontaneously and that heparin and fibrinolytic agents although they may be effective are dangerous. A rigorous search for infection is made and septicaemia and shock are treated with appropriate antibiotics and restoration of fluid and electrolyte balance. Blood pressure is carefully controlled. The anaemia is treated by transfusion and appropriate measures taken to manage renal failure including early peritoneal dialysis. Renal failure may be caused by tubular necrosis in which case spontaneous recovery is likely or by patchy cortical necrosis which may be fatal. We attempt to distinguish the two and assess renal blood flow using gamma camera renal scintillography with $^{99}Tc^m$-DTPA and dimercaptosuccinic acid (DMSA); the former is filtered at the glomerulus and a characteristic picture is seen with tubular necrosis whilst DMSA is concentrated by the tubules and little concentration in the kidney is seen in cortical necrosis. When impending cortical necrosis is suggested a catheter is inserted into the renal artery via the femoral artery and heparin and urokinase are infused locally. Preliminary results are encouraging (Jones et al, 1975) but the important principle is the attempt to reserve the potentially dangerous therapy for the most severely affected children. The difficulty with this policy is that specific treatment is necessarily delayed and this may be undesirable (Stuart et al, 1974). It is hoped that these difficulties in management will be resolved as more experience is obtained and as carefully controlled studies are instituted.

REFERENCES

References are at the end of the next chapter (p. 299).

11
MANAGEMENT AND PROGNOSIS OF RENAL DISEASE IN CHILDHOOD
Renal Failure, Urinary Infections and Hypertension

C. Chantler

ACUTE RENAL FAILURE

The causes and management of acute renal failure in the child especially in the infant are different from those for the adult. Proper care requires knowledge of fluid turnover and nutritional requirements of the infant as well as access to the technology of radiology and nuclear medicine; above all experience is necessary and because acute renal failure is fortunately rare this experience is only likely to be accumulated in regional paediatric nephrology centres.

Management

The requirements for normal kidney function are an adequate blood supply, healthy kidneys and a patent functioning non-obstructed urine collection and excretion system. This is recognised in the division into prerenal, renal and postrenal causes for acute renal failure. The diagnosis and management of renal failure proceed simultaneously (Table 11.1). Certain points need to be emphasised.

In prerenal failure the poor renal perfusion pressure associated with electrolyte depletion or blood loss is associated with the production of a small quantity of highly concentrated urine (Table 11.2). The restoration of renal perfusion by adequate replacement of fluid and electrolytes should proceed without delay. The adequacy of this replacement is best judged clinically by frequent monitoring of pulse, blood pressure and respiratory rate. Measurement of venous pressure either clinically or if possible using manometry with an indwelling central venous catheter is useful. We have found the measurement of central and peripheral temperatures (Aynsley-Green and Pickering, 1974) using a rectal temperature probe and a probe attached to the toe or foot especially valuable and have noted a fall in renal output when the temperature gap has widened to more than 6°C, before an alteration in pulse or blood pressure has been detected. The finding of a raised venous pressure and poor peripheral perfusion with hypotension suggest a falling cardiac output due to myocardial dysfunction which may respond to beta-adrenergic

10

Table 11.1 Management of the child with acute renal failure

Assessment	Action
Resuscitation	
Level of consciousness	
Saline depletion or overload (BP)	i.v. infusion, or i.v. frusemide
Adequacy of airway	? assisted ventilation
Clinical and laboratory evaluation	
History:	
Infection, diet, diarrhoea, vomiting, oliguria, haematuria, urine stream, etc.	
Examination:	
Height, weight, palpable kidneys, bladder, etc.	
Laboratory tests:	
(a) Biochemistry:	
Blood electrolytes, urea, creatinine, bicarbonate, calcium, phosphate, alkaline phosphatase, glucose, proteins, urine electrolytes, osmolality protein	
(b) Haematology:	
Hb, WBC, film, platelets, ?clotting studies	
(c) Bacteriology:	
Urine, blood, stool, routine swabs	
Radiology:	
Chest x-ray, abdomen x-ray, x-ray knee, and wrist for osteodystrophy and bone age	
ECG	
Problems	
Prerenal failure	i.v. fluid, plasma, whole blood or saline 20 ml/kg and measure vital signs and urine output
Renal failure	i.v. frusemide 2–10 mg/kg, dialysis
Hypertension	i.v. hydrallazine 0.5–1.0; mg/kg and frusemide
Pulmonary oedema	i.v. frusemide or dialysis
Hyperkalaemia	i.v. 2.5 per cent calcium gluconate 2 ml/kg; calcium/potassium exchange resin 1 g/kg
Hypocalcaemia	i.v. calcium gluconate
Hypoglycaemia	i.v. dextrose 1 g/kg
Sepsis	i.v. antibiotics but reduce dosage if excreted via kidneys
Acidosis	i.v. $NaHCO_3$ or dialysis
Specific investigations	*Diagnosis*
IVU, micturating cystogram, retrograde pyelography, antegrade pyelography, ultrasound visualisation, gamma camera scan, renal biopsy, renal function tests including GFR, proximal and distal tubular function	Acute tubular necrosis, medullary necrosis, cortical necrosis, hypoplastic or dysplastic kidneys, pyelonephritis, glomerulonephritis, obstructive uropathy, renovascular accidents, nephrotic syndrome, haemolytic uraemic syndrome

stimulation with an isoprenaline drip. When peripheral perfusion is poor with normal or raised central venous pressure and arterial blood pressure, an alpha-adrenergic blocking drug such as intravenous chlorpromazine (0.25 mg/ kg) may cause peripheral vasodilation and increased urine production. Chlorpromazine administration may lead to a fall in blood pressure and therefore should only be given when an adequate i.v. infusion has been set up and all circulatory parameters are being carefully monitored.

Septicaemia is extremely common in both prerenal and renal failure and needs to be treated rigorously. Antibiotics such as streptomycin, kanamycin and gentamycin, which have a primary renal route of excretion, need to be used with care if toxicity is to be avoided. Frequent measurement of plasma levels is essential. A loading dose of gentamycin of 1 mg/kg is followed by doses of 0.5 mg/kg spaced according to the level of renal function. The penicillin group can be given in normal doses, but tetracycline should be avoided at all costs for it is extremely toxic in renal failure. All drugs given to the patient with renal failure should be reviewed bearing in mind the route of

Table 11.2 Composition of urine in prerenal and renal failure

	Prerenal failure	Renal failure
Volume (ml/kg/min)	< 0.5	Variable
Sodium (mmol/litre)	< 10	> 20
Urea (mg/dl)	> 1500	< 600
Urine/plasma osmolality ratio	> 1.3	< 1.1

excretion. We have seen a comatose child who was receiving standard doses of phenobarbitone. Epanutin or diazepam are satisfactory substitutes. Reviews of drug metabolism in renal disease should be consulted (Linton and Lawson, 1970; Reidenberg, 1971).

Oliguria. The borderline between prerenal and renal failure is often obscure and of course acute tubular necrosis is a consequence of delayed treatment of shock. The maintenance of urine flow may protect against tubular necrosis and large doses of frusemide in adults with established renal failure may reduce the duration of oliguria (Cantarovich, 1973). We use a single intravenous dose of 5 to 10 mg/kg and repeat 4 to 6 hourly at a dose of 2 mg/kg if a response is seen. The main complication reported to date in adults is deafness (Brown et al, 1974a) but we have not yet seen this with the above regime. Mannitol is not recommended because it causes volume overload unless excreted. Saline overload causing hypertension and pulmonary oedema in the presence of oliguria is one of the main indications for dialysis.

Electrolyte disturbances. Hyponatraemia is generally due to injudicious fluid replacement. Hypernatraemia is more often seen especially in children with gastroenteritis who have received high solute feeds. It should be corrected slowly to avoid the risk of neurological sequelae (Bannister, Martin-Siddigi and Hatcher, 1975). Dialysis, if required, should utilise solutions with progressively decreasing sodium concentrations. Hyperkalaemia (> 7 mEq/ litre) is extremely dangerous; emergency treatment with i.v. 2.5 per cent calcium gluconate (0.5 mg/kg) given as slow injection using ECG control will antagonise the cardiac effects of the hyperkalaemia. A cation exchange resin which exchanges potassium for calcium should be given orally and rectally at a dose of 1 g/kg. Resin charged with sodium should be avoided as it contributes to the sodium overload. Correction of acidosis will help to lower the plasma potassium also. A severe metabolic acidosis often accompanies acute renal failure in infants and an emergency dose of i.v. sodium bicarbonate (not more than 2 mEq/kg) should be given. The sodium contributes to saline overload and too rapid correction may provoke tetany. Dialysis may be necessary especially if hypertension or saline overload is already manifest.

Hypertension. In acute renal failure hypertension is generally secondary to saline overload and is best treated by salt removal if necessary by dialysis. It is important to bear in mind the normal levels of blood pressure of children at different ages and it is vitally important to reduce severe hypertension before a cerebral haemorrhage or acute pulmonary oedema develops. Hydrallazine i.v. or i.v. diazoxide are effective and may be given whilst preparations are made for dialysis.

Dialysis. A detailed consideration of peritoneal or haemodialysis is beyond the scope of this chapter. Both procedures are useful in the management of renal failure even in small infants. Peritoneal dialysis is generally preferred because it is easier and requires less technology and personnel. Great care to avoid infection should be taken when inserting the peritoneal cannula. The abdomen should be filled with dialysate fluid through a small bore needle before inserting the peritoneal cannula. This is particularly important in infants who cannot tense the abdominal wall muscles and therefore there is an increased risk of the catheter and stylet plunging into a hollow viscus or into a large blood vessel such as the inferior vena cava; a fatal complication frequently recorded. An increased dialysate glucose concentration is used when excess fluid needs to be removed; this should not exceed 3 g/dl for higher concentrations lead to peritoneal irritation and may also cause too rapid removal of fluid. This concentration is easily obtained by mixing the commercially available solutions.

Most solutions contain lactate as the metabolisable anion and a lactic acidosis may occasionally develop in sick anoxic neonates. This can be severe and threaten life. A dialysate containing bicarbonate can be prepared but this should not contain calcium which is precipitated. In one case recently i.m. lipoic acid was effective in enabling the lactate to be metabolised (Curran, Toseland and Chantler, 1975).

Frequent and accurate measurement of fluid balance is essential and there is not substitute for clinical assessment and careful weighing to achieve this. The main complication is infection and the dialysate fluid should be checked daily. Careful technique, changing the site of the catheter at not more than weekly intervals or whenever leakage occurs around the cannula or the use of a subcutaneous tunnel so that the catheter enters the peritoneum at a site remote from the skin incision will help to avoid infection.

Haemodialysis is indicated if peritoneal dialysis becomes impossible because of abdominal complications or surgery. It is also useful in older children after cardiac surgery if peritoneal dialysis is unable to cope with fluid overload. We generally use a femoral artery and vein cannula for babies and have successfully dialysed infants as small as 3.5 kg body wt. Considerable experience of haemodialysis in older children and adults is necessary if the technological problems are to be overcome.

Nutrition. Many infants with acute renal failure are hypercatabolic especially if infected. It is important to maintain nutrition and we generally aim to provide 150 to 200 kcal/kg body weight per day with at least 1 to 2 g/kg of first-class protein. This can be achieved by using a suitable modified cow's milk (SMA or S26 which has a lower potassium content), double cream and glucose or glucose polymer (Caloreen or Calonutrin). Fluid intake needs to be kept low if dialysis is to keep pace with fluid removal. The relatively increased insensible loss of infants compared with adults is helpful but where intravenous feeding is required the fluid load involved may create difficulties, especially during haemodialysis, and necessitate more frequent dialysis.

Diagnosis

The history and physical examination will often point to the diagnosis. Anaemia, short stature or renal osteodystrophy suggest long-standing renal disease, a history of diarrhoea and vomiting indicates saline depletion, maldevelopment of the renal tract may be associated with extrarenal anomalies (Chantler, 1975), a poor urine stream in small infants suggests urethral valves and obstructive uropathy, a palpable bladder and enlarged kidneys indicate infravesical obstruction, bilateral gross enlargement of the kidneys is suggestive of infantile polycystic diseases, and an acute onset of renal failure, haematuria and enlarged kidneys may be caused by renal venous thrombosis in the infant. The history and clinical features may be helpful in the diagnosis of acute nephritic syndrome or haemolytic uraemic syndrome. Haematological examination may reveal a microangiopathic haemolytic anaemia. Blood and urine cultures are essential and the urine must be examined microscopically by the clinician for cells and casts. Other investigations such as C3 complement, ANF, ASOT, etc., may be helpful.

Intravenous urography (IVU) is especially valuable in acute renal failure (Fry and Cattell, 1970). Contrast media (not more than 3 ml/kg of sodium iothalamate, Conray 420, or 4 ml/kg of sodium diatrizoate, Hypaque 45) should be injected slowly over 5 min to avoid an excessive rise in plasma osmolality—tomography is required to show the kidneys and extrarenal urinary passages and the examination should continue for up to 24 h. No child with renal insufficiency should be thirsted before an IVU because of the danger of dehydration from the resultant osmotic diuresis. In anuric states the contrast load may itself lead to fluid overload and precipitate dialysis. The examination will often enable a firm diagnosis to be achieved in an acute tubular necrosis, or acute nephritic syndrome and is invaluable in excluding obstructive uropathy. A micturating cystogram is sometimes more useful than an IVU for if ureteric reflux is present it gives valuable information about the upper tract and kidneys as well as about the lower tract. Dysplastic kidneys in particular are often associated with reflux. Antegrade pyelography (Saxton et al, 1973) retrograde pyelography or ultrasonography (Lyons, Murphy and Arneil, 1972) may be required to reach a firm diagnosis; ultrasonography, which is non-invasive, appears especially promising in determining the structure of a non-functioning kidney and in confirming renal agenesis.

Table 11.3   Clinical diagnosis and associated pathological features of 27 children referred to Guy's Hospital with acute renal failure over 18 months, 1969 to 1970 (from Meadow et al, 1971)

Obstructive uropathy	8	(septicaemia 4)
Acute nephritic syndrome	7	(SLE 1, MCGN 1, Prol. neph. 4)
Nephrotic syndrome with hypovolaemia	5	(MC 3, MCGN 1, FGS 1)
Nephrotic syndrome with infection	1	(MC)
Acute pyelonephritis	2	(septicaemia 1, reflux 1)
Hypoplastic kidneys	1	
Staphylococcal endocarditis	1	
Haemolytic uraemic syndrome	1	
Hypertension	1	(multiple renal arterial stenosis)

SLE, systemic lupus erythematosus; MCGN, mesangiocapillary nephritis; Prol. neph., proliferative nephritis; MC, minimal change; FGS, focal glomerulosclerosis

Recently gamma camera dynamic scintillography using tracer amounts of radioactive materials such as $^{99}Tc^m$-DTPA has become available. The amount of radiation involved is less than with conventional radiology and no osmotic load is given during the examination. Information sometimes equivalent to that obtained from the IVU, may be obtained and the latter examination avoided. In addition information on renal blood flow may be obtained and it may be possible to distinguish between tubular and cortical necrosis.

Renal biopsy may be necessary for diagnosis and whilst it is possible to use a closed needle biopsy technique at all ages, an open biopsy may be preferable in the infant for it allows the structure of the kidney to be inspected.

Final diagnosis in 27 children with acute renal failure referred to Guy's Hospital over an 18-month period is shown in Table 11.3 (Meadow et al, 1971). The generally good prognosis in contrast to adults with acute renal failure is demonstrated by the fact that 18 recovered completely, 1 partially, 6 had end-stage disease and 2 died. Our more recent experience contains a similar range of diagnosis but also includes renal venous thrombosis, dehydration especially with hypernatraemia, poisoning with drugs such as sulphonamides and with chemicals such as ethyleneglycol; burns, postcardiac bypass, interstitial nephritis, haemolytic uraemic syndrome more commonly, cortical necrosis following neonatal blood loss, Wegener's granuloma, acute on previously undiscovered chronic renal failure and acute tubular necrosis after surgical trauma. The importance of septicaemia is evident. The early diagnosis of obstructive uropathy is essential especially when the urine is infected and the infant has septicaemia. Urgent operation after initial resuscitation, may be necessary to relieve obstruction whilst definitive surgery can be delayed. The range of diagnostic possibilities is wide and the need for complex investigation in order to reach a firm diagnosis is obvious.

CHRONIC RENAL FAILURE

Management

The increasing availability of chronic haemodialysis in the home, and renal transplantation means that end state renal failure need not necessarily be fatal. Careful management of the child prior to dialysis is important if the metabolic consequences of the uraemic state are to be prevented from producing permanent damage to the child and if the psychological effects of chronic ill health are to be minimised. Moreover, reasonable life, without dialysis, can often be prolonged if proper conservative care is provided. Frequent outpatient monitoring is essential and attention should be directed at each visit to the items shown in Table 11.4.

Biochemical alterations and nutrition. The kidney can be regarded as an organ of nutrition (Holliday, 1972). In health the intake of food is governed by appetite which is controlled by energy requirements. The food consumed inevitably contains an excess of other nutrients apart from energy and the kidney enables this excess of protein (urea), sodium, phosphate, etc., to be excreted. In renal failure the capacity to excrete these nutrients is limited though a rising plasma concentration may enable a similar quantity to be excreted at a lower GFR. The rising plasma concentration can itself cause serious ill effects thus renal osteodystrophy is partly a consequence of phosphate retention. It is obvious that the lower food intake of uraemic children (Betts and MacGrath, 1974) not only reduces the load of nutrients that the kidney has to excrete but also reduces energy intake sometimes to levels associated with malnutrition in underdeveloped communities. The similarities between the uraemic state and protein energy malnutrition have been noted (Chantler and Holliday, 1974). Proper dietary management is directed towards the provision of nutrients in the quantities necessary for normal health but avoiding excess which requires renal excretion. Children especially toddlers do not respond well to dietary limitation and control and cooperation may be impossible to achieve and the stress placed on the family may be considerable. Our strategy is to provide energy without other nutrients as a medicine taken outside meal times in the form of double cream, corn oil and glucose or glucose polymer (Caloreen or Calonutrin). It is possible to formulate a palatable drink containing as much as 4 kcal/ml. If fluid restriction is not necessary such high concentrations are unnecessary. The energy drink blunts appetite and usually prevents excessive intake of other nutrients. Apart from the energy drink the children are allowed to eat and drink anything else they like and special meals are avoided. Each month a three day diet assessment is analysed and nutrient intake recorded. If excessive amounts of

Table 11.4   Conservative management of renal failure; check list for outpatient care

Items to be considered	Action
Biochemical derangements and nutrition sodium, potassium, calcium, phosphate, protein, (urea) energy, water	Measure plasma electrolytes, urea calcium, phosphate, alkaline phosphatase and plasma proteins Assess food intake regularly, give dietary supplements and advice
Infection: renal, non-renal, therapy	Admit for i.v. therapy if fluid losses are severe Check MSU Care must be taken with drugs which are excreted via the kidneys
Renal osteodystrophy	Three-monthly radiographs of hand and wrist
Hypertension	Measure BP at each attendance
Acidosis	Measure plasma bicarbonate
Anaemia	Full blood picture
Growth and skeletal development Family relationships, schooling and emotional adaptations	Measure height and weight and bone age

other nutrients are being ingested then minor adjustments can usually be undertaken with the aid of an experienced dietician without altering a family's eating habits or causing emotional disturbance to the child. Reasonable sodium intakes (40–60 mEq/day or 1–2 mEq/kg/day in the infant) can usually be allowed and excessive weight gain controlled by using frusemide to remove salt. Fluid limitation is rarely required and it is often dangerous because of the obligatory hyposthenuria of renal failure. The correct response to fluid overload is salt reduction and fluid restriction should only be contemplated if weight gain is excessive in the presence of hyponatraemia. Hyperphosphataemia can be controlled with aluminium hydroxide gel (1 ml/kg/day). Hyperkalaemia is rarely a problem but calcium/potassium exchange resin (1 g/kg/day) is effective if dietary manipulation is not possible. Adequate first-class protein intake (2 g/kg/day under one year, 1 g/kg/day afterwards) should be assured. Protein restriction is rarely necessary if energy intake is adequate and should not be attempted if the blood urea is less than 200 mg/dl. We have one child who has remained extremely well, and grown normally for six years with a blood urea between 190 and 220 mg/dl. Adequate calcium intake (1 g/day) should be provided if necessary by giving calcium gluconate supplements in the form of calcium sandoz syrup; the effervescent tablets contain too much sodium. Energy intake should be *above* recommended daily allowances for a child of the same height/age, and a knowledge of normal intakes (DHSS, 1969) is useful when managing these children; at least 150 kcal/kg/day for infants and 110 to 150 kcal/kg/day for older children is a rough guide.

Children with proximal tubular dysfunction such as cystinosis may lose enormous amounts of water, sodium, potassium, calcium and phosphate, and adequate supplementation whilst ensuring good energy intakes is often impossible.

Infection leads to hypercatabolism and with associated diarrhoea and vomiting may cause considerable acute alterations in body composition precipitating rapid deterioration. Urine infection may cause further damage to the already diseased kidneys. It is important to remember that saline depletion and dehydration may be rapid in the child who cannot concentrate the urine, urgent admission to hospital for intravenous fluid replacement will be necessary. Care should be taken in prescribing drugs with a renal route of excretion.

Renal osteodystrophy is complex and has been recently reviewed (Potter, Wilson and Ozonoff, 1974; Coburn and Norman, 1973). Frequent (three-monthly) radiographs of the hand and wrist and sometimes the knee and determination of the plasma alkaline phosphatase concentration should be undertaken to detect osteodystrophy. Once detected, therapy with vitamin D using the amounts necessary to overcome the resistance caused by the failure of the kidney to convert vitamin D to its active metabolite (1,25-dihydroxy-cholecalciferol), should be instituted: we use dihydrotachysterol 0.25–1 mg daily and check plasma calcium frequently (weekly at the start) to prevent hypercalcaemia.

Hypertension can sometimes be controlled by limiting sodium intake or increasing sodium excretion with frusemide. Antihypertensive drugs may be required.

Acidosis probably affects growth and contributes to the osteodystrophy. Alkali therapy with sodium bicarbonate (2 mEq/kg/day) may be effective but adds to sodium overload. Other alkalis such as calcium gluconate or carbonate are useful but less effective.

The anaemia of chronic renal failure is difficult to treat but may improve when adequate nutrition and sufficient intake of iron is ensured. The children usually adapt surprisingly well to the anaemia and transfusion should be avoided wherever possible because of the risk of inducing circulating antibodies which will affect future renal transplantation.

Growth retardation is common but not inevitable and attention to the details discussed above is the best way of ensuring good growth (Chantler and Holliday, 1973). Skeletal maturity is often delayed by two to four years and allowances for this should be made when assessing growth. Serial radiographs of the hand and wrist (Tanner Whitehouse and Healy, 1962) are useful for assessing bone age.

Attention must be directed to helping with the problems that inevitably arise with this group of chronically handicapped children. We have found that normal school attendance is possible and that special schooling is rarely required.

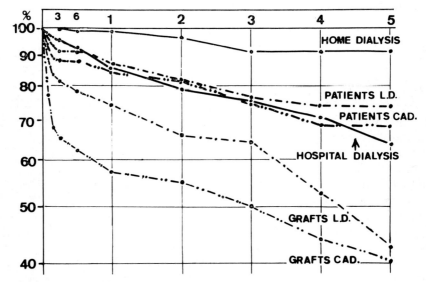

Figure 11.1   Survival of children and renal grafts in Europe on home or hospital dialysis and after live and cadaver donor transplant. (Reproduced with permission from European Dialysis and Transplant Association Register, 1974)

End-stage renal disease

A detailed consideration of dialysis and transplantation is beyond the scope of this article. Figure 11.1 shows the survival of children treated in Europe up to the end of 1974 and a full review of the subject is provided by Cameron (1973). Fisher, Farrow and Johnson (1975) give a detailed analysis of the recent results of transplantation and discuss future prospects. Our personal view is that the present results justify considering therapy for all children over the age of five years but that the impact on the family is considerable and that not all children or all families are able to cooperate sufficiently with the discipline involved, especially in home dialysis, without producing unacceptable stress for themselves or for the other children in the family.

Each case must therefore be assessed carefully by the paediatrician, family doctor, paediatric nephrologist and the dialysis and transplant team. If the aim of therapy is to provide a happy and active life of sufficient duration, say 20 years, then it is unlikely to be achieved on present results without utilising both chronic dialysis and transplantation. The family should therefore be capable of sustaining home dialysis prior to or between renal transplants. Using these criteria and rejecting children with multiple handicaps we have accepted about two-thirds of the children referred to us in the last three years. The decision is taken in conjunction with the parents and we have not had to refuse a child whose parents were enthusiastic for treatment. We have also tried to gauge the parents feelings before advising whether or not treatment

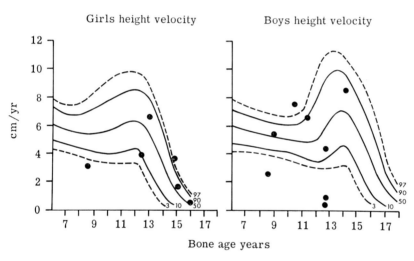

Figure 11.2   Growth velocity in boys and girls on home dialysis in the year ending May 1975

should be offered. It is difficult to judge whether this has been successful but a recent joint survey between Guy's Hospital, Great Ormond Street and the Royal Free Hospital suggests that the proportion of families with severe difficulties is no greater in this group of children than in families with children who have other chronic handicaps (Howarth, 1974, personal communication).

Poor growth on dialysis and after transplantation is another problem related to the management of these children. Recent results at Guy's are encouraging especially in the children taken on to the programme over the last two years. During this time intensive nutritional instruction in order to increase energy intake has been part of the initial training in hospital prior to the commencement of home dialysis. Figure 11.2 shows the growth velocity in the year after starting dialysis in these boys and girls and demonstrates that catch-up growth is possible, though whether it can be sustained is another matter.

It is hoped that over the next few years regional centres for dialysis and transplantation of children will be established throughout the United Kingdom. The reasons for regional centres are given in the report prepared for the British Paediatric Association by the British Association of Paediatric Nephrology and relate to the need to concentrate experience in a small number of highly specialised units with full supporting facilities. It is much easier if decisions about the treatment can be taken before the terminal stages of renal failure and it is suggested that these centres should be contacted and cases discussed with the paediatrician at the regional centre before the terminal phase is reached. The shortage of kidneys for transplantation is widely known and each of us should consider whether or not the parents of a child with terminal illness should be approached concerning possible donation of the kidneys for transplantation. If this is considered desirable the regional transplant centre should be contacted.

MISCELLANEOUS RENAL DISORDERS

Hereditary renal disease, cystic disease and renal involvement in syndromes affecting the whole child

Various types of renal disease may be inherited and all parts of the kidney may be affected. Most structural malformations are not inherited and renal dysplasia is rarely familial. On the other hand cystic disease is often genetically determined and the inheritance of the various types is complex. Many types of inherited renal disease are potentially fatal and constitute a much larger proportion of children reaching terminal renal failure than in an adult population. Juvenile nephronophthisis is a particularly prominent cause of renal failure in children with insidious onset of renal insufficiency (Betts and Forrest-Hay, 1973); other abnormalities may coexist such as liver disease and retinitis pigmentosa. A whole variety of paediatric syndromes may have a renal component which is important in determining prognosis. The importance of hereditary glomerulonephritis in the child with haematuria has been mentioned. Various tubular disorders are hereditary and certain families have a predisposition to the formation of renal calculi.

The following articles are useful reviews: 'Hereditary disorders of the kidney' (Bernstein and Kissane, 1973) covers the whole field of hereditary disorders of the kidney including glomerulonephritis, tubular disorders, cystic disease, other structural malformations, metabolic disease and general paediatric syndromes with a renal component; 'Polycystic disease of the kidneys and liver presenting in childhood' (Blyth and Ockenden, 1971) reviews the various types of cystic disease seen in children; 'Syndromes with a renal component' (Chantler, 1975) lists the general paediatric syndromes where a renal lesion has been described.

Renal damage from vascular insufficiency and renal vessel thrombosis

The newborn kidney is especially susceptible to damage from an acutely diminished blood supply and from renal vessel thrombosis but acute tubular necrosis, and medullary and cortical necrosis can occur at all ages. Blood loss, saline depletion leading to shock, intravascular coagulation as in the haemolytic uraemic syndrome, septicaemia or acute pyelonephritis may lead to tubular necrosis and acute renal failure. Severe cases of tubular necrosis may be accompanied by papillary necrosis (Chrispin et al, 1970) and excessive amounts of contrast media used for intravenous urography may exacerbate this. Residual defects in concentrating and acidifying capacity may follow papillary necrosis which can be recognised by intravenous urography. More extensive damage can occur throughout the medulla and cortex (Bernstein and Meyer, 1961) and the late effects in children who recover from medullary cortical necrosis include chronic renal failure, tubular lesions and hypertension.

Shock, asphyxia, disseminated intravascular coagulation, and cyanotic heart disease are particularly likely to lead to renal venous thrombosis in the infant (Arneil et al, 1973). Haematuria, bilateral or unilateral renal enlargement, oliguria, uraemia and acidosis comprise the clinical syndrome but the absence of these features does not preclude the diagnosis. Intravenous urography is the most helpful investigation but nephrosonography and antegrade or retrograde pyelography may be required to exclude other causes of a non-functioning kidney. Definitive confirmation requires inferior vena caval and selective renal vein venography (Fraley and Najarian, 1970). Spontaneous resolution of the renal failure is possible in about a third of affected children. Heparin anticoagulation is commonly used but no controlled data is available and recovery can occur without it. Thrombectomy for bilateral cases is advocated by some (Lowry et al, 1970) and with increasing experience may be undertaken more widely for many children are left with severely damaged kidneys from cortical necrosis leading to hypertension, renal insufficiency, and tubular abnormalities including the Fanconi syndrome (see also leading article, 1974).

Renal artery thrombosis (Brough and Zuelzer, 1964) is rare and is usually secondary to embolism from bacterial endocarditis, umbilical catheterisation or congenital heart disease. Adrenal haemorrhage (Black and Williams, 1973) is also rare and results in a large mass in the loin pushing the kidney down.

Acidosis

Renal tubular acidosis is most commonly due to damage to the distal tubule which is then unable to maintain a gradient of hydrogen ions between the blood and tubular fluid. Less frequently the acidosis results from the excessive loss of bicarbonate in the urine caused by failure of reabsorption in proximal tubule. This is of course a classical feature of the Fanconi syndrome. Recently an isolated defect of bicarbonate reabsorption has been described in children who present with failure to thrive and short stature (Soriano and Edelmann, 1969). These children have low plasma bicarbonate levels though this may be only intermittently severe; the main clinical feature in the child we have observed was a raised respiratory rate at rest and blood gas analysis showed a low P_{CO_2}. Urine pH is usually greater than 7.0 even in the presence of a low plasma bicarbonate and, unlike distal tubular acidosis, if the plasma bicarbonate is further lowered with ammonium chloride, acid excretion by the kidney may become normal and urine pH will fall below 5.3. The defect appears to be a low renal threshold for bicarbonate reabsorption which can be complete when the plasma concentration falls below this threshold. A careful search for other proximal tubular defects should be made and the Fanconi syndrome excluded. The acidosis is difficult to control and requires much larger doses of bicarbonate (5–10 mEq/kg/day) than in the distal form. Successful therapy will increase growth and the condition usually disappears as the child grows older (Nash et al, 1972).

URINARY TRACT INFECTION (UTI)

This subject is not dealt with in detail because excellent reviews are available (Smellie, 1974; Bailey, 1973). The main advances can be considered under diagnosis, pathogenesis and management.

Diagnosis

The demonstration that dip slide cultures inoculated during voiding in the home are as reliable as carefully taken midstream urine specimens in hospital has made an enormous contribution to the management of urine infection in children (McAllister et al, 1973). The method can be used at all ages and clean catch urines can be collected from small babies negating the need for unreliable bag specimens. The mother should be taught how to collect the specimen into a sterile dish, usually about an hour after a feed whilst the nappy is still dry, and to inoculate the dip slide immediately. False positive cultures and unnecessary investigation are therefore avoided. Suprapubic urine aspiration need only be undertaken if urgency exists or equivocal results have been obtained on dip slide culture.

Recent surveys in normal schoolgirls have shown that 1 to 2 per cent have a urinary infection at any one time, and that about half these children have abnormalities on radiological examination. Up to 20 per cent of girls with UTI will have scarred kidneys by the age of five years but the incidence of scarring does not increase much in older children (Newcastle Asymptomatic Bacteriuria Group, 1975). Because the incidence of *severe* scarring (about 0.05 per cent of the population) is low and because scarring does not increase with age (though of course it may be progressive in the individual child), Savage et al (1973) and the Newcastle group considered that universal adoption of school entry screening was not warranted at the present time. Longitudinal studies from birth to school entry are now required to assess whether earlier screening would prevent the incidence of scarring at five years.

Pathogenesis

It is obvious that the majority of UTI in childhood do not lead to serious renal damage. Hodson (1972) has demonstrated that scarring, identical to classical pyelonephritis, can be produced by vesicoureteric reflux in pigs without infection. The scarring is seen at the site of intrarenal reflux, that is where the urine is extravasated back into the renal tissue by the pressure of the column of urine applied to the renal pelvis during micturition when vesicoureteric reflux is present. Intrarenal reflux is particularly seen in infants and much less common in older children and of course reflux tends to disappear with time. Thus it seems likely that scarred kidneys may be caused by severe vesicoureteric reflux (Bailey, 1973) as well as by recurrent infections in the presence of reflux. Apart from these situations UTI in the absence of pyelonephritis may well be benign.

Management

Our current management is based on the above considerations. Unless the child is ill the presence of infection is carefully confirmed with at least one further urine specimen properly taken. Antibiotics (usually sulphonamides in the first instance) are given for two weeks after which an IVU is arranged. If this is *completely* normal with no evidence of distension of the ureters the child is followed for two years. If a further infection occurs a micturating cystogram is arranged. If reflux is present (usually grade 1 or 2; Smellie, 1974) then prophylactic antibiotics (low dose septrin or furadantin, which are associated with a reduced emergence of resistant strains) is started and follow-up continued for two years. At the end of two years IVU and micturating cystogram is repeated and if normal the child is discharged. Recurrent infections during prophylaxis suggest the need to assess renal growth frequently and consider reimplantation of the ureter if infection cannot be controlled and scarring develops. If the initial IVU is abnormal then a micturating cystogram is carried out. Grade 3 reflux in a child under one year or intrarenal reflux is an indication for surgery. Surgery should also be considered for grade 3 or grade 4 reflux in older children until renal growth has ceased. Other abnormalities such as ectopic ureterocele, pelviureteric junction obstruction, etc., are treated in the usual way (Williams, 1968).

Prognosis

The natural history of untreated UTI is not known but there is evidence that in the absence of structural anomalies the impact of treatment is slight (Savage et al, 1973). On the other hand detailed management can prevent the emergence of scars in children with recurrent infection and anomalies such as vesicoureteric reflux (Smellie, 1974). Among the many unresolved questions is the possible importance of persistence of bacterial antigen in the kidney causing progressive immunological renal damage without obvious infection in some children (MacGregor, 1970; Aoki et al, 1969; Anderson et al, 1973).

HYPERTENSION

Severe hypertension is rare in children but usually has a treatable cause (Table 11.5). It is particularly sad to admit a child following a cerebral vascular accident only to find hypertension which, if it had been discovered earlier, could have been treated and catastrophe averted. We have had this

Table 11.5   Aetiology of hypertension

Renovascular	Renal artery stenosis, extrinsic compression of renal vessels
Parenchymal renal disease	Nephritis, nephrosis, pyelonephritis, trauma, Wilms' tumour, haemangiopericytoma, cystic disease, obstructive uropathy, dysplasia, etc. End-stage renal disease
Cardiovascular	Coarctation of the aorta
Endocrine	Adrenal cortex—congenital adrenal hyperplasia, Cushing's syndrome, Conn's syndrome, dexamethasone suppressible hypertension, 18-hydroxydeoxycorticosterone excess, 1-oxygenated steroid excretion Adrenal medulla—pheochromocytoma, neuroblastoma Thyroid—hyperthyroidism
Metabolic	Porphyria, hypercalcaemia, vitamin D intoxication, heavy metal poisoning, liquorice ingestion, salt and water overload, Liddle's syndrome
CNS	Raised intracranial pressure, convulsions, familial dysautonomia, Gullain–Barre syndrome
Essential	

experience more than once over the last few years and each child had visited their general practitioners or paediatricians on more than one occasion in the previous two to three years but their blood pressure had not been measured. Recently paediatricians have begun to recognise essential hypertension and to consider their responsibility in attempting to prevent the high mortality of vascular disease in later life (Liebermann, 1974).

Blood pressure should be determined with the child lying or sitting in the mother's lap and as relaxed as possible; it is of little value if the child is crying. The cuff must be the appropriate size because small cuffs give falsely high readings. A general rule is to use the widest cuff which still allows auscultation of the brachial artery at the elbow. The systolic pressure determined by palpation is about 10 mm below the true systolic pressure.

The diastolic pressure on auscultation coincides with the muffling of the pressure sounds rather than with disappearance though this may not always be detected. In small infants the Doppler ultrasound method should be used if standard auscultation is not possible. The Doppler method gives readings close to those obtained by direct measurement (Elseed, Shinebourne and Joseph, 1973). The flush method is of little value because it is difficult to perform and underestimates the systolic pressure. The diastolic pressure has generally been considered to be more important in determining morbidity in hypertension but the Framingham data suggest that systolic pressure is no less important (Kannel and Dawber, 1974).

Diagnosis

Normal levels for blood pressure are shown in Table 11.6. It is difficult to know at what level hypertension should be diagnosed. Some workers

Table 11.6   Blood pressure measurement in normal children

Age in years	Mean (mmHg)		Mean +2 s.d. (mmHg)	
	Systolic	Diastolic	Systolic	Diastolic
0– 3	95	55	110	65
4– 7	100	65	120	70
8–10	105	70	130	75
11–15	115	70	140	80

suggest that the mean + 2 s.d. should be regarded as the upper limit of normal (Rance et al, 1974) but this of course defines 5 per cent of the childhood population as hypertensive. The Framingham study (Kannel and Dawber, 1974) suggests that patients with a high normal blood pressure will have an increase incidence of cardiovascular mortality as they grow older. This question has been discussed by Liebermann (1974) who emphasises the importance of checking a single reading again, if necessary in the child's home, and of noting a positive family history which might precipitate earlier investigation and treatment. A number of epidemiological studies are in progress and it is likely that more information will become available over the next few years. My present policy is to recheck a single hypertensive reading again and if necessary ask the general practitioner to measure the BP, usually the pattern will be that although an occasional reading is outside the normal range the majority are not, although they are above the mean. Such a child is not followed up. If the BP is consistently above the normal range then the child is investigated to exclude treatable causes though a renal arteriogram is not performed. If these investigations are normal the hypertension is treated medically and usually responds to relatively small amounts of hypotensive drugs. If control is not easily achieved then renal arteriography may be indicated. Essential hypertension discovered in this way does not seem common in day to day practice, though epidemiological studies may reveal such children.

Hypertension occurring in hospital practice is usually severe and may present with headaches, convulsions, heart failure or CNS signs, such as facial palsy or hemiplegia; often no symptoms are reported. A clue to diagnosis is often found in the history or on physical examination and will direct the investigations accordingly.

Renal causes. Unilateral or bilateral renal artery stenosis may be suspected by the presence of an abdominal bruit. Early films at 1, 3 and 5 min should be requested at intravenous urography (IVU) for the unilateral ischaemic kidney is smaller, and opacifies later and more densely than the normal kidney. Even in severe bilateral renal artery stenosis the IVU may be normal though in such cases filling defects in the ureter, caused by large anastomotic arterial vessels, may be seen. Renal scintillography with the gamma camera or ^{131}I-hippuran renography may reveal an ischaemic kidney. The gamma camera scan can analyse segmental blood flow and may be useful in detecting peripheral branch renal artery stenosis. The scan is also useful in determining the total amount of function contributed by each kidney and this information may aid the decision about the correct surgical treatment. Renal arteriography is necessary to properly delineate stenosis. It is important to include selective injections of contrast media into each renal artery for if aortography alone is performed important information will be missed. The blood pressure should be controlled with drugs before this investigation is undertaken. If propranolol has been used this must be omitted at least 48 h beforehand because its beta-adrenergic blocking action may prevent an increase in heart rate and cardiac output during the anaesthetic, as well as blocking renin release from the ischaemic kidney.

The decision concerning the correct treatment may be difficult. If one kidney is normal and the other is very small with poor function, nephrectomy may be indicated, otherwise the choice lies between medical treatment and arterial reconstructive surgery. Whilst surgery may be performed in unilateral cases, in bilateral cases medical treatment should be tried though it may fail or be associated with severe side effects. Angioplastic reconstruction is difficult and often fails but a saphenous vein graft bypassing the stenosis is easier and more successful (Fry et al, 1973). Autotransplantation, removing the kidney and replacing it in the iliac fossa with anastomosis to the ilial vessels, is also successful (Sinaiko et al, 1973). We have used a saphenous graft in one kidney and autotransplantation on the other side when treating a five-year-old boy with severe hypertension due to bilateral stenosis; one year later off all treatment the BP was normal (Gill, 1975). In young infants hypertension from renal artery stenosis may be secondary to idiopathic generalised arterial calcification (Holm, 1967).

Parenchymal renal disease. The presence of kidney disease will be revealed by urine examination, IVU, renal scintillography, etc. When bilateral but non-uniform renal scarring is revealed, perhaps secondary to pyelonephritis, the problem is often whether one kidney is responsible for the hypertension. Bilateral renal vein renin determinations (Dillon, 1974) may aid in identifying whether one kidney is secreting excess renin whilst the other is suppressed. Renal vein renin levels may also be valuable in revealing an ischaemic kidney even when renal arteriography is normal (Leumann, 1970). A haemangio-pericytoma, a renin secreting tumour, may also be revealed by renal vein renin determinations. Hypertension is a common accompaniment of chronic renal failure and is usually secondary to salt and water overload although renin levels may rise as sodium is removed by diuretics or dialysis.

Endocrine causes. The most useful investigation is a properly performed peripheral plasma renin and aldosterone concentration. This investigation should be undertaken as soon as possible after detection of the hypertension and if possible before treatment is started. A 24 h sodium excretion is useful in evaluating the renin level for salt depletion raises plasma renin concentration. A high plasma renin suggests a renal cause whereas a low renin suggests that the cause of the hypertension should be sought elsewhere. A metabolic alkalosis with or without hypokalaemia suggests oversecretion of mineralo-corticoid, either from secondary aldosteronism from hyperreninaemia or primary endocrine dysfunction if the renin level is normal or low. A plasma potassium concentration of less than 3.8 mEq/litre should initiate a search for an adrenal cause for the hypertension (Robertson, 1974). A 24 h urine for 17-ketosteroid and other steroid metabolites should be obtained along with serum cortisol determinations. This should enable the correct diagnosis of Cushing's syndrome and adrenal hyperplasia as well as the rare 18-hydroxy-deoxycorticosterone excess which responds to suppression with dexametha-zone. This latter syndrome is associated with a normal aldosterone level whereas hypertension suppressible by dexamethasone has also been described in a family with raised plasma aldosterone levels (Sutherland, Ruse and Laidlaw, 1966).

Increased excretion of 1-oxygenated steroids has been described in a neonate with hypertension (Edwards, Harvey and Knight-Jones, 1968). Hypertension and hypokalaemia with normal cortisol and aldosterone levels but raised deoxyaldosterone has been described and this condition is similar to Liddle's syndrome in which the kidneys reabsorb sodium excessively in spite of negligible mineralocorticoid excretion. Both these conditions respond to trimterene but spironolactone is not effective in Liddle's syndrome.

The diagnosis of a phaeochromocytoma is usually suggested by the history and the demonstration of increased secretion of catecholamines and their metabolites (VMA) in the urine. Surgery for these tumours is very specialised and the blood pressure should be controlled with phenoxybenzamine (1 mg/kg/day) and propranolol (1 mg/kg/day) for at least four days beforehand (Barratt, 1973). It is better that the child should be transferred to a unit with the necessary experience and monitoring facilities.

Medical treatment

A full review of antihypertensive agents and their action is given by Nickerson (1970). Laragh (1973) has introduced the concept of volume hypertension and vasoconstrictor hypertension. This recognises that hypertension is related either to excess salt and water retention with increased cardiac output, or to increased peripheral vascular resistance. Obviously both types may coexist, but nevertheless the concept is useful for therapy should be directed towards the prime cause. Thus the child on dialysis, or with end-stage renal failure or with Conn's syndrome may have volume hyper-

Table 11.7   Pharmaceutical agents used in treatment of hypertension

Drug	Principle action	Dosage	
Chlorthiazide	Decreases ECF Lowers peripheral vascular resistance	10 mg/kg/12 h	(oral)
Frusemide	Decreases ECF	0.5–7.5 mg/kg/day 0.5–5 mg/kg	(oral) (i.m.)
Spironolactone	Aldosterone antagonist	1 mg/kg/8 h	(oral)
Propranolol	Beta-adrenergic blocker	0.2–3 mg/kg/8 h	(oral)
Methyldopa	Lowers peripheral vascular resistance Antagonises renin release	2–7.5 mg/kg/6 h	(oral)

Bethanidine	Lowers peripheral vascular
	  resistance due to inhibition of
	  noradrenaline release
		0.1–1 mg/kg/8 h	(oral)

Hydrallazine	Lowers peripheral vascular
	  resistance by direct arteriolar
	  action
		0.2–1 mg/kg/8 h
		500 mg/kg
			(oral)
			(i.m. or i.v.)

Diazoxide	Lowers peripheral vascular
	  resistance by direct arteriolar
	  action
		5 mg/kg/dose	(i.v.)

Minoxidil	Lowers peripheral vascular resistance by direct action	2.5 mg/12 h up to 40 mg/day	(oral)

tension and therapy is directed to removal of sodium either with diuretics or dietary restriction. In fact it is usually easier to use diuretics than to apply strict dietary sodium restriction. In renal failure thiazides are rarely effective though large doses of frusemide may be. Frequent assessment of plasma electrolytes is necessary. Spirolactone should not be used in renal failure because of the danger of hyperkalaemia.

In mild hypertension we generally use a thiazide diuretic but in moderate or severe hypertension methyl dopa is the first choice. It can cause sleepiness and a positive Coombs' test though a haemolytic anaemia is rare. Bethanidine is effective but causes postural hypertension. It is important to start with a small test dose because some children are acutely sensitive to its action

and may experience a severe postural fall in BP. Renin induced hypertension may respond to propranolol. The pulse rate should be monitored, and congestive cardiac failure may occur if the dose is pushed too high. It should be discontinued during a severe febrile illness and before a general anaesthetic. Our policy is to add each drug sequentially until the desired effect is obtained. Oral hydrallazine is especially useful in renal hypertension though a SLE-like syndrome may follow prolonged use; it may also cause sodium retention.

Very severe renal hypertension which is inoperable will respond to oral diazoxide or minoxidil. Both these drugs have severe side effects; diazoxide causes hyperglycaemia, sodium retention, tachycardia and hirsuitism. Minoxidil has similar effects except for the hyperglycaemia and it is our impression that the hirsuitism is worse. Propranolol and frusemide are generally prescribed in addition to control the increased heart rate and sodium retention which occur. In spite of the side effects the use of these drugs can be lifesaving; one of our children presented with malignant hypertension from inoperable ureteric reflux and a GFR of 8 ml/min/1.73 m^2, two years later her blood pressure is controlled on diazoxide and her GFR is 28 ml/min/1.73 m^2.

Hypertensive crises demand immediate action. If volume overload is suspected intravenous frusemide is used. Intramuscular or intravenous hydrallazine or if that fails intravenous diazoxide are effective. A list of drugs with their mode of action and dosage is given in Table 11.7.

REFERENCES

Abramowicz, N., Barnett, H. L., Edelmann, C. M., Greifer, I., Kobayashi, O., Arneil, G. C., Barron, B. A., Gordillo, P. G., Hallmann, N. & Tiddens, H. A. (1970) Controlled trial of azothioprine in children with nephrotic syndrome. *Lancet*, **1,** 959.

Anderson, H. J., Jacobsson, B., Larsson, H. & Winberg, J. (1973) Hypertension, asymmetric renal parenchymal defect, sterile urine high *E. coli* antibody titre. *British Medical Journal*, **3,** 14.

Antoine, B., Symvoulidis, A. & Dardenne, M. (1969) La stabilité évolutive des états de proteinurie. *Nephron*, **6,** 526.

Aoki, S., Imamura, S., Aoki, M. & McCabe, W. R. (1969) Abacterial and bacterial pyelonephritis. *New England Journal of Medicine*, **281,** 1375.

Arneil, G. C., MacDonald, A. M., Murphy, A. V. & Sweet, E. M. (1973) Renal venous thrombosis. *Clinical Nephrology*, **1,** 119.

Aynsley-Green, A. & Pickering, D. (1974) Use of central and peripheral temperature measurements in care of the critically ill child. *Archives of Disease in Childhood*, **49,** 477.

Bailey, R. R. (1973) The relationship of vesicoureteric reflux to urinary tract infection and chronic pyelonephritis-reflux nephropathy. *Clinical Nephrology*, **1,** 132.

Baldwin Gluck, M. C., Schacht, R. G. & Gallo, G. (1974) The long-term course of poststreptococcal glomerulonephritis. *Annals of Internal Medicine*, **80,** 342.

Bannister, A., Martin-Siddigi, S. A. & Hatcher, G. W. (1975) Treatment of hypernatraemic dehydration in infancy. *Archives of Disease in Childhood*, **50,** 179.

Barratt, T. M. (1973) Hypertension in childhood. In *Paediatric Urology*, ed. Williams, D. I., *Encyclopedia of Urology*, 2nd edn, Vol. XV. Heidelberg: Springer Verlag.

Barratt, T. M., Bercowsky, A., Osofsky, S. G., Soothill, J. F. & Kay, R. (1975) Cyclophosphamide treatment in steroid sensitive nephrotic syndrome in childhood. *Lancet*, **1,** 55,

Barratt, T. M. & Chantler, C. (1975) The measurement of renal function. In *Paediatric Nephrology*, ed. Rubin, M. I. & Barratt, T. M. Baltimore: Williams and Wilkins.

Barratt, T. M. & Soothill, J. F. (1970) Controlled trial of cyclophosphamide in steroid sensitive relapsing nephrotic syndrome of childhood. *Lancet*, **2**, 479.

Berger, J. (1969) IgA glomerular deposits in renal disease. *Transplant Proceedings*, **1**, 939.

Bergstrand, A., Bollgren, I., Samuelsson, A., Tornroth, T., Wassermann, J. & Windberg, J. (1973) Idiopathic nephrotic syndrome of childhood: cyclophosphamide induced conversion from steroid refractory to highly steroid sensitive disease. *Clinical Nephrology*, **1**, 302.

Bernstein, J. & Kissane, J. M. (1973) Hereditary disorders of the kidney. In *Perspectives in Paediatric Pathology*, ed. Rosenberg, H. S. & Bolande, R. R., pp. 117. Year Book Publishers Inc.

Bernstein, J. & Meyer, R. (1961) Congenital abnormalities of the urinary system. II. Renal cortical and medullary necrosis. *Journal of Paediatrics*, **59**, 657.

Betts, P. R. & Forrest-Hay, I. (1973) Juvenile nephronophthisis. *Lancet*, **2**, 473.

Betts, P. R. & MacGrath, G. (1974) Growth pattern and dietary intake of children with chronic renal insufficiency. *British Medical Journal*, **2**, 189.

Black, J. & Williams, D. I. (1973) Natural history of adrenal haemorrhage in the newborn. *Archives of Disease in Childhood*, **48**, 183.

Blyth, H. & Ockenden, B. G. (1971) Polycystic disease of kidneys and liver presenting in childhood. *Journal of Medical Genetics*, **8**, 257.

Boulton-Jones, J. M., Sissons, J. G. P., Evans, D. J. & Peters, D. K. (1974) Renal lesions of subacute infective endocarditis. *British Medical Journal*, **2**, 11.

Brough, A. J. & Zuelzer, W. W. (1964) Renal vascular disease. *Paediatric Clinics in America*, **11**, 533.

Brown, C. B., Ogg, C. S., Cameron, J. S. & Bewick, J. S. (1974a) High dose frusemide in acute reversible intrinsic renal failure. *Scottish Medical Journal*, **19**, 35.

Brown, C. B., Wilson, D., Turner, D. R., Cameron, J. S., Ogg, C. S. & Chantler, C. (1974b) Combined immunosuppression and anticoagulation in rapidly progressive glomerulonephritis. *Lancet*, **2**, 1166.

Brzosko, W. J., Krawczynski, K., Nazarewicz, T., Morzyeka, M. & Nowoslawki. A. (1974) Glomerulonephritis associated with hepatitis B surface antigen immune complexes in children. *Lancet*, **2**, 450.

Cameron, J. S. (1968) Histology, protein clearances and response to steroids in the nephrotic syndrome. *British Medical Journal*, **4**, 352.

Cameron, J. S. (1971) Proteinuria. In *Seventh Symposium of Advanced Medicine*, ed. Bouchier, I. A. D. London: Pitman Medical.

Cameron, J. S. (1972) The natural history of glomerulonephritis. In *Renal Disease*, 3rd edn, ed. Black, Sir D. Oxford: Blackwell Scientific Publications.

Cameron, J. S. (1973) The treatment of chronic renal failure in children by regular dialysis and by transplantation. *Nephron*, **11**, 221.

Cameron, J. S., Chantler, C., Ogg, C. S. & White, R. H. R. (1974) Long-term stability of remission in the nephrotic syndrome following treatment with cyclophosphamide. *British Medical Journal*, **4**, 7.

Cantarovich, F., Galli, C., Benedetti, L., Chena, C., Castro, L., Correa, C., Perez Laredo, J., Fernandez, J. C., Locatelli, A. & Tujado, J. (1973) High dose frusemide in established acute renal failure. *British Medical Journal*, **4**, 449.

Chantler, C. (1975) Syndromes with a renal component. In *Paediatric Nephrology*, ed. Rubin, M. I. & Barratt, T. M. Baltimore: Williams and Wilkins.

Chantler, C. & Barratt, T. M. (1972) Estimation of the glomerular filtration rate from the plasma clearance of 51 Chromium edetic acid. *Archives of Disease in Childhood*, **47**, 613.

Chantler, C. & Holliday, M. A. (1973) Growth in children with renal disease with particular reference to the effects of calorie malnutrition: a review. *Clinical Nephrology*, **1**, 230.

Chrispin, A. R., Hull, D., Lillie, J. G. & Risdon, R. A. (1970) Renal tubular necrosis and papillary necrosis after gastroenteritis. *British Medical Journal*, **1**, 410.

Coburn, J. W. & Norman, A. W. (1973) Role of the kidney in the metabolism of calciferol (vitamin D). *Clinical Nephrology*, **1**, 273.

Curran, P., Toseland, P. A. & Chantler, C. (1975) Lipoic acid for acute lactic acidosis (in preparation).

Department of Health and Social Security (1969) Report no. 120, *Recommended Intakes of Nutrients for the United Kingdom*. London: Her Majesty's Staionery Office.

Dillon, M. J. (1974) Renin and hypertension in childhood. *Archives of Disease in Childhood*, **49**, 831.

Dixon, F. J. & Wilson, C. B. (1972) Immunological aspects of glomerulonephritis. In *Renal Disease*, 3rd edn, ed. Black, Sir D., p. 275. Oxford: Blackwell Scientific Publishers.

Dodge, W. F., Spargo, B. H. & Travis, L. B. (1967) Occurrence of acute glomerulonephritis in sibling contacts of children with sporadic acute glomerulonephritis. *Paediatrics*, **40**, 1029.

Edwards, R. W. H., Harvey, D. R. & Knight-Jones, E. (1968) Hypertension and excretion of 1-oxygenated steroids. *Archives of Disease in Childhood*, **43**, 611.

Egan, T. J., Kenny, F. M., Jarra, L. A. & Holliday, M. (1967) Shock as a complication of the nephrotic syndrome. *American Journal of Diseases of Children*, **113**, 364.

Elseed, A. M., Shinebourne, E. A. & Joseph, M. C. (1973) Assessment of techniques for measurement of blood pressure in infants and children. *Archives of Disease in Childhood*, **48**, 932.

Emanuel, B. & Aronson, N. (1974) Neonatal haematuria. *American Journal of Diseases of Children*, **128**, 204.

Epstein, W. V. (1973) Immunologic events preceding clinical exacerbation of systemic lupus erythematosus. *American Journal of Medicine*, **54**, 631.

Fairley, K. J., Barrie, J. U. & Johnson, W. (1972) Sterility and testicular atrophy related to cyclophosphamide therapy. *Lancet*, **1**, 568.

Fisher, D. J. H., Farrow, S. C. & Johnson, D. B. (1975) Renal transplantation: trends and prospects. *British Journal of Hospital Medicine*, **13**, 451.

Fraley, E. D. & Najarian, J. S. (1970) Treatment of renal vein thrombosis in the newborn. *Journal of the American Medical Association*, **212**, 1377.

Fry, I. K. & Cattell, W. F. (1970) The IVP in renal failure. *British Journal of Hospital Medicine*, **3**, 67.

Fry, W. J., Ernst, C. B., Stanly, J. C., Brink, B. & Arbor, A. (1973) Renovascular hypertension in the paediatric patient. *Archives of Surgery*, **107**, 692.

George, C. R. P., Slichters, S. J., Quadracci, L. J., Striker, G. E. & Harker, L. A. (1974) A kinetic evaluation of hemostasis in renal disease. *New England Journal of Medicine*, **291**, 1111.

Gill, D., Chantler, C., Cameron, J. S. & Ogg, C. S. (1975) Anticoagulation and immuno-suppression in the treatment of rapidly and slowly progressive nephritis. Presented at IX Congress of ESPN, Cambridge.

Gill, D. (1975) Bilateral renal artery stenosis in a five year old child. *Proceedings of the Royal Society of Medicine* (in press).

Gill, D., Visy, M. & Chantler, C. (1975) The significance of red cell casts in children with haematuria. Paper presented at British Paediatric Association, Harrogate.

Habib, R. (1970) Classification anatomique des néphropathies glomérulaires. *Päediatrische Fortbildungskurse*, **28**, 3.

Habib, R. & Kleinknecht, C. (1971) The primary nephrotic syndrome of childhood, classi-cation and clinicopathologic study of 406 cases. In *Pathology Annual*, ed. Sommers, S. C., p. 417. Appleton-Century-Crofts.

Habib, R., Kleinknecht, C., Gubler, M. C. & Levy, M. (1973) Idiopathic membrano-proliferative glomerulonephritis in children. Report of 105 cases. *Clinical Nephrology*, **1**, 194.

Hallman, N. (1973) The congenital nephrotic syndrome. *Nephron*, **11**, 101.

Hendler, E. D., Kashgarian, M. & Hayslett, J. P. (1972) Clinicopathological correlations of primary haematuria. *Lancet*, **1**, 458.

Hardwicke, J., Soothill, J. F., Squire, J. R. & Holti, G. (1959) Nephrotic syndrome with pollen hypersensitivity. *Lancet*, **1**, 500.

Hodson, C. J. (1972) A new concept of the pathogenesis of atrophic pyelonephritis. In Abstracts (no. 598) of 5th International Congress of Nephrology, Mexico City.

Holliday, M. A. (1972) Calorie deficiency in children with uremia. Effect upon growth. *Paediatrics*, **50**, 590.

Holm, V. (1967) Arteriopathia calcificans infantum. *Acta paediatrica scandinavica*, **56**, 537.

Hoyer, J. R., Kjellstrand, C. M., Simmons, R. L., Najarian, J. S., Mauer, S. M., Buselmeier, T. J., Michael, A. F. & Vernier, R. L. (1973) Successful renal transplantation in three children with congenital nephrotic syndrome. *Lancet*, **1**, 1410.

Hughes, G. R. V. (1974) Systemic lupus erythematosus. *British Journal of Hospital Medicine*, **12**, 309.

International Study of Kidney Disease in Children (1974) Prospective controlled trial of cyclophosphamide therapy in children with the nephrotic syndrome. *Lancet*, **2**, 423.

Johnston, C. & Shuler, S. (1969) Recurrent haematuria in childhood: a five year follow-up. *Archives of Disease in Childhood*, **44**, 483.

Jones, F. E., Black, P. J., Cameron, J. S., Chantler, C., Gill, D., Maisey, M. N., Ogg, C. S. & Saxton, H. (1975) Local infusion of urokinase and heparin into the renal arteries in impending renal cortical necrosis (submitted for publication).

Joseph, M. C. & Polani, P. E. (1958) The effect of bed rest on acute haemorrhagic nephritis in children. *Guy's Hospital Reports*, **107**, 500.

Kannel, W. B. & Dawber, T. R. (1974) Hypertension as an ingredient of a cardiovascular risk profile. *British Journal of Hospital Medicine*, **11**, 508.

Kaplan, B. S., Bureau, M. A. & Drummond, K. N. (1974) The nephrotic syndrome in the first year of life: Is a pathologic classification possible? *Journal of Paediatrics*, **85**, 615.

Kaufman, D. B. & McIntosh, R. M. (1971) The pathogenesis of the renal lesion in a patient with streptococcal disease, infected ventricularterial shunt cryoglobulinemia and nephritis. *American Journal of Medicine*, **50**, 262.

Laragh, J. H. (1973) Vasoconstriction-volume analysis for understanding and treating hypertension: the use of renin and aldosterone profiles. *American Journal of Medicine*, **55**, 261.

Leading article (1974) Renal vascular damage after birth. *British Medical Journal*, **3**, 296.

Leumann, E. P., Bauer, R. P., Slaton, P. E., Biglieri, E. G. & Holliday, M. A. (1970) Renovascular hypertension in children. *Paediatrics*, **46**, 362.

Lewy, J. E., Salimas-Madrigal, L., Herdson, P. B., Pirani, C. L. & Metcoff, J. (1971) Clinico-pathologic correlations in acute post-streptococcal glomerulonephritis. *Medicine*, **50**, 453.

Liebermann, E. (1972) Haemolytic-uremic syndrome. *Journal of Paediatrics*, **80**, 1.

Liebermann, E. (1974) Essential hypertension in children and youth: a paediatric perspective. *Journal of Paediatrics*, **85**, 1.

Linton, A. L. & Lawson, D. H. (1970) Antibiotic therapy in renal failure. *Proceedings of the European Dialysis and Transplant Association*, **7**, 371.

Lowry, M. F., Mann, J. R., Abrams, L. D. & Chance, G. W. (1970) Thrombectomy for renal venous thrombosis in infant of diabetic mother. *British Medical Journal*, **3**, 687.

Lyons, E. D., Murphy, A. V. & Arneil, G. C. (1972) Sonar and its use in kidney disease in children. *Archives of Disease in Childhood*, **47**, 777.

MacGregor, M. (1970) Pyelonephritis. Consideration of childhood urinary infection as the forerunner of renal insufficiency in later life. *Archives of Disease in Childhood*, **45**, 159.

McAdams, A. J., McEnery, P. T. & West, C. D. (1975) Mesangiocapillary glomerulonephritis: changes in glomerular morphology with long-term alternate day prednisone therapy. *Journal of Paediatrics*, **86**, 23.

McAllister, T. A., Arneil, G. C., Barr, W. & Kay, P. (1973) Assessment of plane dipslide quantitation of bacteruria. *Nephron*, **11**, 111.

McDonald, J., Murphy, A. V. & Arneil, G. C. (1974) Long-term assessment of cyclophosphamide therapy for nephrosis in children. *Lancet*, **2**, 980.

Meadow, S. R. (1975) Post-streptococcal nephritis—a rare disease? *Archives of Disease in Children*, **50**, 379.

Meadow, S. R., Cameron, J. S., Ogg, C. S. & Saxton, H. M. (1971) Children referred for acute dialysis. *Archives of Disease in Childhood*, **46**, 221.

Meadow, S. R., Glasgow, E. F., White, R. H. R., Moncrieff, M. W., Cameron, J. S. & Ogg, C. S. (1972) Schonlein–Henoch nephritis. *Quarterly Journal of Medicine*, **41**, 241.

Monnens, L., Kleynen, F., Van Munster, P., Schvetlen, E. & Bonnermann, A. (1972) Coagulation studies and streptokinase therapy in the haemolytic uremic syndrome. *Helvetica paediatrica acta*, **27**, 45.

Nash, M. A., Torrado, A. D., Greifer, I., Spitzer, A. & Edelmann, C. M. (1972) Renal tubular acidosis in infants and children. *Journal of Paediatrics*, **80**, 738.

Newcastle Asymptomatic Bacteriuria Research Group (1975) Asymptomatic bacteriuria in school children in Newcastle upon Tyne. *Archives of Disease in Childhood*, **50**, 90.

Niall, J. F. (1965) Prolonged survival in the nephrotic syndrome. *Medical Journal of Australia*, **1**, 843.

Nickerson, M. (1970) Acute hypertensive agents and the drug therapy of hypertension. In *The Pharmacological Basis of Therapeutics*, ed. Goodman, L. S. & Gillman, A., p. 728. New York: Macmillan & Company.

Pennisi, A. J., Grushkin, C. M. & Liebermann, E. (1975) Gonadal function in children with nephrosis treated with cyclophosphamide. *American Journal of Diseases of Children*, **129**, 315.

Perlman, L. V., Herdman, R. C., Kleinman, H. & Vernier, R. L. (1965) Poststreptococcal glomerulonephritis. A ten-year follow-up of an epidemic. *Journal of American Medical Association*, **194**, 175.

Peters, D. K., Gwyn Williams, D., Charlesworth, J. A., Boulton Jones, J. M., Sissons, J. G. P. & Evans, D. J. (1973) Mesangiocapillary nephritis, partial lipodystrophy and hypocomplementaemia. *Lancet*, **3**, 535.

Popovic-Rolovic, M. (1973) Serum C3 levels in acute glomerulonephritis and postnephritic children. *Archives of Disease in Childhood*, **48**, 622.

Potter, D., Wilson, C. J. & Ozonoff, M. B. (1974) Hyperparathyroid bone disease in children undergoing long-term haemodialysis treatment with vitamin D. *Journal of Paediatrics*, **85**, 60.

Powell, H. R., Rotenberg, E., Williams, A. L. & McCredie, D. A. (1974) Plasma renin activity in acute poststreptococcal glomerulonephritis and the haemolytic-uraemic syndrome. *Archives of Disease in Childhood*, **49**, 802.

Raitt, J. W. (1972) Wegener's granulomatosis—treatment with cytoxic agents and adrenocortocoids. *Annals of Internal Medicine*, **74**, 344.

Rance, C. P., Arbus, G. S., Balfe, J. W. & Kooh, S. W. (1974) Peristent hypertension in infants and children. *Paediatric Clinics of North America*, **21**, 801.

Reidenberg, M. M. (1971) *Renal Function and Drug Action*. Philadelphia: W. B. Saunders.

Robertson, J. B. (1974) Endocrine aspects of hypertension. *British Journal of Hospital Medicine*, **11**, 707.

Row, P. G., Cameron, J. S., Turner, D., Evans, D. J., White, R. H. R., Ogg, C. S., Chantler, C. & Brown, C. B. (1975) Membranous nephropathy, long-term follow-up and association with neoplasia. *Quarterly Journal of Medicine*, **44**, 207.

Savage, D. C. L., Wilson, M. I., McHardy, M., Dewar, D. A. E. & Fee, W. M. (1973) Covert bacteriuria of childhood. A clinical and epidemiological study. *Archives of Disease of Childhood*, **48**, 8.

Saxton, H. M., Cameron, J. S., Chantler, C. & Ogg, C. S. (1973) Renal puncture in infancy. *British Medical Journal*, **3**, 267.

Siegel, N. J., Goldberg, B., Krassner, L. S. & Hayslett, J. P. (1972) Long-term follow-up of children with steroid responsive nephrotic syndrome. *Journal of Paediatrics*, **81**, 251.

Simenhoff, M. L., Guild, W. R. & Dammin, G. J. (1968) Acute diffuse interstitial nephritis. *American Journal of Medicine*, **44**, 618.

Sinaiko, A., Najarian, J., Michael, A. F. & Mirkin, B. L. (1973) Renal autotransplantation in the treatment of bilateral renal artery stenosis: relief of hypertension in an eight year old boy. *Journal of Paediatrics*, **83**, 409.

Singer, D. B., Hill, L. L., Rosenberg, H. S., Marshall, J. & Swenson, R. (1968) Recurrent haematuria in childhood. *New England Journal of Medicine*, **279**, 7.

Sissons, J. G. P., Evans, D. J., Peters, D. K., Eisinger, A. J., Boulton Jones, J. M., Simpson, I. J. & Macanovic, M. M. (1974) Glomerulonephritis associated with antibody to glomerular basement membrane. *British Medical Journal*, **3**, 11.

Sissons, J. G. P. & Woodrow, D. F. (1975) Recurrent haematuria. *Lancet*, **2**, 275.

Smellie, J. M. (1974) Urinary tract infection in childhood. *British Journal of Hospital Medicine*, **12**, 485.

Soriano, J. R. & Edelmann, C. M. (1969) Renal tubular acidosis. *Annual Revue of Medicine*, **20**, 363.

Stuart, J., Winterborn, M. H., White, R. H. R. & Flinn, R. M. (1974) Thrombolytic therapy in haemolytic-uraemic syndrome. *British Medical Journal*, **3**, 217.

Sutherland, D. J. A., Ruse, J. L. & Laidlaw, J. C. (1966) Hypertension, increased aldosterone secretion and low plasma renin activity relieved by dexamethasone. *Canadian Medical Association Journal*, **95**, 1109.

Tanner, J. M., Whitehouse, R. H. & Healy, M. J. R. (1962) A new system for estimating skeletal maturity from the hand and wrist with standards derived from the study of 2600 healthy British children. Centre International de L'Enfance, Paris.

Travis, L. B., Dodge, W. F., Beathard, G. A., Spargo, B. H., Lorentz, W. B., Carrajal, H. F. & Berger, M. (1973) Acute glomerulonephritis in children: a review of the natural history with emphasis on prognosis. *Clinical Nephrology*, **1,** 169.

Tune, B. M., Leavitt, T. J. & Gribble, T. J. (1973) The haemolytic-uraemic syndrome in California: a review of 28 non-heparinised cases with long-term follow-up. *Journal of Paediatrics*, **82,** 304.

Wegmann, W. & Leumann, E. P. (1973) Glomerulonephritis associated with (infected) ventriculo-arterial shunt. *Virchows Archiv; Abteilung A; pathologische Anatomie*, **359,** 185.

White, R. H. R. (1970) Glomerulonephritis in children. *British Journal of Hospital Medicine*, **3,** 746.

Wiggelin-Khuizen, J., Kaschula, R. O. C., Uys, C. J., Kuijten, R. H. & Dale, J. (1975) Congenital syphilis and glomerulonephritis with evidence for immune pathogenesis. *Archives of Disease in Childhood*, **48,** 375.

Williams, D. I. (1968) *Pediatric Urology*. London: Butterworths.

12
OBESITY

June K. Lloyd   Otto H. Wolff

DEFINITION AND MEASUREMENT

Although obesity is strictly defined as a condition in which the whole adipose organ is enlarged out of proportion to other body tissues (Wolff and Lloyd, 1974), this definition is of limited practical value because of the difficulty of assessing the size of the adipose organ. Thus obesity has usually been defined in terms of relative body weight or of skinfold thickness. Each method has its technical limitations but whatever method is used to estimate the amount of body fat there is a lack of agreed ideal values. Data on patients are compared with data obtained from populations of healthy children, but within the range of values recorded in such populations there are no criteria by which to judge what is desirable in health terms. In presenting revised standards for skinfold measurements in British children, Tanner and White-house (1975) emphasise that the standards represent 'what is, not what ought to be'. If paediatricians and other health workers are to play a more active role in the prevention and early detection of obesity, some agreement must be reached on definition and standards. Methods of measurement should be chosen which give a reliable index of body fatness and can be used both in the community and in hospital. Some of the methods, with their advantages and disadvantages, will be discussed.

Inspection

Inspection, the easiest and least expensive of all methods, still has a place in the assessment of obesity. Visual assessment has long been used for the appraisal of carcass traits in animals and correlates well with measurements of body composition (Orme, 1963). An experienced doctor is seldom in doubt of the diagnosis of obesity when he sees the child undressed. Crawford et al (1974), in a study designed to determine the most useful indices for the definition of obesity in babies, in fact, used the visual appraisal of three paediatricians as the reference standard. Rauh and Schumsky (1969) found visual ratings made by highly trained observers to be of value in the assessment of school children, and showed a strong positive relationship between the visual rating of fatness on the one hand and body weight, estimates of body fat, and triceps skinfold measurements on the other. Visual assessment should not be ignored; a child who looks too fat probably is too fat and conversely a child who looks lean is unlikely to have significant enlargement of his adipose tissue mass. Inspection is of particular value in the recognition of the child in whom an unusual degree of muscular development results in above average weight for height.

Weight

Marked overweight usually indicates some degree of obesity, and the statement that children whose weight exceeds the standard for their height, age and sex by 20 per cent are likely to be obese provided they are not oedematous (Wolff, 1965) has provided a working basis for the definition of obesity. Newens and Goldstein (1972), reviewing three methods of deriving weight-for-height standards, conclude that neither a power type index nor a relative weight index should be used in place of centile standards of weight-for-height, and that in calculating standards of weight-for-height in children, age should be taken into account. Unfortunately such standards are not readily available and in practice centile charts are used which give height and weight separately. These have limitations when used for assessing overweight; weight centiles are skewed upwards especially at puberty in girls, and in many obese children overnutrition has accelerated their growth in height. We suggest that quantification of obesity based on weight-for-height measurements is not sufficient on its own, though of course weight and height measurements should still be made and are of particular value in monitoring progress.

Skinfold Thickness

Skinfold measurements estimate the amount of fat in the subcutaneous compartment and give a useful index of obesity. It is essential to use standard equipment (Harpenden calipers, obtained from Holtain Ltd, Crymmych, Pembrokeshire) at standard sites, and centile charts for triceps and subscapular skinfolds are available (Tanner and Whitehouse, 1975). For babies aged six months a single triceps skinfold measurement was found to correlate better with the clinical assessment of fatness than the more traditional weight-for-length ratios (Crawford et al, 1974). A committee on nutrition of the American Academy of Pediatrics recommended in 1968 that triceps skinfold measurements should be used in conjunction with height and weight standards in the assessment of body fatness. We would agree that skinfold calipers should become part of the standard measuring equipment in paediatric clinics. When, however, obesity is extreme it may not be possible to apply the caliper.

Skinfold measurements can also be used to estimate the total amount of body fat. Durnin and Rahaman (1967) correlated body density (estimated by underwater weighing) with the sum of skinfold measurements taken over the biceps, triceps, subscapular and suprailiac sites in adolescent boys and girls, and produced regression equations which enable body fat to be calculated. Brook (1971a) showed that similar skinfold measurements can be used to estimate total body fat in children over the age of one year. Haisman (1970) showed that, in young adults, a single abdominal skinfold measurement correlates with total body fat as well as does the sum of several skinfold measurements from different sites.

The error of prediction of total body fat from skinfold measurements is considerable (Brook, 1971a) and is contributed to by differences in the compressibility of the skinfold and in the thickness of the skin. In epidemiological studies variability between observers and between instruments will add to the magnitude of the error which may then be as high as 20 per cent.

Body Fat

In addition to the estimation of body fat from skinfold measurements, there are three other well-established and more accurate methods. These are measurements of total body water, total body potassium, and body density. The techniques are all relatively complex, require specialised laboratory facilities, and cannot be used for routine clinical purposes or for epidemiological studies. They are, however, useful for validating simpler methods. 'Normal' values for body fat in children have not been established but from the limited data available it seems likely that total body fat in excess of 25 per cent of body weight is 'abnormal'.

Combined Measurements

For six-month-old babies Crawford et al (1974) have evaluated a large number of anthropometric measurements and have found a three variable linear equation using weight gain since birth, waist circumference, and suprailiac skinfolds to give the most discriminating measure of obesity. Similar combined indices (apart from multiple skinfold measurements) have not been worked out for older children.

PREVALENCE AND INCIDENCE

Although obesity is said to be the most common nutritional disorder of children in industrialised societies and its incidence is thought to be increasing, few studies of its prevalence and incidence have been made. Comparison between studies is hampered by differences in definition and lack of agreed standards of normality. Most observations have been on infants under one year of age or on school children, and little information is available on the preschool child.

Infancy

Hutchinson-Smith (1970) found that 35 per cent of 200 babies followed throughout the first year exceeded their expected weight for length by 20 per cent or more; Taitz (1971) in a study of 240 babies during the first six weeks of life found that 59 per cent had exceeded the ninetieth centile for weight; and Shukla et al (1972), in a cross-sectional study of 300 infants up to one year old, found 16 per cent to be 'obese' (20 per cent above standard weight-for-length) and a further 27 per cent to be 'overweight' ($>10<20$ per cent above standard weight). The difference in the prevalence of obesity between the babies in the studies of Hutchinson-Smith and Shukla et al may be due in part to the fact that Hutchinson-Smith used the standards of Tanner and Whitehouse of 1959 whereas Shukla et al used those of Tanner et al of 1966. Recently, Tanner and Whitehouse (1975) have produced revised standards for skinfold measurements which show that today's infants are fatter than those of 12 years ago. It is in the first six months of life that the most marked increase in the incidence of fatness, as judged by triceps skinfolds, has occurred, so that the ninetieth centile measurement has now become the fiftieth centile measurement.

Childhood

Estimates of the prevalence of obesity in school children, in the age range of 6 to 14 years, in various countries vary between 2 and 15 per cent with the prevalence increasing at adolescence. Obesity is more common amongst girls than boys especially in the older age groups; Colley (1974) in a study of 6 to 14 year old children in Buckinghamshire found 32 per cent of 14 year old girls to be obese (triceps skinfold >25 mm) whereas only 3 per cent of the boys were obese by the same criterion. From a comparison of his findings with those (Scott, 1961) obtained by similar methods in London school children in 1959, he concludes that obesity has become more frequent in the older girls.

In adults of industrialised countries obesity is more common in the lower socio-economic groups (Moore, Stunkard and Srole, 1962; Silverstone, Gordon and Stunkard, 1969). The same probably applies to children. White-law (1971), in a study of skinfold thickness in London schoolboys, found between 8 and 11 per cent (depending on the method of definition) of boys from social classes IV and V to be obese compared with 5 to 7 per cent of boys from classes I and II. He found obesity to become less frequent with increasing number of siblings. Wilkinson (1975) found similar social class differences in Newcastle upon Tyne.

Adolescence

In many studies of 'adolescent' obesity the term adolescence is not precisely defined and boys and girls from 12 up to 18 or even 20 years are included. Interpretation of the findings is made more difficult because reference is rarely made to the stage of pubertal development, which of course includes a spurt of growth of the adipose organ. Nevertheless there is agreement that obesity becomes more common in adolescence and the high prevalence in adolescent girls reported by Huenemann (1968) has recently been confirmed by Colley (1974).

NATURAL HISTORY

Recently the concept that fat babies grow into fat children who in turn become fat adults has been widely, and perhaps too easily, accepted. As a result there is a growing concern to prevent obesity in infancy together with a tendency to adopt a defeatist attitude towards the treatment of the obese older child. It is therefore important to examine the evidence upon which our present beliefs about the natural history of obesity in childhood are based.

Infancy

Two studies in England (Asher, 1966; Eid, 1970) showed that babies who, at the age of six months, were overweight and probably obese, were more likely to be overweight at the age of five to seven years than were infants whose weight at six months was normal. However, despite a statistically significant difference in the prognosis between the groups of obese and non-obese infants, the majority (80 per cent) of the children who had been overweight as babies, were no longer overweight at school entry. This conclusion, which is not usually emphasised, is in keeping with the accepted figures for the prevalence of obesity in the two age groups (25–30 per cent in babies, and 3–6 per cent during the school years). That weight gain in early infancy is not a strong indicator of obesity at school entry is also shown by the large and careful longitudinal study of Mellbin and Vuille (1973) in Sweden. They found only a weak correlation between velocity of weight gain in infancy and weight at seven years; only 10 per cent of the overweight school children had been obese as babies. Correlation between infant and later obesity was almost wholly confined to the boys. The age at which most obese babies lose their excess fat is not known.

It has been suggested that fat babies are more likely to become fat again at adolescence. A retrospective study of a group of obese adolescent girls in the USA (Heald and Hollander, 1965) supports this idea by showing that this group had gained weight more rapidly during the first year of life, and had been heavier at the age of one year, than their non-obese peers. A prospective study of children in Switzerland showed little correlation between skinfold measurements at one year of age and at puberty (Hernesniemi, Zachmann and Prader, 1974). The conclusions of these two studies are not necessarily at variance because the Swiss workers studied an unselected population of children and their findings may not apply to obese children.

Childhood

Children who are referred to hospital clinics on account of obesity are likely to remain obese as adults (Haase and Hosenfeld, 1956; Lloyd, Wolff and Whelen, 1961; Hammar, Campbell and Wooley, 1971). In the study of Lloyd et al 80 per cent of their patients were obese when re-examined nine years after their original attendance at a special clinic, even though most of them had initially lost weight. There was a tendency for the degree of obesity to increase with increasing age so that the group of individuals over 20 years at follow-up was more overweight than the younger group aged 17 to 19 years. Mullins (1958) in a study of obese adults attending an outpatient clinic reported that in one-third of his patients the obesity had started in childhood.

A limitation of most studies of the prognosis of obesity in children is that they are based on a hospital or clinic population. Such children may not be representative of the situation in the community.

AETIOLOGY

The increased storage of fat in obesity is due to an energy intake in the form of food in excess of the individual's requirements, including, in the case of children, requirements for growth. Many factors can disturb this energy balance and they differ in their importance, not only between individuals but also in the same individual at different times. Although we shall discuss the various aetiological factors separately they seldom occur in isolation. Furthermore the aetiology of obesity is complicated by the development of certain vicious circles. To give two examples, physical inactivity may cause obesity which then further restricts activity; emotional disturbance may cause overeating and the resulting obesity then worsens the emotional upset. In the individual child it may be impossible to distinguish between cause and effect and a search for the primary event can be logically meaningless and practically unhelpful.

Genetic Factors

Although it is accepted that there is a genetic component in the aetiology of obesity it is difficult to separate the effects of heredity from those of the common family environment and, therefore, to estimate the size of the genetic influence. This difficulty applies for instance to the interpretation of the classical study of Gurney (1936) who found that if both parents are obese, two-thirds of their children will be obese, whereas if one of the parents is obese only half of their children will be obese.

Accurate measurements of heritability (that is the proportion of the total variance of a characteristic in a population due to genetic causes) can only be derived from studies of twins. Studies based on weight show a close correlation between the weights of identical twins (Newman, Freeman and Holzinger, 1937; Bakwin, 1973). Even in identical twins reared in dissimilar environments the primary factor determining body weight appears to be genetic (Von Verschuer, 1927). Recently Brook, Huntley and Slack (1975) examined the relative contributions of genetic and environmental factors in determining skinfold thicknesses in 222 pairs of like-sex twins of whom 78 were monozygotic and 144 dizygotic. The conclusions reached were that taking all ages together and for both sexes genetic factors appeared more important in determining trunk fat (estimated by subscapular skinfolds) than limb fat (estimated by triceps skinfolds). Genetic factors played a greater part in determining limb fat in girls than in boys. Above 10 years of age it was found that heritability was high for both trunk and limb fat in boys and girls, but for younger children environmental influences appeared to be of greater importance, and only in the trunk fat of younger boys was the degree of heritability high. The study contained only a few twins who were obese and no special investigation of these was possible; the results of the study, therefore, strictly apply only to heritability of skinfold thickness over the normal population range, and could be different for individuals who are obese. Similar caution is needed in the interpretation of the other reported twin studies. The mechanisms whereby genetic factors influence fat deposition are not known.

Food Consumption

Energy is consumed as food. The composition of the food, and the periodicity with which it is eaten, as well as the absolute amount of energy derived from it, are all relevant to the aetiology of obesity.

Few data are available on the role of individual nutrients in food in causing obesity. Carbohydrates are generally considered to be 'fattening', and the increased prevalence of obesity of children in the lower socio-economic groups has been attributed to increased consumption of these relatively cheap foods (Whitelaw, 1971). Cook et al (1973) found that children from the lower social classes and larger families had a higher proportion of their energy intake from carbohydrate and added sugar; however, they also found that the heavier children in their study had a lower sugar intake than the lighter children but considered that some of the restriction by the heavier children may have been intentional.

Periodicity of eating may be important in the regulation of energy balance, with a correlation between obesity and infrequent meals. Nibbling (the taking of small frequent meals) appears less likely to lead to obesity than gorging (the taking of large infrequent meals). Studies in adults have given discrepant findings (Garrow, 1974); in school children between 10 and 16 years one study has shown that those who ate three meals daily were fatter than those who ate five or seven meals a day (Fabry et al, 1966). There is a clinical impression that many obese children do not eat breakfast; in Bristol the Chief Medical Officer of the Ministry of Education (1962) reported that 8 per cent of children had no breakfast before coming to school, and these children were more likely to be from lower social classes or to have mothers going out to work.

In normal individuals, at all ages in both sexes, there is a large variation in energy intake (Widdowson, 1962), but the reasons for this wide range of nutritional requirements are not understood. The concept of nutritional individuality needs to be stressed and its neglect may result in the over-feeding of some children whose needs happen to be less than the 'average standard requirement'.

Infants

Excess energy intake is more likely to occur in babies who are artificially fed than in those who are breast fed, and in practice the latter are less likely to be overweight (Fomon et al, 1971; Shukla et al, 1972). The reasons for the difference are not fully understood. One reason is that artificially fed infants are more likely to have their nutritional individuality ignored by being urged to consume a predetermined volume of feed. Overconsumption of nutrients in cow's milk feeds can also arise because of inaccuracies in the reconstitution of the feed (Wilkinson et al, 1973). A further cause of increased energy intake in infancy is the giving of non-milk solids at an early age. There is a tendency to start these foods, usually in the form of cereals, during the first three months and often before the age of one month (DHSS, 1974). Hutchinson-Smith (1970) found that early introduction of cereals was equally common amongst breast-fed infants and those bottle fed.

There is some evidence in normal babies (Fomon et al, 1971) and in malnourished children (Ashworth, 1974) that appetite can be adjusted to the nutritional status. Possibly the mechanism for this adjustment fails in some individuals; for instance, studies in heavy newborn infants have suggested that they have an appetite regulating system which is relatively insensitive to internal cues of hunger and satiety (Nisbett and Gurwitz, 1970). Hall (1975) postulated that in the newborn the appetite control mechanism is sensitive to the change in the composition of breast milk which occurs during the feed. This mechanism cannot operate in babies fed on cow's milk preparations whose composition does not alter during the feed.

Older children

For older children there is little evidence that obese children as a group consume more energy than their non-obese peers. Population studies have shown that heavier children have a higher average daily intake than lighter children (Cahn, 1968; Cook et al, 1973), but the heavy children were not necessarily fat. In groups of 14 year old children Durnin et al (1974) found that between 1964 and 1971 body fat had increased in the boys whilst over the same period there had been a decrease in daily energy intake of between 200 and 250 kcal. Amongst the girls, the fattest consumed consistently less energy than the thinnest. This study suggests that, at least in this age group, decreased energy output is of greater importance in determining fatness than excess energy intake.

Energy Output

Reduced energy output is probably more important in the aetiology of obesity than used to be thought. The finding of Durnin et al (1974) that adolescent boys in Glasgow were fatter than a comparable group studied seven years previously, despite a reduced energy consumption, suggests that children in our society are becoming less active. Bradfield, Paulos and Grossman (1971) showed that adolescent girls in the USA spend on average less than 1 h a day in moderate or strenuous physical activity, and of the remaining 15 waking hours 9 are spent in light activity such as sitting whilst being transported to school, whilst at school, or when at home watching television. A similar pattern probably applies to younger children though perhaps to a lesser extent to boys.

Ideally methods of measuring energy expenditure should assess the expenditure during normal activities and over periods sufficiently long to give a meaningful reflection of the average daily output. Three main methods have been used in field studies. First, the documentation of all activity by keeping a diary card and then calculating the energy value for each task from published tables. Unfortunately documentation of energy values for children's activities is limited. The method has the further disadvantage that it requires an unusual degree of cooperation from the child. Second, the continuous measurement of oxygen uptake with portable equipment. This cannot be applied to children over long periods. Third, the use of continuous heart rate monitoring equipment (socially acceptable monitoring instruments, SAMI) over long periods. For each individual, heart rate has to be correlated with measurements of oxygen consumption and, particularly for children, there are serious technical difficulties in applying this method under conditions of everyday life. Changes in posture and emotional state influence the relationship between heart rate and energy consumption and may invalidate results. Whatever method is used the coefficient of variation is likely to be around 20 per cent.

Reduced energy expenditure and/or physical activity in an obese child does not necessarily imply aetiological importance. In order to clarify the role of diminished energy expenditure in the causation of obesity children should be studied when no longer obese, or ideally even before becoming obese.

In conditions in which physical activity is grossly limited, for example meningomyelocoele and myopathy, obesity is common and the contribution of low energy output to its causation is clear.

Emotional Factors

The relative importance of emotional factors in the aetiology of obesity may be difficult to assess in the individual child. In cases of extreme obesity the role of such factors is usually great and often obvious. Once obesity has developed the child's appearance which often leads to teasing, and in adolescents to lack of attractiveness to the opposite sex, perpetuates the emotional problems and may set up a vicious circle.

There are several psychological mechanisms whereby emotional disturbance can lead to a food intake in excess of physiological requirements. In early infancy the giving and taking of food is central to the mother–infant relationship. Normally, as the child grows older, the psychological significance of food becomes less, though even in the older child food continues to have important psychological meaning, in addition to satisfying physiological needs. For obese children, eating may be a means of dealing with ungovernable or undesirable emotions such as frustration or anxiety because they are unable to deal with them in more mature and realistic ways, and because their parents may be unable to help them to find more desirable means. The child may subconsciously wish to revert to babyhood, a stage of life when food was of prime importance in the mother–infant relationship. In some children, food may have the psychological significance of a 'transitional object', and take the place of the more usual rag or teddy bear. Overeating may be a symptom of depression in childhood as it is in adult life.

Some adolescent girls may eat more than they need because subconsciously they believe that they will be more attractive to boys if they are not too thin. Others, who do not want to attract boys, overeat because they believe that fatness is unattractive. Possibly a disturbance of body image may play a role in the aetiology of obesity similar to that which may occur in anorexia nervosa (Slade and Russell, 1973). In different cultures, and in the same culture at different periods of time, the concepts of beauty and attractiveness to the other sex are not necessarily the same. What may have appeared attractive in the days of Rubens would not be regarded as attractive in the more recent days of Modigliani. Boredom is a common cause of overeating particularly in older children.

Family eating patterns are also relevant and excessive eating may be part of the pattern. In the life of some families eating together has an unusually important place and in these families, whose members also often have a close and complex relationship, any attempt, however minor, to change the eating pattern is likely to meet deep resistance.

Psychological disturbance in the parents, and especially in the mother, is particularly likely to be present when the obesity is gross. Some mothers feel themselves most adequate in their maternal role when their children are still babies, and may use food subconsciously as a means of maintaining the kind of relationship which existed when the child was an infant. Other mothers feel guilty because they believe that they do not love their child sufficiently and subconsciously give food in place of love. Whether the primary emotional disturbance is in the mother or child, it is bound to have secondary effects on the mother–child relationship and may also affect other members of the family.

Metabolic and Endocrine Factors

Although the pathways involved in the storage and release of triglyceride in the adipose cell have been extensively studied (Galton, 1971), in the great majority of obese patients it has not proved possible to establish a primary metabolic defect in either the mechanisms responsible for triglyceride synthesis or lipolysis. The various metabolic abnormalities which occur in obese individuals tend to be corrected by weight loss and are, therefore, likely to be results rather than causes of the obesity. In one family a defect of lipolysis has been described which may constitute the basic abnormality causing triglyceride storage (Gilbert, Galton and Kay, 1973).

In hypothyroidism and Cushing's syndrome obesity may be the presenting feature. These conditions are also associated with short stature and their diagnosis should be considered when an obese child is found to be below average height or below that expected for his family. Children receiving long-term therapy with corticosteroids will usually become obese unless preventive measures are taken. Children with growth hormone deficiency tend to be heavier than expected for their height and have increased skinfold thickness; loss of body fat occurs during treatment with growth hormone (Brook, 1973).

In the Prader–Willi syndrome (Dunn, 1968) obesity is associated with mental retardation, short stature and hypogonadism. In infancy hypotonia and feeding difficulties are the outstanding features and obesity does not usually develop until the second year of life. During the later years of childhood or adolescence diabetes mellitus may occur. The primary abnormality is unknown. Treatment of the condition is complicated by the fact that a low calorie diet may further slow down growth in height. Even rarer conditions which are associated with obesity are pseudo-hypoparathyroidism and the Laurence–Moon–Biedl syndrome.

EFFECTS

Adipose Tissue Cellularity

The increase in adipose tissue, which characterises obesity, is associated with either an increase in the number of adipose cells or enlargement of existing cells, or a combination of both processes. Methods of estimating cell size and number were first applied in experimental animals, mainly using the epididymal fat pad of the rat, and it is not certain to what extent the results

apply to the human. In the epididymal fat pad of the developing rat enlargement of adipose tissue is associated with an increase in cell numbers up to the
age of 14 to 15 weeks. Thereafter the total number appears to be fixed and
further enlargement of the tissue takes place only by an increase in cell size
(Hirsch and Han, 1969; Johnson et al, 1971). It is important to note that the
rat becomes skeletally mature at about 15 weeks (Hughes and Tanner, 1970)
and the corresponding age in the human is about 16 years. An excess food
intake in the young rat leads to an accelerated rate of cell multiplication
with a resulting increase in the ultimate number of cells; a deficient intake
slows down multiplication and the ultimate number is reduced (Knittle and
Hirsch, 1968). Studies of the effects of dietary deficiency in the lactating
mother rat on the adipose cellularity of her offspring suggest that a deficiency
in protein has a permanent effect on cell number whereas the effects of a
deficiency in calories may be reversible (Knittle, 1972a). In the rat genetic
factors may influence cellularity independently of nutrition. Thus strains with
genetic obesity increase their cell number up to 26 weeks of age, whereas
genetically non-obese rats made hyperphagic by hypothalamic lesions at 14
weeks develop obesity by cellular enlargement (Johnson et al, 1971). Exercise
may also affect cellularity, and in the young rat results in a reduction in cell
number as well as in cell size (Oscai et al, 1972). Insulin increases cell size
independently of the age of the animal and does not affect cell number (Salans,
Zarnowski and Segal, 1972).

In children studies of adipose tissue cellularity have been made on small
fragments of tissue obtained by needle aspiration or on material obtained
during a surgical procedure or at autopsy. Three main methods have been
used to determine the number and size of adipose cells in a small sample of
tissue. The cells may be fixed by osmium tetroxide and then freed from the
stroma and finally counted manually or in a Coulter counter; the lipid content
of a separate piece of the tissue is determined and the mean cell size can then
be expressed as the mean weight of lipid per cell (Hirsch and Gallian, 1968).
Disadvantages of the method are that very small fat cells (less than 10 μm)
will not be counted, and only the mean size of the cells and not the range is
obtained (Widdowson and Shaw, 1973). Recently, Boulton, Dunlop and Court
(1974) have described a modification of the method which may overcome
these difficulties. The second method of cell counting involves separation of
the cells from the stroma by collagenase and then counting the cells in
suspension and measuring their diameter (Bray, 1970). Great care is needed
to avoid rupture of the larger cells. The third method consists of micro-
scopical examination of thin frozen sections of adipose tissue (Björntorp and
Martinsson, 1966); it requires careful attention to the preparation of the
section and is time consuming, but of the three methods is probably least
subject to error.

Estimates of the total number of fat cells in the body have been derived
from a calculation based on the number of cells in the biopsy sample and the

total body fat. Such estimates must be interpreted with caution because, in addition to the difficulties and inaccuracies involved in measurements of total body fat in children, differences in the cellularity of adipose tissue have been demonstrated between subcutaneous and deep sites (Brook, 1971b), and between different subcutaneous sites in the same individual (Salans, Cushman and Weismann, 1973).

Dauncey and Gairdner (1975) examined adipose tissue, taken at autopsy, operation, or by subcutaneous aspiration from premature and full-term newborns and infants up to the age of 18 months. They reported an increase in mean cell size from about 40 μm at 25 weeks gestation to 50 to 80 μm at full term. The adipose cells from the buttocks were larger than those from the abdominal wall. After birth adipose cell size continued to increase with a mean size of about 90 μm at three months. The rate of increase in adipose cell size appeared to be the same whether development was intra- or extrauterine.

Boulton et al (1974) found differences in the distribution of cell size between infants of different ages. In fetal life the majority of cells had a diameter of about 11 μm. Thereafter cells increased in size to reach a modal value of around 60 μm but the distribution varied between individuals, some tending to have a persistence of cells of small size whereas others had lost the small cells which had presumably filled out with fat.

No studies have been reported of adipose tissue cellularity of obese babies. The study of obese children by Brook, Lloyd and Wolff (1972) suggested that the children who had already been obese at one year of age had a greater total cell number than those in whom the obesity had developed later. Brook (1972a) postulated the existence of a sensitive period for multiplication of adipose cells during which the basic complement of cells is determined, and suggested that this period extends from approximately 30 weeks of gestation to about one year of age. Dobbing (1975), however, has cast some doubt on the validity of this concept.

Throughout childhood the number of adipose cells increases, the full complement probably being reached around puberty. Opinions differ about the rate of multiplication at different ages. The studies of Brook et al (1972) suggested a continuous increase between the age of one year and puberty whereas Knittle (1972b) found little change between 2 and 10 years followed by a rapid increase between 9 and 12 years. More recently Brook (1975) has suggested that growth in the number of fat cells follows a similar pattern to that of the thickness of skinfolds with a spurt at puberty; he postulates that during the periods of most rapid growth cells are particularly sensitive to nutritional influences. Cell size and its distribution appear to stay relatively constant throughout childhood after infancy. No major differences in size or number have been documented between the sexes but, in view of the methodological difficulties, it is possible that minor differences may have been missed.

In obese children mean cell size is increased in comparison with that found in non-obese children (Brook et al, 1972; Knittle, 1972b), and Bonnet et al

(1970) have shown that the distribution of cell size is wider. Studies of cell number in obese children have given varying results. Knittle (1972b) found that obese children at all ages had a greater number of adipose cells and distinguished two groups, those with marked hypercellularity and a small increase in cell size, and those with less marked hypercellularity and a large increase in cell size. Brook et al (1972) also found two groups of obese children who differed in their cellularity; those with an onset of the obesity before the age of one year had a markedly increased cellularity, whereas those with an onset later in childhood had cell numbers which did not differ significantly from the normal (Brook, 1972a). Wilkinson and Parkin (1974) found a positive correlation between the degree of obesity and the total number of fat cells irrespective of the age of onset of the obesity. In short-term studies of the effect of weight loss on adipose cellularity in obese children, Brook and Lloyd (1973) showed that mean cell size decreased but total number was unaltered. These conclusions must, however, be interpreted with caution because of the methodological difficulties (Ashwell and Garrow, 1973). Even if hypercellularity persists there is no evidence that this influences the prognosis. Brook, Lloyd and Wolff (1974) found no correlation between adipose cell size or number and the rate of weight loss in obese children.

Growth and Puberty

Overnutrition accelerates linear growth and thus the height of obese children tends to be above that expected for their family. Brook (1972b) suggested that the effect on height is most marked when overnutrition occurs during the early years of childhood, that is at a period of growth when the rate of cell multiplication may be particularly susceptible to nutritional influences. Skeletal development tends to be advanced and on average the bone age is about one year ahead of the chronological age (Mossberg, 1948). In both sexes the onset of puberty also occurs about one year earlier (Wolff, 1955). In boys, this fact has clinical importance because it enables reassurance to be given that the impression that obesity is associated with delayed or abnormal pubertal development is mistaken. The early onset of puberty is associated with early cessation of growth and the ultimate height of obese children is normal or even slightly below average (Lloyd et al, 1961).

Emotional Effects

Obese children tend to be teased about their appearance at school and sometimes also at home. Many dislike sports and other physical activities, not only because their performance is likely to be poor, but also because they may be embarrassed at changing in front of their peers. Around the years of puberty obese boys are particularly embarrassed by the size of their penis which may be buried in rolls of fat and thus appears small. The accumulation of fat on the chest of boys may give the impression of breast development and this also causes distress, and anxiety that pubertal development may be abnormal. Many obese children deny that they are embarrassed by their appearance, and insist that they do not mind being teased or indeed that they are not teased. Beneath such denial, there usually hides much unhappiness which may show itself as aggression, depression or withdrawal. Underachievement at school is probably common and leads to further emotional problems. School refusal may occur.

Lack of attractiveness, especially to the opposite sex, and difficulties in finding 'fashionable' clothes aggravate the emotional problems for the adolescent.

Metabolic Effects

Amongst the many metabolic changes which have been described in obese individuals are abnormalities of glucose tolerance and hyperinsulinaemia, deficient secretion of growth hormone, increased secretion of cortisol with the appearance of excess of metabolites in the urine, and abnormalities of serum lipids and lipoproteins. All these abnormalities can be reversed by weight reduction. Changes in glucose tolerance and serum insulin, and in serum lipids, may play a role in the later development of diabetes mellitus or atherosclerosis.

Glucose tolerance and serum insulin

In 16 to 28 per cent of obese children oral glucose tolerance tests show abnormalities in blood glucose response which can be classified as 'chemical diabetes' (Chiumello et al, 1969; Martin and Martin, 1973). Virtually all obese children show hyperinsulinaemia after oral glucose; a positive correlation has been reported between the degree of insulin response on the one hand and the age of the children and duration of the obesity on the other (Parra et al, 1971; Martin and Martin, 1973). The relationship between the hyperinsulinaemia and the abnormality of blood glucose response is less clear; Paulsen, Reichenderfer and Ginsberg-Fellner (1968) and Martin and Martin (1973) found the hyperinsulinaemia to be most marked in the children with the most abnormal blood glucose response, but Chiumello et al (1969) found the opposite relationship. There is, however, agreement that insulin resistance is present in obese children.

Studies in adults have shown a strong positive correlation between the size of adipose cells and the hyperinsulinaemia (Stern et al, 1972). Because weight loss is associated with a fall in serum insulin and a return of glucose tolerance to normal, and also with a decrease in the size of adipose cells, it has been inferred that large adipose cells are responsible for the insulin resistance. In obese children, Brook and Lloyd (1973) found only a weak correlation between the degree of hyperinsulinaemia and the adipose cell size. During treatment with a low-calorie diet the hyperinsulinaemia lessened rapidly and before any significant reduction in cell size occurred. Reduced serum insulin response was only maintained whilst weight was being lost on the low-calorie diet. Even after considerable reduction in adipose cell size, hyperinsulinaemia still occurred as soon as the intake of calories and carbohydrates was increased. These findings suggest that the enlargement of the adipose cells in obesity is not the cause of the hyperinsulinaemia but rather that both abnormalities may be due to excess carbohydrate ingestion.

In adults the relationship between obesity and clinical diebates mellitus is established. Obese children, many of whom may become obese adults, are therefore predisposed to the later development of diabetes and the risk is greatest for the grossly overweight children (Abraham, Collins and Nordsieck, 1971). Thus the prevention and treatment of obesity in childhood will play a part in the prevention of diabetes mellitus in the adult, although as Mann (1974) has pointed out such measures will only have a small effect on the overall incidence of diabetes in the community.

Serum lipids

In obese children serum concentrations of non-esterified fatty acids (NEFA) in the fasting state are higher than in non-obese children (Theodoridis, Albutt and Chance, 1971; Fosbrooke, Brook and Lloyd, 1971). Fosbrooke et al (1971) found an increased proportion of palmitoleic acid in the serum NEFA as well as in serum and adipose tissue triglyceride and regard this finding as evidence for increased lipogenesis.

Serum cholesterol and triglyceride concentrations are usually within the normal range (Spahn and Plenert, 1968; Fosbrooke et al, 1971). A significant positive correlation has been found between serum cholesterol and obesity in a population study of 9 to 12 year old school children in Holland (Uppal, 1974). A similar correlation has been reported in obese adults (Montoye, Epstein and Kjelsberg, 1966).

Treatment of gross obesity with a 350 kcal diet results in a fall in serum cholesterol concentration, probably due to the reduction in dietary fat intake (Fosbrooke et al, 1971). We have found that when familial hypercholesterol-aemia occurs in association with obesity, treatment of the obesity by restriction of calories and dietary fat often also reduces the serum cholesterol level.

Cardiorespiratory Failure

The most dangerous effect of obesity is cardiorespiratory failure. This complication, which occurs more often in adults than in children, is also known as the Pickwickian, or obesity-hypoventilation, syndrome. The typical features as described in adults with gross and long-standing obesity are breathlessness on exertion, somnolence, cyanosis, tachycardia, raised central venous pressure, cardiac dilatation, hepatomegaly, and peripheral oedema (Howell, 1971). Periodic breathing during sleep may occur.

All children with gross obesity probably have a low chest wall compliance and reduced functional residual capacity, and a high oxygen cost of breathing. The lungs empty more completely than normal at the end of each breath, and as a result there is a high closing volume with some shunting of blood through poorly ventilated alveoli. This may cause intermittent but easily reversed cyanosis at rest. In some patients secondary alveolar hypoventilation supervenes with retention of carbon dioxide and a reduced ventilatory response to the increased partial pressure of carbon dioxide. Eventually secondary cardiac failure occurs, and deaths have been reported in childhood (Ward and Kelsey, 1962). This situation is a medical emergency, demanding hospitalisation, and its treatment consists of measures to relieve heart failure and reduce weight. Care must be exercised in the use of oxygen which may lead to severe underbreathing and oxygen narcosis. Respiratory function may not return to normal until a near normal weight has been achieved.

TREATMENT

Obesity is a difficult and disappointing condition to treat. About 80 per cent of treated cases relapse in the long term (Lloyd et al, 1961) and the outcome for untreated obesity is unknown. As 'cure' is uncommon the question should be posed whether or not an attempt should be made to treat *all* obese children. Because of the role of obesity in the pathogenesis of much adult disease and disability including diabetes mellitus, osteoarthritis and cardiovascular disorders, and because of the potentially serious emotional and cardiopulmonary consequences in childhood, we consider that an attempt at treatment is always indicated. It could be argued that for some children with associated defects, such as mental retardation, primary psychological disorders, meningomyelocoele, or myopathy, treatment of the obesity imposes an additional and unnecessary burden on the child and his family. In our experience with such severely handicapped children, the obesity makes management of the primary condition more difficult, especially as they grow older, and we feel that it is justifiable to institute treatment of the obesity. More difficult, in our opinion, is the decision whether to abandon treatment in those children in whom it is unsuccessful, or is found to pose an intolerable burden.

In the management of the obese child, before explaining the details of treatment, reassurance should be given to the child and parents that no primary endocrine abnormality is present; such reassurance can usually be given without the need for special investigations if the child is above average height, taking into account the parents' height, and physical examination shows no abnormality which is not directly attributable to the obesity Knock-knee is common at all ages and striae occur frequently in adolescents. An explanation of the probable causes of the obesity in the individual child should be given, and the concept of nutritional individuality explained with the corollary that not all obesity is due to gluttony.

The principle of treatment is to ensure that intake of energy is less than the output. A reduction in food intake is the mainstay of treatment but an increase in energy output through increasing physical activity is also important, and the two approaches should be combined. Psychiatric help may be required. The practice of weight reduction is difficult; many methods have been described and successes claimed. No method can be regarded as entirely satisfactory for all patients, and there is need for a critical evaluation of current practice as well as of new methods. For any method it is necessary to know in what proportion of children weight loss is achieved, how much of the excess weight is lost, for how long satisfactory weight is maintained, what proportion of children relapse and at what interval after starting treatment, and how many children fail to attend follow-up appointments. Many reports purporting to show success of a particular treatment regime do not fulfil these criteria.

Diet

Diets must be adjusted to individual needs. The amount and type of food allowed will depend on the age, the degree of the obesity, and individual requirements and preferences. Helpful information can be obtained by taking a careful dietary history. If this is done by a dietitian a more accurate assessment will be obtained, but even a record obtained by a doctor will indicate whether the child has been eating excessively, or if his intake has been relatively small. When taking a dietary history enquiries must be made about drinks as well as about foods and about the number and frequency of meals and snacks.

For most obese school children a diet providing 800 to 1000 kcal/day results in weight loss. Such a diet should contain approximately 60 g of protein and 40 g of fat; the main restriction will fall on the carbohydrate intake which will be reduced to about 100 g. The food should be divided between not less than three meals, and children who do not eat breakfast should be encouraged to do so. Within the limits of the prescribed energy intake, diets should allow as much choice as possible, and rigid diet sheets which suggest foods the child does not like and the family cannot afford should be avoided. As the ultimate aim is to achieve a pattern of eating which will enable the child, after the excess weight has been lost, to maintain a normal rate of weight gain, education of child and family in the principles involved should start as early as possible. The contribution of a dietitian, preferably with paediatric experience, is invaluable.

In many children satisfactory weight loss occurs initially with dietary treatment but ceases after some weeks. It is then usually assumed that the failure to continue to lose weight is due to failure to follow the diet. Although this assumption is often correct it may not be true for all children. In some obese adults it has been shown that prolonged reduction in energy intake may depress the basal metabolic rate (Miller and Parsonage, 1975). If this effect of a low calorie diet can be shown to occur also in children, it will be necessary in some children to reduce further the energy intake to 600 to 800 kcal/day.

There is less experience in the treatment of preschool children but a diet providing 600 to 800 kcal/day is probably suitable. For the obese toddler between the age of one to two years the aim should be to prevent further weight gain unless the obesity is gross. Because children at this age are growing rapidly in height, it is possible for an obese toddler whose weight is kept stable by moderate dietary restriction to 'grow into his height' and 'out of his fatness' in about 6 to 12 months. Obese infants present a special problem; because many will in any case lose their fatness spontaneously, rigid diets need not be used. Advice is given about the general principles of infant feeding, and a diet suitable for a normal infant of that age is described with the aim of preventing further weight gain rather than achieving weight loss.

For children whose obesity is associated with another disability which further limits physical activity, for example meningomyelocoele or myopathy, very low calorie intakes may be needed to achieve weight loss. Children requiring intakes as low as 350 kcal/day should probably be admitted to hospital, as such diets are difficult to provide at home. For obese children without associated handicaps such very low calorie diets have probably only a limited place in therapy. Although rapid weight loss can be achieved in hospital, relapse will occur in the majority on return home (Stark, Lloyd and Wolff, 1975).

During a period of rapid weight loss, children are likely to grow in height at less than the normal rate and lose some lean body mass (Wolff, 1955; Brook et al, 1974). With slower weight loss a normal height velocity is maintained and there is little loss of lean body mass (Brook et al, 1974). For obese children of above average height a small reduction in height velocity is unimportant, but for obese children of short stature a reduction in height velocity may result in undesirable ultimate stunting of growth. It is our impression that, even when such children relapse and gain weight at an excessive rate, catch-up growth does not take place and height velocity may not even return to normal. We, therefore, suggest caution in the use of very low calorie diets for obese children of below average height, and recommend that growth in height is charted as part of the management of all obese children.

An initial period of total starvation has been tried in the treatment for obese adults, but long-term results have been disappointing (Maagøe and Mogensen, 1970). Starvation continued until normal weight is achieved has also been attempted (Forbes, 1970; Rooth and Carlström, 1970; Munro et al, 1970). Such treatment can only be carried out in hospital, may have undesirable side effects, and even result in death (Spencer, 1968; Lloyd-Mostyn et al, 1970); it cannot be recommended for children.

Ileal-bypass operations, which result in malabsorption of food, have been used in the treatment of gross obesity unresponsive to ordinary treatment. In adults encouraging results have been reported with the patients losing weight without the need for severe dietary restriction, and often deriving much psychological and social benefit (Gazet et al, 1974; Solow, Silberfarb and Swift, 1974). Side effects can, however, be serious especially in the immediate postoperative period and deaths have been reported (McGill et al, 1972). Experience with children is limited but in carefully selected cases considerable weight loss has been achieved, and maintained during the first postoperative year, without impairment of growth in height (Randolph, Weintraub and Rigg, 1974).

The use of drugs to curb appetite and thereby reduce food intake is not, in our opinion, advisable during childhood and adolescence. All available drugs have some effect on the central nervous system and may be habit forming. In any case their therapeutic effect is limited and usually of short duration.

Physical Activity

Encouragement to become physically more active should be part of the management. Regular daily exercise, taken as part of normal life, for example walking to school and walking up stairs, is more likely to be effective than short and irregular bursts of more energetic activities. In the individual child details of physical activities obtained during the taking of the history may suggest ways in which energy output can be increased.

Psychiatric Treatment

Many obese children need psychiatric help, irrespective of whether they have a primary emotional disturbance playing a role in the aetiology, or a secondary disturbance resulting from the obesity. At the initial interview it is often possible to decide whether formal psychiatric help is needed. When the obesity is gross, with the weight in the region of double the expected, the associated emotional disturbance is usually also gross and requires urgent help. The relationship between mother and child is often severely disturbed and the mother may not be able to cooperate in efforts to reduce the child's weight. Irrespective of whether or not a psychiatrist is involved in the treatment, the paediatrician should be aware of the emotional problems, and should not regard the child who, despite dietary advice, fails to lose weight as 'naughty' or 'uncooperative'.

Psychotherapy, although often successful in helping with the emotional problems and in improving the family relationships, is not necessarily effective in achieving weight reduction. The value of behaviour modification in the treatment of obesity has not yet been critically assessed. Short-term studies in adults suggest that it deserves further evaluation (Stuart, 1967; Penick et al, 1971; Levitz and Stunkard, 1974), and trials of behaviour modification in children, as well as evaluation of other forms of treatment such as group therapy, including groups for the parents, are needed.

PREVENTION

Because treatment of obesity is difficult and the long-term results disappointing, prevention should be the aim. We are suggesting the adoption of certain preventive measures although we realise that proof of their efficacy is not yet available. Such measures may be instituted in the prenatal period, in infancy, and in later childhood.

Prenatal Period

The avoidance of excessive weight gain during pregnancy is desirable from the obstetric point of view and may also play a role in preventing foetal overnutrition. Antenatal care should include advice on infant feeding (DHSS, 1974). The advantages of breast feeding should be emphasised; amongst these is the fact that obesity is less common in breast-fed babies than in those artificially fed. The mother's intention to breast feed, and the encouragement of her advisors, are probably the most important factors in ensuring successful breast feeding. The disadvantages of overfeeding are stressed and the concept of nutritional individuality is explained; what is an adequate intake for one baby may be excessive for another of the same age. Other points to be made are that a baby may cry because of thirst rather than hunger, and that it is usually unnecessary to give foods other than milk before the age of four to five months.

Infancy

Weight records are kept by all infant clinics and many mothers; the original aim was the prevention of underfeeding, and in the developing world the weight chart is still an important tool in the prevention of malnutrition (Morley, 1971). Because in Britain and other developed countries undernutrition has become uncommon, it has been suggested that there is no longer a need for routine weight records. We believe that the value of weight charts in the prevention of overnutrition deserves investigation. If an infant is found to be gaining weight at an excessive rate his mother can be given appropriate advice, for example to make up more dilute feeds or give less solid food, especially cereals.

Childhood

In childhood prevention of obesity consists mainly in establishing sensible eating habits and encouraging regular physical activity. When nutritional advice is given, cultural and social differences in eating patterns must be respected, and the expense and time involved in the provision and preparation of meals remembered. In the prevention of obesity broad guidelines can be suggested for all children and are not out of place for the rest of the family. Meals should be spaced throughout the day, and excess of carbohydrate, especially of refined products such as sweets, biscuits and the various proprietory sweetened drinks, should be avoided. For children in families with a high incidence of obesity, and for those who are beginning to become too fat, additional advice may include the avoidance of snacks between meals, and encouragement to satisfy appetite with vegetables and fruit rather than with chips and pudding.

Prevention of obesity is particularly important for children with a disorder which interferes with physical activity, such as meningomyelocoele, myopathy, or cerebral palsy other than the athetoid variety. Children with severe emotional disorders and mental retardation also carry a special risk for the development of obesity. Another group at risk are those in whom normal feeding is introduced after a long period of undernutrition (Ashworth, 1969) or of a restrictive diet, such as that used for phenylketonuria. Preventive measures should be instituted routinely for children on long-term corticosteroid treatment.

Regular weight checks are indicated for all children at special risk including those with a family history of obesity. The role of school medical examinations in the prevention and early detection of obesity in the community needs to be evaluated.

Education in Nutrition

Health education should include the important subject of nutrition; and because obesity is such a common nutritional disorder a discussion of its prevention is appropriate. Such education should start in childhood and continue through adolescence into adult life. During the antenatal period, and when their children are young, parents are likely to be particularly receptive of advice aimed at ensuring the good health of their children.

At present doctors and nurses often find themselves ill-prepared to give either specific dietary advice to patients, or education in nutrition in the community. The subject of nutrition deserves greater emphasis in undergraduate and postgraduate training. Dietitians, in addition to their involvement with individual patients, contribute to the education in nutrition of other health workers as well as of the community. The dietetic services in hospitals and community need strengthening.

ACKNOWLEDGEMENTS

We are grateful to Drs Bryan Lask and H. H. O. Wolff for helpful discussions on the emotional aspects of obesity, and to Dr E. Hey for advice on the section on cardiorespiratory complications.

REFERENCES

Abraham, S., Collins, G. & Nordsieck, M. (1971) Relationship of childhood weight status to morbidity in adults. *Public Health Reports*, **86**, 273–284.

Asher, P. (1966) Fat babies and fat children. *Archives of Disease in Childhood*, **41**, 672–673.

Ashwell, M. & Garrow, J. S. (1973) Full and empty fat cells. *Lancet*, **2**, 1036–1037.

Ashworth, A. (1969) Growth rates in children recovering from protein-calorie malnutrition. *British Journal of Nutrition*, **23**, 835–845.

Ashworth, A. (1974) Ad libitum feeding during recovery from malnutrition. *British Journal of Nutrition*, **31**, 109–112.

Bakwin, H. (1973) Body-weight regulation in twins. *Developmental Medicine and Child Neurology*, **15**, 178–183.

Björntorp, P. & Martinsson, A. (1966) Composition of human subcutaneous adipose tissue in relation to its morphology. *Acta medica scandinavica*, **179**, 475–480.

Bonnet, F., Gosselin, L., Chantraine, J. & Senterre, J. (1970) Adipose cell number and size in normal and obese children. *Revue Française d'Etude Cliniques et Biologique*, **15**, 1101–1104.

Boulton, T. J. C., Dunlop, M. & Court, J. M. (1974) Adipocyte growth in the first two years of life. *Australian Paediatric Journal*, **10**, 301–305.

Bradfield, R. B., Paulos, J. & Grossman, L. (1971) Energy expenditure and heart rate of obese high school girls. *American Journal of Clinical Nutrition*, **24**, 1482–1488.

Bray, G. A. (1970) Measurement of subcutaneous fat cells from obese patients. *Annals of Internal Medicine*, **73**, 565–569.

Brook, C. G. D. (1971a) Determination of body composition of children from skinfold measurements. *Archives of Disease in Childhood*, **46**, 182–184.

Brook, C. G. D. (1971b) Composition of human adipose tissue from deep and subcutaneous sites. *British Journal of Nutrition*, **25**, 377–380.

Brook, C. G. D. (1972a) Evidence for a sensitive period in adipose cell replication in man. *Lancet*, **2**, 624–627.

Brook, C. G. D. (1972b) *Obesity in Childhood*. M.D. thesis, University of Cambridge.

Brook, C. G. D. (1973) Effect of human growth hormone treatment on adipose tissue in children. *Archives of Disease in Childhood*, **48**, 725–728.

Brook, C. G. D. (1975) Fat cells and childhood obesity. *Lancet*, **1**, 224.

Brook, C. G. D. & Lloyd, J. K. (1973) Adipose cell size and glucose tolerance in obese children and effects of diet. *Archives of Disease in Childhood*, **48**, 301–304.

Brook, C. G. D., Lloyd, J. K. & Wolff, O. H. (1972) Relation between age of onset of obesity and size and number of adipose cells. *British Medical Journal*, **2**, 25–27.

Brook, C. G. D., Lloyd, J. K. & Wolff, O. H. (1974) Rapid weight loss in children. *British Medical Journal*, **3**, 44–45.

Brook, C. G. D., Huntley, R. M. C. & Slack, J. (1975) Influence of heredity and environment in the determination of skinfold thickness in children. *British Medical Journal*, **2**, 719–721.

Cahn, A. (1968) Growth and calorie intake of heavy and tall children. *Journal of the American Dietetic Association*, **53**, 476–480.

Chief Medical Officer of the Ministry of Education (1962) Report on the Health of the School Child. London: HMSO.

Chiumello, G., Guercio, M. J. Del, Carnelutti, M. & Bidone, G. (1969) Relationship between obesity, chemical diabetes, and beta pancreatic function in children. *Diabetes*, **18**, 238–243.

Colley, J. R. T. (1974) Obesity in schoolchildren. *British Journal of Preventive and Social Medicine*, **28**, 221–225.

Committee on Nutrition of American Academy of Pediatrics (1968) Measurement of skinfold thickness in childhood. *Pediatrics*, **42**, 538–543.

Cook, J., Altman, D. G., Moore, D. M. C., Topp, S. G., Holland, W. W. & Elliott, A. (1973) A survey of the nutritional status of schoolchildren. *British Journal of Preventive and Social Medicine*, **27**, 91–99.

Crawford, P. B., Keller, C. A., Hampton, M. C., Pacheco, F. P. & Huenemann, R. L. (1974) An obesity index for six-month-old children. *American Journal of Clinical Nutrition*, **27**, 706–711.

Dauncey, M. J. & Gairdner, D. (1975) Size of adipose cells in infancy. *Archives of Disease in Childhood*, **50**, 286–290.

Department of Health and Social Security (1974) Present Day Practice in Infant Feeding. Reports on Health and Social Subjects, 9. London: HMSO.

Dobbing, J. (1975) Fat cells and childhood obesity. *Lancet*, **1**, 224.

Dunn, H. G. (1968) The Prader–Labhart–Willi syndrome: review of the literature and report of nine cases. *Acta paediatrica scandinavica*, Suppl. **186**, 1–38.

Durnin, J. G. V. A. & Rahaman, M. M. (1967) The assessment of the total amount of fat in the human body from measurements of skinfold thickness. *British Journal of Nutrition*, **21**, 681–689.

Durnin, J. G. V. A., Lonergan, M. E., Good, J. & Ewan, A. (1974) A cross sectional nutritional and anthropometric study with an interval of 7 years, on 611 young adolescent school children. *British Journal of Nutrition*, **32**, 169–179.

Eid, E. E. (1970) Follow-up study of physical growth of children who had excessive weight gain in first 6 months of life. *British Medical Journal*, **2**, 74–76.

Fabry, P., Hejda, S., Cerny, K., Osancora, K. & Pechar, J. (1966) Effect of meal frequency in school children: changes in weight:height proportion and skinfold thickness. *American Journal of Clinical Nutrition*, **18**, 358–361.

Fomon, S. J., Thomas, L. N., Filer, L. J., Ziegler, E. E. & Leonard, M. T. (1971) Food consumption and growth of normal infants fed milk based formulas. *Acta paediatrica scandinavica*, Suppl., **223**.

Forbes, G. B. (1970) Weight loss during fasting: implications for the obese. *American Journal of Clinical Nutrition*, **23**, 1212–1219.

Fosbrooke, A. S., Brook, C. G. D. & Lloyd, J. K. (1971) Plasma lipids in obese children treated with 350 kcal diets. *Postgraduate Medical Journal* (June suppl.), 444–446.

Galton, D. J. (1971) *The Human Adipose Cell*. London: Butterworth.

Garrow, J. S. (1974) In *Energy Balance and Obesity in Man*, p. 150. Amsterdam: North-Holland Publishing Company.

Gazet, J.-C., Pilkington, T. R. E., Kalucy, R. S., Crisp, A. H. & Day, S. (1974) Treatment of gross obesity by jejunal bypass. *British Medical Journal*, **4**, 311–314.

Gilbert, C., Galton, D. J. & Kaye, J. (1973) Triglyceride storage disease: a disorder of lipolysis in adipose tissue in two patients. *British Medical Journal*, **1**, 25–27.

Gurney, R. (1936) Hereditary factor in obesity. *Archives of Internal Medicine*, **57**, 557.

Haase, K.-E. & Hosenfeld, H. (1956) Zur Fettsucht im Kindesalter. *Zeitschrift für Kinderheilkunde*, **78**, 1–27.

Hall, B. (1975) Changing composition of human milk and early development of appetite control. *Lancet*, **1**, 779–781.

Haisman, M. F. (1970) The assessment of body fat content in young men from measurements of density and skinfold thickness. *Human Biology*, **42**, 679–688.

Hammar, S. L., Campbell, V. & Wooley, J. (1971) Treating adolescent obesity: long-range evaluation of previous therapy. *Clinical Pediatrics*, **10**, 46–52.

Heald, F. P. & Hollander, R. J. (1965) The relationship between obesity in adolescence and early growth. *Journal of Pediatrics*, **67**, 35–38.

Hernesniemi, I., Zachmann, M. & Prader, A. (1974) Skinfold thickness in infancy and adolescence. *Helvetica paediatrica acta*, **29**, 523–530.

Hirsch, J. & Gallian, E. (1968) Methods for the determination of adipose cell size in man and animals. *Journal of Lipid Research*, **9**, 110–119.

Hirsch, J. & Han, P. W. (1969) Cellularity of rat adipose tissue: effects of growth, starvation and obesity. *Journal of Lipid Research*, **10**, 77–82.

Howell, J. B. L. (1971) Cardiorespiratory failure of extreme obesity. In *Textbook of Medicine* (Cecil-Loeb), 13th edn, ed. Beeson, P. B. & McDermott, W., p. 880. Philadelphia: W. B. Saunders Co.

Huenemann, R. L. (1968) Consideration of adolescent obesity as a public health problem. *Public Health Reports*, **83**, 491–495.

Hughes, P. C. R. & Tanner, J. M. (1970) The assessment of skeletal maturity in the growing rat. *Journal of Anatomy*, **106**, 371–402.

Hutchinson-Smith, B. (1970) The relationship between the weight of an infant and lower respiratory infection. *Medical Officer*, **123**, 257–262.

Johnson, P. R., Zucker, L. M., Cruce, J. A. F. & Hirsch, J. (1971) Cellularity of adipose depots in the genetically obese Zucker rat. *Journal of Lipid Research*, **12**, 706–714.

Knittle, J. L. (1972a) Maternal diet as a factor in adipose tissue cellularity and metabolism in the young rat. *Journal of Nutrition*, **102**, 427–434.

Knittle, J. L. (1972b) Obesity in childhood: a problem in adipose tissue cellular development. *Journal of Paediatrics*, **81**, 1048–1059.

Knittle, J. L. & Hirsch, J. (1968) Effect of early nutrition on the development of rat epididymal fat pads: cellularity and metabolism. *Journal of Clinical Investigation*, **47**, 2091–2098.

Levitz, L. S. & Stunkard, A. J. (1974) A therapeutic coalition for obesity: behaviour modification and patient self help. *American Journal of Psychiatry*, **131**, 423–427.

Lloyd, J. K., Wolff, O. H. & Whelen, W. S. (1961) Childhood obesity: a long-term study of the height and weight. *British Medical Journal*, **2**, 145–148.

Lloyd-Mostyn, R. H., Lord, P. S., Glover, R., West, C. & Gilliland, I. C. (1970) Uric acid metabolism in starvation. *Annals of Rheumatic Disease*, **29**, 553–555.

Maagøe, H. & Mogensen, E. F. (1970) Effect of treatment on obesity: a follow-up of material treated with complete starvation. *Danish Medical Bulletin*, **17**, 206–209.

Mann, G. V. (1974) The influence of obesity on health. *New England Journal of Medicine*, **291**, 226–232.

Martin, M. M. & Martin, A. L. A. (1973) Obesity, hyperinsulinism, and diabetes mellitus in childhood. *Journal of Pediatrics*, **82**, 192–201.

McGill, D. B., Humphreys, S., Baggenstoss, A. & Dickson, E. R. (1972) Cirrhosis and death after jejunoileal shunt. *Gastroenterology*, **63**, 872–877.

Mellbin, T. & Vuille, J.-C. (1973) Physical development at 7 years of age in relationship to velocity of weight gain in infancy with special reference to the incidence of overweight. *British Journal of Social and Preventive Medicine*, **27**, 225–235.

Miller, D. S. & Parsonage, S. (1975) Resistance to slimming: adaptation or illusion? *Lancet*, **1**, 773–775.

Montoye, H. J., Epstein, F. H. & Kjelsberg, M. O. (1966) Relationship between serum cholesterol and body fatness. *American Journal of Clinical Nutrition*, **18**, 397–406.

Moore, M. E., Stunkard, A. & Srole, L. (1962) Obesity, social class and mental illness. *Journal of American Medical Association*, **181**, 962–966.

Morley, D. C. (1971) The use of weight charts in the promotion of adequate nutrition. *Proceedings of Nutrition Society of India*, **10**, 104.

Mossberg, H. O. (1948) Obesity in children: a clinical-prognostical investigation. *Acta paediatrica scandinavica*, **35**, Suppl. 2, 1–22.

Mullins, A. G. (1958) The prognosis in juvenile obesity. *Archives of Disease in Childhood*, **33**, 307–314.

Munro, J. F., Maccuish, A. C., Goodall, J. A. D., Fraser, J. & Duncan, L. J. P. (1970) Further experience with prolonged therapeutic starvation in gross refractory obesity. *British Medical Journal*, **4**, 712–714.

Newens, E. M. & Goldstein, H. (1972) Height, weight and the assessment of obesity in children. *British Journal of Preventive and Social Medicine*, **26**, 33–39.

Newman, H. H., Freeman, F. N. & Holzinger, K. J. (1937) *Twins, a Study of Heredity and Environment*. Chicago: University of Chicago Press.

Nisbett, R. E. & Gurwitz, S. (1970) Weight, sex and eating behaviour of human newborns. *Journal of Comparative Physiology and Psychology*, **73**, 245–253.

Orme, L. E. (1963) Estimating composition from linear measurements, live probe, and body weight. *Annals of New York Academy of Sciences*, **110**, 307–317.

Oscai, L. B., Spirakis, C. N., Wolff, C. A. & Beck, R. H. (1972) Effects of exercise and of food restriction on adipose tissue cellularity. *Journal of Lipid Research*, **13**, 588–592.

Parra, A., Schultz, R. B., Graystone, J. E. & Cheek, D. B. (1971) Correlative studies on obese children and adolescents concerning body composition and plasma insulin and growth hormone levels. *Pediatric Research*, **5**, 605–613.

Paulsen, E. P., Reichenderfer, L. & Ginsberg-Fellner, F. (1968) Plasma glucose, free fatty acids and immunoreactive insulin in sixty-six obese children. *Diabetes*, **17**, 261–269.

Penick, S. B., Filion, R., Fox, S. & Stunkard, A. J. (1971) Behaviour modifications in the treatment of obesity. *Psychosomatic Medicine*, **33**, 49–55.

Randolph, J. G., Weintraub, W. H. & Rigg, A. (1974) Jejunal bypass for morbid obesity in adolescents. *Journal of Pediatric Surgery*, **9**, 341–345.

Rauh, J. L. & Schumsky, D. A. (1969) Relative accuracy of visual assessment of juvenile obesity. *Journal of American Dietetic Association*, **55**, 459–464.

Rooth, G. & Carlström, S. (1970) Therapeutic fasting. *Acta medica scandinavica*, **187**, 455–463.

Salans, L. B., Zarnowski, M. J. & Segal, R. (1972) Effects of insulin upon the cellular character of rat adipose tissue. *Journal of Lipid Research*, **13**, 616–623.

Salans, L. B., Cushman, S. W. & Weismann, R. E. (1973) Adipose cell size and number in non-obese and obese patients. *Journal of Clinical Investigation*, **52**, 929–936.

Scott, J. A. (1961) Report on heights and weights (and other measurements) of school pupils in the County of London in 1959. London County Council.

Shukla, A., Forsyth, H. A., Anderson, C. M. & Marwah, S. M. (1972) Infantile overnutrition in the first year of life: a field study in Dudley, Worcestershire. *British Medical Journal*, **4**, 507–515.

Silverstone, J. T., Gordon, R. & Stunkard, A. J. (1969) Social factors in obesity in London. *Practitioner*, **202**, 682–688.

Slade, P. D. & Russell, G. F. (1973) Awareness of body dimensions in anorexia nervosa: cross sectional and longitudinal studies. *Psychological Medicine*, **3**, 188–189.

Solow, C., Silberfarb, P. M. & Swift, K. (1974) Psychosocial effects of intestinal bypass surgery for severe obesity. *New England Journal of Medicine*, **290**, 300–304.

Spahn, W. & Plenert, W. (1968) Investigations on the treatment of obesity in childhood by total starvation. III. Serum lipid patterns during drastic calorie restriction and total starvation. *Zeitschrift für Kinderheilkunde*, **103**, 13–27.

Spencer, I. O. B. (1968) Death during therapeutic starvation for obesity. *Lancet*, **1**, 1288–1290.

Stark, O., Lloyd, J. K. & Wolff, O. H. (1975) Long-term results of hospital in-patient treatment of obese children. *Recent Advances in Obesity Research: 1* (Proceedings of First International Congress on Obesity). ed. Howard, A. pp. 289–290. London: Newman Publishing Co.

Stern, J. S., Batchelor, B. R., Hollander, N., Cohn, C. K. & Hirsch, J. (1972) Adipose cell size and immunoreactive insulin levels in obese and normal weight adults. *Lancet*, **2**, 948–951.

Stuart, R. B. (1967) Behavioural control of overeating. *Behaviour Research and Therapy*, **5**, 357–365.

Taitz, L. S. (1971) Infantile overnutrition among artificially fed infants in the Sheffield region. *British Medical Journal*, **1**, 315–316.

Tanner, J. M. & Whitehouse, R. H. (1959) Standards for height and weight of British children from birth to maturity. *Lancet*, **2**, 1086–1088.

Tanner, J. M. & Whitehouse, R. H. (1962) Standards for subcutaneous fat in British children. Percentiles for thickness of skinfolds over triceps and below scapula. *British Medical Journal*, **1**, 446–450.

Tanner, J. M., Whitehouse, R. H. & Takaishi, M. (1966) Standards from birth to maturity for height, weight, height velocity and weight velocity: British children in 1965. *Archives of Disease in Childhood*, **41**, 454–471.

Tanner, J. M. & Whitehouse, R. H. (1975) Revised standards for triceps and subscapular skinfolds in British children. *Archives of Disease in Childhood*, **50**, 142–145.

Theodoridis, C. G., Albutt, E. C. & Chance, G. W. (1971) Blood lipids in children with the Prader–Willi syndrome: a comparison with simple obesity. *Australian Paediatric Journal*, **7**, 20–23.

Uppal, S. C. (1974) *Coronary Heart Disease, Risk Pattern in Dutch Youth.* Leiden: New Rhine Publishers.

Von Verschuer, O. (1927) Die vererbungsbiologische Zwillingsforschung. Ihre biologischen Grundlagen studien an 102 eineiigen und 45 gleichgeschlechtlichen zwillings—und an 2 Drillingspaaren *Ergebnisse Innerern Medizin Kinderheilkunde*, **31**, 35–120.

Ward, W. A. & Kelsey, W. M. (1962) The Pickwickian syndrome. *Journal of Pediatrics*, **61**, 745–750.

Whitelaw, A. G. L. (1971) The association of social class and sibling number with skinfold thickness in London schoolboys. *Human Biology*, **43**, 414–420.

Widdowson, E. M. (1962) Nutritional individuality. *Proceedings of Nutrition Society*, **21**, 121–128.

Widdowson, E. M. & Shaw, W. T. (1973) Full and empty fat cells. *Lancet*, **2**, 905.

Wilkinson, P. W. (1975) Obesity in Childhood. A community study in Newcastle upon Tyne. *Archives of Disease in Childhood*, **50**, 826.

Wilkinson, P. W., Noble, T. C., Gray, G. & Spence, O. (1973) Inaccuracies in measurements of dried milk powders. *British Medical Journal*, **2**, 15–17.

Wilkinson, P. W. & Parkin, J. M. (1974) Fat cells in childhood obesity. *Lancet*, **2**, 1522.

Wilkinson, P. W., Parkin, J. M., Phillips, P., Pearlson, G. & Sykes, P. (personal communication).

Wolff, O. H. (1955) Obesity in childhood: a study of the birth weight, the height, and the onset of puberty. *Quarterly Journal of Medicine*, **24**, 109–123.

Wolff, O. H. (1965) Obesity in childhood. In *Recent Advances in Paediatrics*, 3rd edn, ed. Gairdner, D. G., Ch. 9, p. 216. London: J. & A. Churchill Ltd.

Wolff, O. H. & Lloyd, J. K. (1974) Obesity. *Medicine*, **27**, 1583–1593.

13

HYPERLIPOPROTEINAEMIA AND ATHEROSCLEROSIS

June K. Lloyd

Atherosclerosis involving the coronary, cerebral and peripheral arteries and the aorta is a major cause of death and disability in the industrialised countries of the world. Ischaemic heart disease (IHD) resulting from involvement of the coronary arteries is the most extensively studied of the clinical manifestations of the disorder, and most of the current concern about the prevention of atherosclerosis centres on this aspect. The World Health Organisation has described IHD as the 'greatest epidemic mankind has faced' (Stamler, 1971) and the figures for death rates from IHD in the UK between 1950 and 1971 (DHSS, 1974) show a considerable rise in the rates for men, with the most marked and rapid increase occurring in the youngest age group (35–44 years); for women the increase occurred later, was less marked, and was confined to the youngest age group (Fig. 13.1).

Pathological lesions of sufficient severity to result in death by the age of about 40 years are likely to have been developing over a considerable period, and a number of studies have indicated that they may be present already in childhood. Autopsy studies on American soldiers killed at the age of about 20 years in the Korean and Vietnamese wars (Enos, Holmes and Beyer, 1953; McNamara et al, 1971) showed coronary atheroma, in some instances extensive, to be present in a substantial proportion of these young men. In a detailed study of children and young adults from different geographical and ethnic groups Strong and McGill (1969) found fatty streaks in the aortas of almost all boys and girls aged 10 to 11 and coronary artery fatty streaks in most persons aged 20 to 29 years. Although it is accepted that not all fatty streaks progress to atheromatous lesions, Strong and McGill found this process to occur at an earlier age in populations with high morbidity and mortality from coronary heart disease. Jaffé and her colleagues (1971) in Toronto in a study of coronary arteries from birth onwards have built up a picture of gradually developing intimal thickening and fatty infiltration occurring from the earliest months of life. Structural changes in coronary arteries in early life, which differ between ethnic or geographical groups whose susceptibility to IHD is different, have also been reported (Vlodaver, Kann and Neufeld, 1969; Pesonen, Norio and Sarna, 1975).

The accumulation of pathological evidence that lesions which may progress to IHD have their origin in the childhood years, has focused attention on the possibility of prevention of atherosclerosis at this age. Studies in adults have indicated a number of risk factors which predispose to the development of IHD. There is general agreement regarding the importance of hyperlipidaemia (which includes both hypercholesterolaemia and hypertriglyceridaemia), hypertension, cigarette smoking, and physical inactivity (Kannel et al, 1971; Carlson and Böttiger, 1972), but obesity probably only has a minor independent contribution (Keys, Aravanis and Blackburn, 1972). Kannel and Dawber

Percentage change in death rates of males and females in three age groups (from 35 to 64 years) from ischaemic heart disease* in England and Wales, 1950-71. (Three-year moving averages with 1950-52=100)

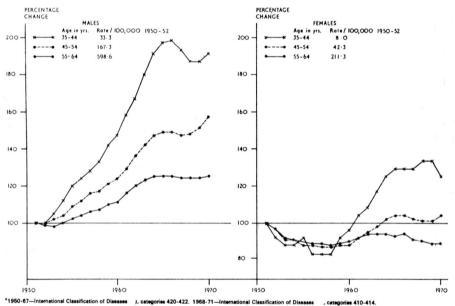

*1950-67—International Classification of Diseases), categories 420-422. 1968-71—International Classification of Diseases , categories 410-414.

Figure 13.1   Increase in death rate from ischaemic heart disease in England and Wales, 1950 to 1071. (Reproduced from *Diet and Coronary Heart Disease*, HMSO, by permission)

(1972) reviewed the relevance of risk factors in childhood and concluded that paediatricians should be actively concerned with the prevention of atherosclerosis in children, and should approach this (1) by preventing and treating obesity, (2) by diagnosing and treating hyperlipidaemia, (3) by diagnosing and treating hypertension, (4) by discouraging cigarette smoking, and (5) by encouraging physical activity. In this chapter hyperlipidaemia in children will be discussed with the object of providing a foundation on which the diagnosis and treatment of the various disorders which may accelerate the development of atherosclerosis may be based.

SERUM LIPIDS AND LIPOPROTEINS

Four major classes of lipid are found in human serum: cholesterol and its esters, triglyceride, the phospholipids, and non-esterified fatty acids. All exist in combination with protein in the form of lipoproteins. Although epidemiological studies have tended to relate concentrations of individual lipids with the risk of IHD, the nature of the lipoprotein abnormality is probably of greater relevance, and identification of the type of hyperlipoproteinaemia is a prerequisite to diagnosis and treatment.

Terminology

A large number of different terms are used to describe the same lipoprotein molecule; this confusion arises from the fact that different methods can be used to separate and identify lipoproteins. The classical and best known method is electrophoresis, and classification of the hyperlipoproteinaemias is usually based on the pattern obtained by this technique (Beaumont et al, 1970). The four major classes of lipoprotein identified by electrophoresis are known as chylomicrons, betalipoprotein, pre-betalipoprotein and alphalipoprotein. The major disadvantage of the method is that it yields qualitative information only; the staining techniques generally show only the lipid portion of the molecule and dye uptake varies according to the type of lipid. Because lipoproteins differ from each other both in the ratio of lipid to protein, and in the proportions of the individual lipids in the molecule, measurements based on intensity of staining of the lipoprotein bands do not accurately estimate the amount of lipoprotein present. This is not to deny that simple inspection of the strip can on occasion give useful information about the likely concentration, but the technique should never be used alone and without some quantitative measure of at least cholesterol, and preferably of both cholesterol and triglyceride.

Methods used for quantitative study of the lipoproteins include analysis after ultracentrifugation, precipitation techniques, immunochemical determinations, and physical estimations of particle size. Preparative ultracentrifugation which enables lipoprotein species to be isolated and their constituents chemically determined remains the most satisfactory method for detailed study; it is, however, expensive and time consuming and uses relatively large volumes of serum. Precipitation and immunochemical methods suffer from the disadvantage that they do not distinguish between betalipoprotein and pre-betalipoprotein, and can therefore only be used in conjunction with other techniques. Physical determination of particle size is the basis of the method devised by Stone and Thorpe (1966); filtration is used to separate different sized lipoproteins (chylomicrons being the largest and betalipoproteins the smallest) whose concentration is then measured by the intensity of light scattering (nephelometry). Because this method is relatively simple and quick it is used in many laboratories; distinction between chylomicrons and pre-betalipoproteins is not absolute because there is overlap in particle size. Alphalipoproteins cannot be measured by this technique as they are too small to scatter light.

Simple inspection of the serum, which can be made by the clinician can also yield useful information. Both chylomicrons and pre-betalipoprotein render the serum turbid. If the sample is allowed to stand overnight in a refrigerator at 4°C chylomicrons will form a cream layer on the surface and if there is no excess of pre-betalipoprotein the infranatant fluid will remain clear. If, however, pre-betalipoprotein is increased the infranatant will be opalescent. If only excess of beta- or alphalipoprotein is present the serum will remain clear. This manoeuvre is known as the 'standing plasma' test (Beaumont et al, 1970).

Table 13.1 Methods used for separation of serum lipoproteins and interrelationship of terminologies

Electrophoresis (paper, agarose, celulose acetate)	Preparative ultracentrifuge[a]	Analytical ultracentrifuge (S_f[b]-value)	Nephelometry[c]
Chylomicrons	Chylomicrons	> 400	Large (L)
Pre-betalipoprotein	Very low-density lipoprotein (VLDL)	20–400	Medium (M)
Betalipoprotein	Low-density lipoprotein (LDL)	0–20	Small (S)
Alphalipoprotein	High-density lipoprotein (HDL)	—	—

[a] Chylomicrons are usually removed before preparative ultracentrifugation

[b] S_f value is the flotation rate of the lipoprotein in a sodium chloride medium of density 1.063 g/ml at 26°C expressed in Svedberg units (10^{-13} cm/s/dyn/g).

[c] Nephelometry by method of Stone and Thorpe (1966)

A summary of the main methods used, and the interrelationship of the various terminologies is given in Table 13.1. It is essential for the clinician faced with the interpretation of laboratory reports on lipoproteins to know the method employed and to appreciate its limitations. In this chapter terminology based on electrophoretic separation will be used wherever possible.

Composition

All lipoproteins contain the three major lipids (cholesterol and its esters, triglyceride, and phospholipids) though in different and distinctive proportions. Very small amounts of non-esterified fatty acids (NEFA) are also associated with the lipoproteins but most of the serum NEFA is carried in association with albumin.

The protein moiety of the lipoproteins, known as apoprotein, is also distinctive. Apoproteins are at present named according to the amino acid residue at the carboxyl end of the molecule (C-terminal amino acid) and it is possible that in the future determination and classification of lipoproteins may be more related to apoproteins than to lipids.

The composition of the four main lipoprotein classes is given in Table 13.2. With a knowledge of the composition of specific individual lipoproteins, considerable information about the lipoprotein pattern in an individual can, for practical purposes, be obtained by estimation of total serum cholesterol and triglyceride, together with the qualitative information given by inspection of an electrophoretic strip. For example, if serum cholesterol is raised but triglyceride is normal, the excess cholesterol can only be in beta- or alphalipo-protein as increased pre-betalipoprotein or chylomicrons must give rise to appreciable increase in triglyceride in addition. The increase required in alphalipoprotein to elevate total serum cholesterol is proportionately greater than that required for betalipoprotein, and inspection of the strip should

Table 13.2   Average percentage composition of lipoproteins (by weight)

Lipoprotein	Protein	Chol.	Trig.	Phos.
Chylomicrons	2	7	83	8
Pre-betalipoprotein	7	23	52	18
Betalipoprotein	21	47	9	23
Alphalipoprotein	46	19	8	27

Chol. = total cholesterol including cholesterol ester
Trig. = triglyceride
Phos. = total phospholipid

indicate whether alphalipoprotein is likely to be greatly increased or whether, as is more common, the excess cholesterol is in betalipoprotein.

Metabolism

Knowledge of the metabolism of lipoproteins is helpful in planning therapy, but much remains to be learnt about their formation, functions and fate. Present views can be summarised as follows.

Chylomicrons are formed in the intestinal absorptive cell and provide the transport vehicle for dietary triglyceride; they also carry dietary cholesterol although some of their cholesterol is endogenously synthesised in situ. They reach the systemic blood stream via the thoracic duct. The triglyceride is hydrolysed by lipoprotein lipase, probably acting at cell surfaces, and the fatty acids thus liberated are used for energy or storage. The residue of the molecule follows a similar pathway to that of pre-betalipoprotein.

Pre-betalipoprotein is largely synthesised in the liver although some may arise in the intestine. The triglyceride is of endogenous origin, as is the cholesterol and phospholipid. This lipoprotein therefore provides the trans-port vehicle for endogenous triglyceride which like exogenous chylomicron triglyceride, is hydrolysed by lipoprotein lipase. Removal of lipid from the molecule is accompanied by loss of apoproteins and a so-called 'intermediate' lipoprotein is formed. This undergoes further degradation with loss of lipid and apoprotein and finally results in the formation of betalipoprotein.

Betalipoprotein thus arises in the serum from the catabolism of chylomicrons and pre-betalipoprotein. Nevertheless the original sources of its lipid and protein are the liver, and to a lesser extent the intestine. It is the major carrier of serum cholesterol. The mechanisms responsible for its degradation, which probably occurs at cell surfaces, are poorly understood and its fate is unknown.

Alphalipoprotein is synthesised in the liver. It provides the substrates for the esterification of serum cholesterol and is associated with the enzyme responsible for this reaction. It also plays a part in the activation of lipoprotein lipase. As is the case for betalipoprotein little is known about the mechanisms of its catabolism.

Normal Values

A definition of normality is essential before abnormality can be identified. For children, current concepts of normality for serum lipids and lipoproteins tend to be based on scanty and inadequate information. Studies of serum cholesterol and triglyceride have in general been made on relatively small and selected groups, and virtually no data is available for normal concentrations of lipoproteins.

Normal ranges are usually defined on a statistical basis as a result of estimations carried out on supposedly healthy individuals; in the case of children such investigations are limited by ethical and practical considerations. Variations in the values reported from different studies can be due to many factors: the analytical methods used, the timing of the sample (especially important in relation to triglyceride), and environmental factors such as diet, about which exact information is often not available. Furthermore, standards obtained in this way 'represent what *is*, not what ought to be' (Tanner and Whitehouse, 1975). What is *normal* for serum lipids in a community is not necessarily *desirable* in terms of the development of atherosclerosis and the subsequent risk of IHD. Precise information is lacking on which to base decisions regarding the appropriate upper cut-off limits for either cholesterol or triglyceride, and at present it is not even clear whether serum lipid levels in adult life can be predicted from estimations made during infancy and childhood (*British Medical Journal*, 1973).

Serum cholesterol

There is a good agreement between various studies that mean serum cholesterol concentrations in umbilical cord blood are around 75 mg/dl, and that there is no correlation between the level of cholesterol on the one hand

and the gestational age, birth weight, ethnic origin, or degree of maternal hyperlipidaemia on the other. Estimations of serum lipoproteins at birth have shown that betalipoprotein is reduced (in comparison with adult values) to a greater degree than alphalipoprotein; thus there is a proportionately greater amount of the total serum cholesterol carried by alphalipoprotein at birth than at other ages. The practical application of this fact lies in the recognition that total cholesterol at birth may give misleading information about the probable concentration of betalipoprotein.

After birth cholesterol concentrations rise rapidly, about doubling by the end of the first week of life and thereafter increasing more slowly, with values equivalent to those of later childhood being achieved by the end of the first year (Darmady, Fosbrooke and Lloyd, 1972) (Table 13.3).

Table 13.3   Serum cholesterol concentration during first year of life

| Age | Serum cholesterol (mg/dl, mean ± 1 s.d.) | | | | | |
	No.	Total	No.	Boys	No.	Girls
Birth	302	78 ± 23	155	76 ± 22^a	147	81 ± 25^a
1 week	300	155 ± 31	156	149 ± 31^b	144	162 ± 29^b
6 weeks	257	155 ± 31	134	152 ± 29	123	159 ± 32
4 months	265	184 ± 36	140	182 ± 32	125	186 ± 41
8 months	60	195 ± 37	31	188 ± 36	29	203 ± 38
1 year	273	191 ± 36	143	189 ± 35	130	192 ± 38

[a] $P < 0.05$
[b] $P < 0.001$

Reproduced from Darmady, Fosbrooke and Lloyd (1972) by permission of the authors and editors

The type of milk fed can have a marked effect on serum cholesterol concentrations in infancy. In general babies receiving human milk have the highest concentrations, and those fed on cow's milk based preparations, in which the fat has been replaced by polyunsaturated oils (for example, S-M-A), have the lowest (Darmady et al, 1972). There is no evidence that the amount of dietary cholesterol or polyunsaturated fat fed to babies during the first six months affects their serum cholesterol response to dietary cholesterol or saturated fat in later infancy (Glueck et al, 1972). Indeed, by the age of one year, when a 'normal infant diet' had been established, Darmady, Fosbrooke and Lloyd (unpublished) found no significant difference between the serum cholesterol concentrations of the various groups of babies fed different milks in early infancy.

There is as yet no convincing evidence to suggest that, in normal infants, serum cholesterol concentrations in early life are related either to subsequent cholesterol concentrations at a later age or to the development of atherosclerosis.

During childhood up to puberty in industrialised societies serum cholesterol concentrations probably stay relatively stable with mean values of around 180 ± 25 mg/dl (1 s.d.) (Table 13.4). Some studies have, however, shown a gradual rise in mean values in school children with a preadolescent peak (Hames and Greenberg, 1961; Godfrey et al, 1972), whereas our own observations indicate a possible slight fall in mean values in later childhood as compared with those found at the age of one year (Roberts, Fosbrooke and Lloyd, unpublished). Girls tend to have somewhat higher mean values than boys at all ages.

Table 13.4   International comparison of mean serum cholesterol levels (mg/dl) in school children

Age (years)	Country	Mean cholesterol	% of children with cholesterol levels > 200 mg/dl
10–14	Mexico	100	0
Teenagers	Masai, Africa	130	—
9–12	New Guinea	139	—
9–19	Arizona, USA	156	10
Teenagers	Iowa, USA	167	14
10–14	Tecumseh, USA	174	—
9–12	Busselton, Australia	175	5
9–12	Westland, Holland	180	33
10–14	Wisconsin, USA	185	33
10	Leuven, Belgium	178	—

Adapted from Uppal, S. C. (1974) *Coronary Heart Disease, Risk Pattern in Dutch Youth.* Leiden: New Rhine Publishers; by permission of the author and publishers

At puberty changes in cholesterol concentration occur, but their magnitude and the timing of the changes in relationship to the stage of puberty have not been adequately documented. The studies of Lee (1967), and our own observations (Roberts, Fosbrooke and Lloyd, unpublished) indicate that concentrations fall in both sexes during the adolescent growth spurt.

Serum triglyceride

Even less data is available for serum triglyceride in healthy children than for serum cholesterol, and the collection of information is hampered by the need to standardise the timing of blood specimens in relation to meals. Whereas there is little diurnal variation in serum cholesterol concentration, triglyceride varies greatly during fat absorption, and blood should therefore be taken in the fasting state; for older children a 12 h fast is desirable but for younger children and babies an 8 h period is probably adequate.

In umbilical cord blood mean values for serum triglyceride are around 35 mg/dl and levels rise rapidly with the start of feeding. At one year of age fasting levels between 37 to 111 mg/dl were found in a small group of London infants, and values for children between 2 and 13 years ranged from 31 to

87 mg/dl (Fosbrooke and Darmady, unpublished data). The suggested upper limit for American children aged 1 to 19 years is 140 mg/dl (Fredrickson and Levy, 1972) and this figure is supported by more recent data from Cincinnati (Glueck et al, 1973).

Implications

The implications of defining *normality* are that children with *abnormal* concentrations will be selected for further investigation and possible treatment, and the justification for treatment designed to lower serum lipids in terms of prevention of IHD has yet to be established. Drash (1972) in an editorial entitled 'Atherosclerosis, cholesterol, and the paediatrician' suggested that upper cut-off limits might be set by epidemiological rather than statistical criteria. He proposed that 200 mg/dl be accepted as the upper limit for serum cholesterol in children and adolescents until studies firmly establish whether there is in fact a cholesterol risk factor for the child. Support for the use of this figure can be found in the epidemiological study of Godfrey et al (1972) in Western Australia; these workers concluded that serum cholesterol of 200 mg/dl in a 6-year-old boy may represent a risk equivalent to that predicted by a level of 238 mg/dl in an adult. The latter value was chosen because it was the lowest limit of the second highest quartile in the study of London busmen by Morris et al (1966), and significantly more men in this group had IHD than in the groups with lower cholesterol concentrations.

Adoption of the criteria suggested by Drash (1972), who further recommends that dietary therapy be instituted for all children with serum cholesterol above 235 mg/dl and probably also for those with values above 200 mg/dl, would have far-reaching consequences in terms of the number of children involved and the need to introduce a screening programme. An international comparison of mean serum cholesterol concentrations in school children (Table 13.4) suggests that in our society as many as one-third of children might become subject to some form of intervention. Until we have further evidence that such intervention is both feasible and effective, the criteria proposed are probably too rigid, and routine screening of serum cholesterol (or any other lipid) during childhood cannot at the moment be justified. For the present the approach summarised in Table 13.5 is probably an acceptable compromise (Lloyd, 1975).

HYPERLIPOPROTEINAEMIA

Classification

The classification of hyperlipoproteinaemia into five types which was originally proposed by Fredrickson, Levy and Lees (1967), and later adopted with minor modifications by the World Health Organisation (Beaumont et al, 1970), is widely used and is as applicable to children as to adults. It must be emphasised, however, that the definition of a type only describes a particular electrophoretic lipoprotein pattern; it does not of itself constitute the diagnosis of a disease (Fredrickson, 1975). Furthermore, the typing system is not applicable unless there is chemical evidence of hyperlipidaemia; for example, a lipoprotein electrophoretic strip showing a prominent betalipoprotein band cannot be designated as a type II pattern if the serum cholesterol concentration is normal.

Hyperlipoproteinaemia may occur as the result of a primary genetically determined disorder or may be found as a secondary manifestation in a variety of diseases. Figure 13.2 gives a simplified classification of the main

Table 13.5   Suggested basis for diagnosis of hyperlipidaemia in children

Age	Cholesterol mg/dl	Fasting triglyceride mg/dl	Conclusion
Under 1 year			Defer diagnostic tests until about one year unless gross hyperlipid-aemia present
1 year to puberty	< 200	< 120	Normal
	200–230	< 140	No action indicated at present; treat as 'normal'
	231–250	< 140	Repeat; normals will tend to be lower. For those still 'high' consider family studies
	> 250	> 140	Abnormal until proved otherwise. Repeat with full lipoprotein studies, exclusion of other diseases, and probably family investigation
Puberty			Consider individuals empirically; insufficient data available for firm recommendations

Reproduced from Lloyd (1975) *British Heart Journal*, by permission of the editor and publishers

conditions in which hyperlipoproteinaemia occurs in childhood, and also indicates the relative magnitude of the elevation of serum cholesterol and triglyceride associated with the various types. It will be appreciated that the same lipoprotein type can be found in different disorders. Treatment may also result in a change in the lipoprotein type within the individual. Diagnostic terminology should not, therefore, consist simply of the type number; at the very least it must be made clear whether the condition is primary or secondary, and it is preferable to describe the actual lipoprotein abnormality.

Secondary Hyperlipoproteinaemias

Although secondary hyperlipoproteinaemias may not appear to be as important as the primary disorders in relation to the subsequent development of atherosclerosis, they should be considered for two reasons. First, they must always be excluded before the diagnosis of a primary disorder is made and second, the possibility of atheroma complicating a chronic disease in which hyperlipoproteinaemia is a feature should be remembered in the overall management.

In children the cause of secondary hyperlipoproteinaemia is usually obvious and the diagnosis already established by the time the lipid abnormality is defined. Occasionally, however, hyperlipoproteinaemia may be the presenting feature. The type of lipoprotein abnormality is seldom diagnostic for a specific disease; indeed the pattern may differ between individuals with the

ELECTROPHORETIC PATTERN	SERUM LIPIDS Chol. Trig.	TYPE	PRIMARY	SECONDARY
CHYLOMICRONS		I	HYPERCHYLOMICRONAEMIA (Fat-induced or exogenous hypertriglyceridaemia)	(DIABETES MELLITUS)
β		II	HYPER β LIPOPROTEINAEMIA (Familial hypercholesterolaemia)	HYPOTHYROIDISM NEPHROTIC SYNDROME OBSTRUCTIVE JAUNDICE
broad-β		III	BROAD-β DISEASE	(HYPOTHYROIDISM)
pre-β		IV	HYPER-PREβLIPOPROTEINAEMIA (Endogenous or CHO-induced hypertriglyceridaemia)	DIABETES MELLITUS NEPHROTIC SYNDROME GLYCOGENOSIS (TYPE I) HYPERCALCAEMIA (HYPOTHYROIDISM)
CHY. pre-β		V		DIABETES MELLITUS NEPHROTIC SYNDROME PANCREATITIS

Figure 13.2   Classification of hyperlipoproteinaemias. (Adapted from Lloyd, J. K. (1972) *Australian Paediatric Journal*, **8**, 264–272, by permission of the editor and publishers)

same disorder, and also in the same individual at different stages of the disease. Because all secondary hyperlipoproteinaemias tend to be reversed by treatment of the underlying disease, serial observations of serum lipids and lipoproteins may sometimes be helpful in assessing progress. Treatment of the hyperlipoproteinaemia in its own right may be necessary in rare instances either because the basic abnormality cannot be treated, or because treatment has not resulted in restoration of a normal lipid pattern and continuing hyperlipidaemia is judged to be harmful.

The disorders most commonly associated with secondary hyperlipoproteinaemia are: poorly controlled diabetes mellitus, hypothyroidism, the nephrotic syndrome, the hepatic glycogenoses, and obstructive liver disease. In addition, populations of industrialised countries who tend to have, amongst other things, a high consumption of saturated fats have higher mean serum cholesterol concentrations than populations in less developed countries who eat less saturated fat; for such a situation the term 'hyperlipoproteinaemia of affluence' could perhaps be used, and this form of secondary hyperlipoproteinaemia also merits discussion.

Poorly controlled diabetes mellitus

In adults, diabetes mellitus is known to increase the risk of IHD (Garcia et al, 1974), and for children with diabetes mellitus the chance of developing some type of vascular complication in early adult life is high. The role of hyperlipoproteinaemia in the pathogenesis of the vascular lesions is still not clear, but it is likely that it contributes to the increased risk of large blood vessel disease including IHD. Attention has therefore been focused on the control of hyperlipoproteinaemia as well as of hyperglycaemia in diabetic children (Lloyd, 1966).

The most common lipoprotein abnormality in poorly controlled diabetes mellitus is an increase in pre-betalipoprotein (type IV pattern) with resulting hypertriglyceridaemia and less marked hypercholesterolaemia. This is mainly due to increased endogenous hepatic synthesis of triglyceride caused by high circulating NEFA levels, but some delay in catabolism may also occur due to deficiency of lipoprotein lipase. In some children, there may be hyperbetalipo-proteinaemia or even hyperchylomicronaemia and a small proportion of children will have a normal pattern despite poor diabetic control. With adequate insulin treatment the lipoprotein pattern in the majority of children will become normal (Chance, Albutt and Edkins, 1969a). Because diabetic control is unlikely to remain perfect throughout the months and years, Salt et al (1960) started a prospective trial of a diet low in ordinary (largely saturated) fat and rich in polyunsaturated fat in an attempt to prevent hyper-lipoproteinaemia and thus the later development of vascular disease. Although during the first six years of this study significantly lower levels of serum choles-terol and betalipoprotein were achieved in children in the diet treated group compared with those in a control group (Lloyd, 1966), further follow-up showed that by the end of 10 years the difference had not been maintained (Chance, Albutt and Edkins, 1969b). Adherence to the regime in the long-term was poor, and some children even developed an excess of pre-betalipoprotein possibly provoked by the relatively high carbohydrate content of the low-fat diet. At present therefore strict control of dietary fat cannot be recommended for diabetic children as a measure designed to prevent the development of IHD.

Hypothyroidism

Hyperlipoproteinaemia is common, but not invariable, in children with untreated hypothyroidism. It is due to decreased catabolism of betalipo-protein and the usual abnormality is an increase in betalipoprotein (type II pattern), although occasionally increase in the intermediate lipoprotein (broad-beta, type III pattern) may occur. Serum lipids and lipoproteins rapidly revert to normal on treatment with thyroxine.

Renal disease

Most children with the nephrotic syndrome have hyperlipoproteinaemia. Elevation of betalipoprotein with hypercholesterolaemia is common and there is a strong negative correlation between the concentrations of serum cholesterol and serum albumin. Increased levels of pre-betalipoprotein and hence of serum triglyceride as well as of cholesterol may also occur, but there appears to be no correlation between concentrations of serum triglyceride and serum albumin. The mechanism responsible for the hyperlipoproteinaemia is not fully understood. It has generally been assumed that hepatic synthesis of betapoprotein is increased along with synthesis of albumin in response to that hypoalbuminaemia, and it has also been suggested that the accumulation of triglyceride rich pre-betalipoprotein may be due to deficiency of lipoprotein lipase (Yamada and Matsuda, 1970), perhaps caused by renal loss of the latter protein. The lipoprotein pattern can be expected to return to normal when proteinuria has been controlled and serum albumin levels restored.

Hyperlipoproteinaemia in association with other forms of renal disease in children is not well documented, although it is recognised that children dying in renal failure may have extensive atheroma. The need to give children on renal dialysis high-fat diets in order to provide sufficient calories for growth may itself result in secondary hyperlipoproteinaemia and acceleration of atherosclerotic processes; this aspect of management requires further investigation.

Hepatic glycogenoses

Hyperlipoproteinaemia is usual in children with any of the forms of hepatic glycogenosis, and the finding of hyperlipidaemia in a child with hepatic enlargement (who does not have obvious cirrhosis) should always arouse suspicion of this diagnosis. Although the type of hyperlipoproteinaemia tends to vary with the nature of the glycogenosis (in glucose-6-phosphatase deficiency there is predominately an increase in pre-betalipoprotein, and in the debrancher and phosphorylase deficiencies the increase is mainly in betalipoprotein), the distinction is not absolute and the lipoprotein pattern cannot be used as an aid to the diagnosis of the type of glycogen storage disease. As there is no specific treatment for the glycogenoses, and as most affected children can be expected to survive into adult life, control of the hyperlipoproteinaemia, if severe, should probably be considered and Fernandes and Pikaar (1969) have described the use of different dietary regimes for the different enzyme variants. They suggest that for children with glucose-6-phosphatase deficiency fat intake should be reduced to about 15 to 35 per cent of calories and given mainly as polyunsaturated fat, and that the carbohydrate be given mainly as starch, and glucose. Meals should be eaten at frequent intervals. Control of hyperlipidaemia is most difficult in this type. For children with deficiency in the debrancher or phosphorylase enzyme systems dietary fat can provide 30 to 40 per cent of calories, but again should be mostly polyunsaturated, and the carbohydrate source should be mainly starch. Long-term evaluation of such therapeutic approaches either in relation to control of serum lipids, or to the development of atheroma is not yet available.

Obstructive liver disease

Children with obstructive liver disease commonly have hyperlipoprotein-aemia until liver failure supervenes when lipoprotein levels tend to be sub-normal, presumably due to depressed synthesis of apoproteins. The type of hyperlipoproteinaemia is variable, although in intrahepatic biliary atresia a specific variety of hyperlipoproteinaemia is often present due to accumulation of so-called lipoprotein X (Seidel, Agostini and Muller, 1972). This lipo-protein has high proportions of unesterified cholesterol and phospholipid in the molecule; as a result there is usually gross hypercholesterolaemia, with the majority of the cholesterol unesterified, and even more marked hyperphos-pholipidaemia. Extensive xanthomataosis of skin and mucous membranes can occur from an early age; treatment of the hyperlipoproteinaemia by a low-fat diet and drugs such as cholestyramine are often successful in alleviating this distressing clinical feature. It is likely that such children will also develop premature atherosclerosis and, if more radical treatment of the hepatic disorder were to become possible, control of hyperlipoproteinaemia could become even more important in management.

'Hyperlipoproteinaemia of affluence'

Epidemiological studies in populations of adults have shown that there is a strong positive correlation between what might be termed affluence (at least in dietary terms) on the one hand and levels of serum cholesterol and the incidence of IHD on the other (Keys, 1970; Findanza, 1972). Similar well-designed studies with comparable methodology are not available for popula-tions of children, but from the limited data available (Table 13.4) Uppal (1974) concluded that children in the so-called developed countries have the highest serum cholesterol levels. Although it is not known to what extent serum lipid levels in childhood predict adult values, significant correlations between the serum cholesterol concentrations of children and those of their parents have been demonstrated (Deutscher, Ostrander and Epstein, 1970; Godfrey et al, 1972). Patterson and Slack (1972), in a study of serum lipids in survivors of myocardial infarction, found that in the majority of those with hyperbetalipoproteinaemia the disorder was polygenically determined, and they suggested that environmental factors such as diet made a major contri-bution.

As a result of the epidemiological studies linking serum cholesterol, diet, and IHD, recommendations regarding dietary modifications for the population have been made by official and semi-official bodies in several countries. Only some of these will be reviewed in this chapter.

For the United Kingdom, the Department of Health and Social Security (1974) recommended that the amount of fat in the United Kingdom diet (which has been steadily rising over the past 20 years), should be reduced. The reduction should apply particularly to saturated fat from both animal and plant sources, but high intakes of polyunsaturated fats were not recommended. Recognising that dietary changes adopted by adults are likely to affect the whole family, it was specifically stated that these recommendations could also safely apply to children.

In Australia, a committee of the National Heart Foundation of Australia (1974) recommended dietary modification for those subjects (adults) whose serum cholesterol exceeds 250 mg/dl or whose serum triglyceride exceeds 160 mg/dl. The diet suggested limited total fat intake to 30 to 35 per cent of calories, increased the proportion of polyunsaturated fat, and restricted cholesterol to 300 mg/day. In their report the committee emphasised the early development of atherosclerosis, and sought to encourage a trend in the national diet away from the current high intake of calories and fat. They were satisfied that diets providing 30 to 35 per cent of calories from fat were adequate for the nutritional needs of growing children and they advocated that dietary education for the community should begin at school.

For New Zealand, the National Heart Foundation of New Zealand (1971) considered it 'premature to advocate a sweeping change in diet for the New Zealand populace, old or young, men or women, Maori or European, regardless of habits or state of health'. However, they did state that 'eventually diet manipulation may prove to be one of the most effective ways in which to modify the course of the disorder (IHD), particularly in those who cannot yet be recognised as potential sufferers'. Thus they suggested that for the population as a whole reasonable restriction of saturated fat intake could be advised with reduction of total calories from fat to 35 per cent, and of cholesterol to 300 to 600 mg/day. They did not consider the use of polyunsaturated fats needed to be especially encouraged. They also comment that these measures should be introduced as habits in childhood rather than as modifications of diet later in life. For individuals identified as being at high risk (serum cholesterol of 250 mg/dl or greater at age 40) dietary modification should be actively promoted.

In the United States of America, the Inter-Society Commission for Heart Disease Resources (1970) recommended diets for all children which provided less than 35 per cent of calories from fat equally divided among saturated, monounsaturated and polyunsaturated sources, and restricted dietary cholesterol to 150 mg/day. However, the Committee on Nutrition of the American Academy of Pediatrics (1972) could not support this recommendation and they proposed that dietary intervention should be restricted to those children with a known high risk for IHD, namely those with familial hyperbetalipoproteinaemia.

Faced with official indecision and conflict of opinion it is difficult to give clear-cut instructions about either the quantity or the type of fat that should be eaten by the average child in order to prevent hypercholesterolaemia and delay the development of atherosclerosis. It is even more difficult to advise about dietary cholesterol, the role of which in producing hypercholesterolaemia is less firmly established than is that of dietary fat. Unless a diagnosis of familial hyperbetalipoproteinaemia has been firmly established dogmatic instructions should be avoided. Parents can, however, be advised that some reduction in fat intake, especially from butter, cream and highly saturated fats such as those in most meats will do no harm, and they can also be reassured that one egg daily (about 250 mg cholesterol) is unlikely to be harmful.

Controlled epidemiological studies in populations of children to determine the range of serum cholesterol (and triglyceride) concentrations, and whether such concentrations can indeed be modified by acceptable dietary changes, seem justifiable and would yield important information. However, population screening of children to detect hyperlipoproteinaeima, whether genetically determined or environmentally induced, cannot be recommended at the present time.

Primary Hyperlipoproteinaemia

Of the five types of primary hyperlipoproteinaemia (Fig. 13.2), primary hyperchylomicronaemia (familial type I) and combined hyperchylomicronaemia and pre-betalipoproteinaemia (familial type V) do not appear to carry an increased risk for the early development of atherosclerosis and will therefore not be discussed. Familial hyperbetalipoproteinaemia (familial type II) is a common condition with a high risk of developing IHD. The other two types, broad-beta disease (familial type III) and primary pre-betalipoproteinaemia (familial type IV) are rarely expressed during childhood and will only be mentioned briefly.

Familial hyperbetalipoproteinaemia (familial hypercholesterolaemia; FH; familial type II)

GENETICS

This is a monogenic disorder inherited as an autosomal dominant (Khachadurian, 1972; Kwiterovich, Fredrickson and Levy, 1974). Homozygous individuals have a more severe disease both clinically and biochemically. Heterozygotes show variable clinical manifestations. Myant and Slack (1973) suggest that it is possible that the mutant gene for FH is not the same in all kindreds and in all parts of the world, though they admit that there is as yet no positive evidence for this.

BASIC DEFECT

The basic defect probably involves the mechanisms for removal of beta-lipoprotein from the serum, and recent work by Brown and Goldstein (1974) suggests there may be deficiency of cell surface receptors for betalipoprotein.

PREVALENCE

At present diagnosis of the heterozygous state is based on an increased concentration of serum cholesterol and/or betalipoprotein, and because it is impossible to define precise cut-off points (Fredrickson, 1971) for either of these determinants, the prevalence cannot be accurately calculated. Carter, Slack and Myant (1971) have estimated the proportion of heterozygotes in England and Wales by making an assumption about the number of homozygous individuals; they suggest a figure of about 1 in 280 which is comparable with that of 1 in 225 reported by Tsang, Fallat and Glueck (1974) from the USA. Whatever the exact figure, the disorder is clearly common.

RISK OF PREMATURE IHD

Homozygous individuals usually develop clinical evidence of IHD in mid or late childhood and seldom live beyond adolescence or early adult life (Fredrickson and Levy, 1972).

Heterozygotes have a considerably increased risk for the development of IHD at an early age in comparison with that of individuals without the lipoprotein disorder; and at all ages the risk for males is greater than that for females. Slack (1969) found that 51 per cent of heterozygous males, but only 12 per cent of heterozygous females, had had a heart attack by the age of 50 years, and Stone et al (1974), in a large study of over 1000 individuals from 116 families with FH, came to essentially similar conclusions. They found IHD occurred in 30 per cent of affected persons but in only 10 per cent of normal relatives ($P < 0.001$) and that there was no difference in the incidence of other risk factors (hypertension, smoking, obesity) between those with FH and those without. The cumulative probability of IHD by age 60 for males with FH in their series was 52 per cent, whereas the normal males had a risk of 13 per cent and were lagging some 20 years behind their affected relatives. For females the risks were 33 per cent for those with FH and 9 per cent for normals.

The incidence of IHD in heterozygous FH is also considerably higher than the incidence expected in people with a comparable degree of hypercholesterolaemia in the general population (Myant and Slack, 1973). This may be due, at least in part, to the fact that the lipoprotein abnormality in FH has been present throughout life, and this reinforces the need to establish the diagnosis and introduce preventive measures at an early age.

CLINICAL PRESENTATION

Homozygous children usually develop tuberous and tendon xanthomata within the first few years of life. Evidence of coronary artery disease commonly appears by puberty and death from IHD often occurs in later childhood or adolescence.

Heterozygous children usually have no clinical evidence of the disorder. In a small proportion, however, xanthomata or corneal arcus may be found. In a study of 70 affected children aged 1 to 19 years Kwiterovich et al (1974) reported five with tendon and/or tuberous xanthomata, and two with corneal arcus; none of the children had any history suggestive of myocardial ischaemia.

The majority of children with heterozygous FH will therefore only present as a result of family studies.

DIAGNOSIS

Homozygous FH does not usually present any diagnostic problem. The serum cholesterol concentration is very high, often of the order 600 to 1000 mg/dl and there is a corresponding increase in the level of beta-lipoprotein. Depending upon the age, xanthomata may already be present. Both parents will have the heterozygous form of the disease. Occasionally, however, diagnostic difficulty may be encountered; secondary hyperlipo-proteinaemia can present with gross hypercholesterolaemia and xanthomata, although usually in this case the underlying disease should be obvious. More problems are likely to arise from the recently described condition of pseudo-homozygous type II hyperlipoproteinaemia (Morganroth et al, 1974). In this disorder clinical and biochemical features compatible with homozygous FH were present but no abnormality could be demonstrated in any first-degree relatives; furthermore, the patients responded remarkably well to treatment, unlike the usual situation in homozygous FH. This emphasises the need for family studies before making a diagnosis of FH.

Heterozygous FH can often be diagnosed with comparative ease on the basis of raised serum cholesterol and betalipoprotein concentrations, and the demonstration of a similar abnormality in a parent or other first-degree relative. In the majority of affected children pre-betalipoprotein is not increased and serum triglyceride concentrations are normal. Kwiterovich et al (1974) have estimated that only about 10 per cent of heterozygous children have slight increase in pre-betalipoprotein with modest hypertriglyceridaemia, the so-called type IIB pattern (Beaumont et al, 1970).

Because there is as yet no specific diagnostic test for FH, and no precise value for serum cholesterol which will differentiate normals from abnormals, problems will be encountered with children whose serum cholesterol concentration falls in the 'borderline' range. Repeat analyses, and determination of betalipoprotein cholesterol, may help to resolve the difficulty, and these estimations should always be made in any doubtful cases. Nevertheless in some instances empirical decisions may have to be taken. Such decisions will be influenced by whether it is intended to follow a positive diagnosis by treatment, and this decision will in turn be affected by the sex of the child, the degree of IHD already manifest in the family, and the amount of anxiety likely to be engendered by diagnosis and treatment. Until the long-term feasibility of treatment is better established it is probably wise to err on the side of diagnosing 'normality' in doubtful cases.

Neonatal diagnosis of FH, and the possibility of neonatal screening, continue to be a subject for debate (Kwiterovich, 1974). If a parent is known to have FH, and if betalipoprotein cholesterol and not simply total serum cholesterol is estimated in cord blood, the diagnosis can be established with reasonable certainty at birth (Kwiterovich, Levy and Fredrickson, 1973). Determination of cord serum cholesterol alone in unselected populations of babies has not, however, proved helpful (Darmady et al, 1972). In the study of Darmady et al the only infant out of a total of 300 who was subsequently shown to have FH at the age of one year, had a normal cord cholesterol value. The majority of babies diagnosed as having 'neonatal hypercholesterolaemia' (cord serum cholesterol greater than 100 mg/dl) in the study of Tsang et al (1974) did not have FH, and neither did they have hypercholesterolaemia at the age of one year. Thus cord blood screening of serum cholesterol as a means of diagnosis of FH on a population basis cannot be recommended.

Diagnosis during the first year of life may be difficult because of the marked effect of diet on serum cholesterol at this age. Babies who are breast fed tend to have the highest cholesterol levels, and those fed on infant formulas containing polyunsaturated fat have the lowest values. In individual infants concentrations can vary considerably depending on the type of feed. Thus it is usually wiser to defer making a definitive diagnosis until the child is about one year of age and established on ordinary cow's milk and normal infant foods (Darmady et al, 1972).

MANAGEMENT

Homozygous children present a major therapeutic challenge. Combined use of diet (low saturated fat supplemented with polyunsaturated fat), cholestyramine, and nicotinic acid in large doses appears to be the most effective medical regime for lowering serum cholesterol and betalipoprotein, and xanthomata have regressed with such treatment (Segall et al, 1970a; Levy et al, 1972). In most cases, however, serum cholesterol has not been lowered beyond about 500 mg/dl, and the effect of such treatment on the development of atheroma has not been evaluated. Because of the poor prognosis for the untreated disease, many other procedures have been tried; these include plasmapheresis (Apstein et al, 1974), ileal bypass (Balfour and Kim, 1974) and portacaval shunt (Starzl et al, 1974). All these forms of treatment require critical evaluation and, owing to the rarity of the disorder, it has been suggested that a Central Registry should be kept at the National Institutes of Health, USA, in order to collect and disseminate information and to initiate collaborative studies.

For heterozygous children the only certainty about treatment is that it will need to be continued for a long time, probably for life. There is as yet no evidence that treatment initiated in childhood will prevent or delay the development of atherosclerosis and IHD. Trials of lipid lowering therapy in adults in whom the magnitude of the hyperlipoproteinaemia has varied and its type not been defined, have tended to give encouraging but inconclusive results; controlled studies of therapy in adults with FH have only recently been initiated (Rifkind and Levy, 1974). The degree of reduction in serum cholesterol necessary for optimum effect has likewise not been evaluated; on epidemiological grounds it would seem that any reduction is better than none, and that the lower the ultimate levels achieved the better. It is of great importance that all children with FH who are being treated should be carefully followed so that answers to these and other questions may be obtained.

Current treatment relies on diet or drugs or a combination of both:

Diet involves a reduction in ordinary fat intake (largely saturated fat) to about 15 to 20 g/day. Such a diet is likely to be boring and can be made more palatable by the use of oils and margarines rich in polyunsaturated fat. Polyunsaturated fat itself has, however, no specific hypocholesterolaemic effect in FH (Segall et al, 1970a). Limitation of dietary cholesterol to below 300 mg/day is stressed by some investigators (Levy et al, 1972), but as most dietary cholesterol consumed by children is in the form of eggs or other foods rich in saturated fat, a strict low-fat diet effectively limits cholesterol intake and formal instructions regarding this component seem unnecessary. The description of the diet as a low-cholesterol diet should be discouraged as this fails to emphasise that a most important aspect of the diet is the reduction in saturated fat.

Dietary treatment alone may be expected to achieve a reduction in serum cholesterol of about 20 per cent of the pretreatment value. If the aim of treatment is to achieve cholesterol levels below 250 mg/dl, diet by itself is unlikely to be adequate therapy for children whose initial values are over 350 mg/dl. In the long term, dietary treatment, even when initially effective, is likely to prove difficult to maintain. In our experience 80 per cent of children were no longer adequately controlled after the first $1\frac{1}{2}$ to 2 years of dietary treatment (West, Fosbrooke and Lloyd, 1975). For those children with good long-term compliance, however, diet continued to achieve reasonable control of serum cholesterol with levels around 250 mg/dl.

The advisability of diet during the first year of life for those infants who, in the course of family studies, have been diagnosed at this age has been questioned and recently reviewed (McBean and Speckmann, 1974). It has been suggested that dietary 'cholesterol challenge' during early infancy might be necessary in order to stimulate the development of the enzyme systems responsible for cholesterol homeostasis, and artificial lowering of serum cholesterol in young animals has been reported to lead to higher values in later life (Reiser, 1971). A study in human infants has, however, failed to show any influence of dietary cholesterol or type of milk fat during the first year of life, on the subsequent serum cholesterol levels (Glueck et al, 1972). There does not therefore appear to be any valid reason for avoiding the use of infant formulas known to have a high polyunsaturated fat content in the feeding of infants with FH. Equally there is no evidence that treatment at such an early age is beneficial, and breast feeding should certainly not be discouraged because of its effect on serum cholesterol concentrations.

Drugs are likely to be needed for the control of hypercholesterolaemia in the majority of children with FH either because diet produces inadequate lowering of serum cholesterol, or because it is not adhered to over the years. Clofibrate has only a weak hypocholesterolaemic effect in FH; furthermore it has to be given in conjunction with diet and for these reasons it probably has no place in the management of children (West et al, 1975). Nicotinic acid and D-thyroxine have potential side effects which limit their use in paediatric practice.

Cholestyramine (Questran brand, Bristol Laboratories), a non-adsorbable ion exchange resin which binds bile acids in the intestine, is currently the drug of choice. It has been shown to be effective without the need for dietary fat restriction, and can be given in twice daily dosage. The amount of cholesterol lowering is proportional to the size of the dose and reduction of about 35 per cent in serum cholesterol can be achieved with a mean daily dose of about 0.6 g/kg body weight (West and Lloyd, 1973). Compliance with this treatment is better than for any regime involving a strict diet, but even so only 57 per cent of a group of 36 children remained satisfactorily controlled after a three-year period (West et al, 1975). The major reason for non-adherence was unpalatability of the resin, and studies with more palatable and less bulky preparations are clearly indicated.

Side effects of cholestyramine are limited to those caused by discomfort due to the bulk of the resin, or due to interference with absorption. In our experience gastrointestinal discomfort has been rare in children. Folate deficiency occurs due to binding of folic acid to the resin, and can be corrected by additional oral folate which should always be given to children on long-term therapy. Steatorrhoea and progressive lowering of serum concentrations of vitamins A, E and inorganic phosphate have also been observed over a two-year period, though without any obvious clinical consequences (West and Lloyd, 1975). Long-term studies for possible adverse effects need to be continued on all children receiving resin therapy.

Compliance with any treatment regime is likely to decline with the passage of time. Blackwell (1973) has defined patients at special risk of non-compliance as those with chronic illnesses requiring long-term maintenance with suppressive or preventive treatment, and in whom the ill effects of stopping treatment are not obvious. Children with FH clearly come into this group. Compliance can be improved if the doctor is familiar to the patients and takes time to discuss the various problems; it is also improved if the number of drugs and their frequency of administration is reduced, and if the side effects are minimal. Until more acceptable therapy is available for children with FH, and reasonable long-term compliance can be expected, it would seem appropriate to confine treatment to those children from families in which early IHD has already occurred and motivation is therefore high. It may also be argued that girls should not be treated as their risk is substantially less than that for boys; whilst this distinction may be epidemiologically correct, its application can be practically difficult especially in a family where a female relative has already had a premature IHD event, or in which there are both affected boys and girls.

Psychological effects of treating outwardly healthy and symptom-free children with a restricted diet or unpleasant drugs have not been critically evaluated. Our experience with high-risk families who have themselves requested help suggests that, in this highly selected group, the need for treatment is well accepted and general family anxiety may be allayed, at least in the short term.

Control of other risk factors is important in overall management. A combination of risk factors is known to greatly enhance the risk of IHD and investigations of children with FH should include assessment of fatness and measurement of blood pressure, as well as enquiry about family smoking and exercise patterns. Obesity and hypertension should be treated and the risks of cigarette smoking explained. Parents should be told that the likelihood of children smoking becomes much greater if their parents smoke. A parent who has FH, with or without clinical IHD, should in any case stop smoking, but parents in general may be prepared to give up smoking for the sake of their children's health even when they would not do it for their own.

Broad beta disease (familial type III)

This type of lipoprotein disorder is rare during childhood. Fredrickson and Levy (1972) failed to find evidence of the disease under the age of 20 years in the course of extensive family studies of 36 kindreds; Fuhrmann et al reported one family with affected children in 1971; and we have recently seen one girl aged eight years who first developed xanthomata behind her knees at the age of six years.

In adults xanthomata are common and are usually of the tubero-eruptive variety and occur in palmar creases; occurrence of the latter is virtually characteristic of this particular lipoprotein abnormality. Both IHD and peripheral vascular disease may occur at an early age. The mode of inheritance has not yet been completely established; in some families it appears to be an autosomal dominant. Response of the hyperlipidaemia to treatment is usually good and some evidence has been obtained that peripheral arterial disease may actually regress (Zelis et al, 1970). If the patient is obese, weight should be reduced by a diet in which calories, saturated fat and cholesterol are restricted; thereafter it is recommended that the diet contains about 40 per cent of calories from fat with cholesterol reduced to about 300 mg/day. If drug treatment is required, clofibrate is the drug of choice (Levy, Morganroth and Rifkind, 1974).

The metabolic abnormality is an accumulation of intermediate lipoprotein (Fig. 13.2) which has more cholesterol than pre-betalipoprotein and more triglyceride than betalipoprotein. The serum thus contains excess cholesterol and triglyceride in about equal amounts. Lipoprotein electrophoresis usually, but not invariably, shows a broadened beta band but the diagnosis has to be established by ultracentrifugation and demonstration of betalipoprotein of abnormally low density (intermediate lipoprotein).

Primary pre-betalipoproteinaemia (familial type IV)

This condition also appears to be uncommon under the age of 21 years (Glueck, Tsang and Fallat, 1972) and originally only a few isolated cases were reported around the age of puberty (Segall et al, 1970b; Fredrickson and Levy, 1972). More recently Glueck et al (1973) in an investigation of 33 families with pre-betalipoproteinaemia found abnormal lipoprotein patterns in 32 of the 77 children under the age of 21. In only nine of these, however, was the type IV pattern present, and of these nine children three were under 12 years and five over 19 years. Seventeen of the 32 children had hyperbetalipoproteinaemia (type II) and six had hyperbetalipoproteinaemia with slight elevation of pre-betalipoprotein (type IIB). This study therefore also emphasises the rarity of the condition before puberty, and further illustrates the confusion about its mode of inheritance. Glueck et al comment that it will be interesting to see how many of the children in their study who have the type II pattern will eventually develop a type IV pattern.

The serum lipid concentrations reflect the increase of pre-betalipoprotein with moderate to marked elevation of serum triglyceride and relatively modest increase in cholesterol.

Obesity and impaired carbohydrate tolerance are often associated with pre-betalipoproteinaemia; xanthomata both tuberous and eruptive can occur; and premature atherosclerosis is common. Treatment is by weight reduction if indicated, by restriction of dietary carbohydrate, and by the use of clofibrate if dietary measures do not control the hyperlipoproteinaemia.

REFERENCES

Apstein, C. S., George, P. K., Zilversmit, D. B., Feldman, H. A. & Lees, R. S. (1974) Cholesterol reduction with intensive plasmapheresis. *Clinical Research*, **22**, 459A.

Balfour, J. F. & Kim, R. (1974) Homozygous type II hyperlipoproteinaemia treatment; partial ileal bypass in two children. *Journal of American Medical Association*, **227**, 1145–1151.

Beaumont, J. L., Carlson, L. A., Cooper, G. R., Fejfar, Z., Fredrickson, D. S. & Strasser, T. (1970) *Bulletin of the World Health Organisation*, **43**, 891–915.

Blackwell, B. (1973) Drug therapy; patient compliance. *New England Journal of Medicine*, **289**, 249–252.

British Medical Journal (1973) Serum cholesterol in children. **1,** 690–691.

Brown, M. S. & Goldstein, J. L. (1974) Expression of the familial hypercholesterolaemia gene in heterozygotes: mechanism for a dominant disorder in man. *Science,* **185,** 61–63.

Carlson, L. A. & Böttiger, L. E. (1972) Ischaemic heart disease in relation to fasting values of plasma triglycerides and cholesterol. *Lancet,* **1,** 865–868.

Carter, C. O., Slack, J. & Myant, N. B. (1971) Genetics of hyperlipoproteinaemias. *Lancet,* **1,** 400–401.

Chance, G. W., Albutt, E. C. & Edkins, S. M. (1969a) Serum lipids and lipoproteins in untreated diabetic children. *Lancet,* **1,** 1126–1128.

Chance, G. W., Albutt, E. C. & Edkins, S. M. (1969b) Control of hyperlipidaemia in juvenile diabetes. Standard and corn oil diets compared over a period of 10 years. *British Medical Journal,* **3,** 616–618.

Committee on Diet and Heart Disease of the National Heart Foundation of Australia (1974) Dietary fat and coronary heart disease: a review. *Medical Journal of Australia,* **1,** 575–579, 616–620, 663–668.

Committee on Nutrition (1972) Childhood diet and coronary heart disease. *Pediatrics,* **49,** 305–307.

Darmady, J. M., Fosbrooke, A. S. & Lloyd, J. K. (1972) Prospective study of serum cholesterol levels during first year of life. *British Medical Journal,* **2,** 685–688.

Department of Health and Social Security (1974) Diet and coronary heart disease. *Report on Health and Social Subjects,* 7. London: HMSO.

Deutscher, S., Ostrander, L. D. & Epstein, F. H. (1970) Familial factors in premature coronary heart disease—a preliminary report from the Tecumseh community health study. *American Journal of Epidemiology,* **91,** 233–237.

Drash, A. (1972) Atherosclerosis, cholesterol, and the paediatrician. *Journal of Pediatrics,* **80,** 693–696.

Enos, W. F., Holmes, R. H. & Beyer, J. (1953) Coronary artery disease among United States soldiers killed in action in Korea. *Journal of the American Medical Association,* **152,** 1090–1093.

Fernandes, J. & Pikaar, N. A. (1969) Hyperlipemia in children with liver glycogen disease. *American Journal of Clinical Nutrition,* **22,** 617–627.

Findanza, F. (1972) Dietary studies and the epidemiology of heart disease. In *Proceedings of the First Asian Congress of Nutrition,* ed. Tulpule, P. G. & Rao, K. S. J., pp. 757–772. Nutrition Society of India.

Fredrickson, D. S. (1971) Mutants, hyperlipoproteinaemia, and coronary heart disease. *British Medical Journal,* **2,** 187–192.

Fredrickson, D. S. (1975) It's time to be practical. *Circulation,* **51,** 209–211.

Fredrickson, D. S. & Levy, R. I. (1972) Familial hyperlipoproteinaemia. In *Metabolic Basis of Inherited Disease,* 3rd edn, ed. Stanbury, J. B., Wyngaarden, J. B. & Fredrickson, D. S., pp. 545–614. New York: McGraw-Hill Book Co. Inc.

Fredrickson, D. S., Levy, R. I. & Lees, R. S. (1967) Fat transport in lipoproteins: an integrated approach to mechanisms and disorders. *New England Journal of Medicine,* **276,** 33–44, 94–103, 148–156, 215–226, 273–281.

Fuhrmann, W., Schoenborn, W., Huth, H. & Reimers, H. J. (1971) Familial hyperlipoproteinaemia, type III. In *Proceedings of XIII International Congress of Pediatrics,* **7,** 199–204. Wiener Medizinschen Akademie.

Garcia, M. J., McNamara, P. M., Gordon, T. & Kannel, W. B. (1974) Morbidity and mortality in diabetics in the Framingham population. Sixteen year follow-up study. *Diabetes,* **23,** 105–111.

Glueck, C. J., Tsang, R. & Fallat, R. (1972) Pediatric familial type IV hyperlipoproteinaemia. *Transactions of Association of American Physicians,* **35,** 139–150.

Glueck, C. J., Tsang, R., Balistreri, W. & Fallat, R. (1972) Plasma and dietary cholesterol in infancy: effects of early low or moderate dietary cholesterol intake on subsequent respones to increased dietary cholesterol. *Metabolism,* **21,** 1181–1192.

Glueck, C. J., Fallat, R., Buncher, C. R., Tsang, R. & Steiner, P. (1973) Familial combined hyperlipoproteinaemia: studies in 91 adults and 95 children from 33 kindreds. *Metabolism,* **22,** 1403–1428.

Godfrey, R. C., Stenhouse, N. S., Cullen, K. J. & Blackman, V. (1972) Cholesterol and the child: studies of the cholesterol levels of Bussleton schoolchildren and their parents. *Australian Paediatric Journal*, **8**, 72–78.

Hames, C. G. & Greenberg, B. G. (1961) A comparative study of serum cholesterol levels in schoolchildren and their possible relation to atherogenesis. *American Journal of Public Health*, **51**, 374–385.

Inter-Society Commission for Heart Disease Resources (1970) Primary prevention of the atherosclerotic diseases. *Circulation*, **42**, A-53–A-95.

Jaffé, D., Hartcroft, W. S., Manning, M. & Eleta, G. (1971) Coronary arteries in newborn children. *Acta paediatrica scandinavica*, Suppl. 219.

Kannel, W. B., Castelli, W. P., Gordon, T. & McNamara, P. M. (1971) Serum cholesterol, lipoproteins, and the risk of coronary heart disease. *Annals of Internal Medicine*, **74**, 1–12.

Kannel, W. B. & Dawber, T. R. (1972) Atherosclerosis as a pediatric problem. *Journal of Pediatrics*, **80**, 544–554.

Keys, A. (1970) Coronary heart disease in seven countries. *Circulation*, **41**, Suppl. 1, 1–211.

Keys, A., Aravanis, C. & Blackburn, H. (1972) Coronary heart disease: overweight and obesity as risk factors. *Annals of Internal Medicine*, **77**, 15–27.

Khachadurian, A. K. (1972) A general review of clinical and laboratory features of familial hypercholesterolaemia (type II hyperbetalipoproteinaemia). In *Protides of the Biological Fluids*, Proceedings of the IXX Colloquium, Bruges, ed. Peeters, H., pp. 315–318. Oxford: Pergamon Press.

Kwiterovich, P. O. (1974) Neonatal screening for hyperlipidaemia. *Pediatrics*, **53**, 455–457.

Kwiterovich, P. O., Levy, R. I. & Frederickson, D. S. (1973) Neonatal diagnosis of familial type II hyperlipoproteinaemia. *Lancet*, **1**, 118–122.

Kwiterovich, P. O., Frederickson, D. S. & Levy, R. I. (1974) Familial hypercholesterolaemia (one form of familial type II hyperlipoproteinaemia): a study of its biochemical, genetic, and clinical presentation in childhood. *Journal of Clinical Investigation*, **53**, 1237–1249.

Lee, V. A. (1967) Individual trends in total serum cholesterol of children and adolescents over a ten-year period. *American Journal of Clinical Nutrition*, **20**, 5–12.

Levy, R. I., Fredrickson, D. S., Shulman, R., Bilheimer, D. W., Breslow, J. L., Stone, N. J., Lux, S. E., Sloan, H. R., Krauss, R. M. & Herbert, P. N. (1972) Dietary and drug treatment of primary hyperlipoproteinaemia. *Annals of Internal Medicine*, **77**, 267–294.

Levy, R. I., Morganroth, J. & Rifkind, B. M. (1974) Drug therapy: treatment of hyperlipidaemia. *New England Journal of Medicine*, **290**, 1295–1301.

Lloyd, J. K. (1966) Control of dietary fat in relation to diabetic complications in children. *Proceedings of the Nutrition Society*, **25**, 74–83.

Lloyd, J. K. (1972) Hyperlipoproteinaemia in childhood. *Australian Paediatric Journal*, **8**, 264–272.

Lloyd, J. K. (1975) Hyperlipidaemia in children. *British Heart Journal*, **37**, 105–114.

McBean, L. D. & Speckmann, E. N. (1974) An interpretive review: diet in early life and the prevention of atherosclerosis. *Pediatric Research*, **8**, 837–842.

McNamara, J. J., Molot, M. A., Stremple, J. F. & Cutting, R. T. (1971) Coronary artery disease in combat casualties in Vietnam. *Journal of the American Medical Association*, **216**, 1185–1189.

Morganroth, J., Levy, R. I., McMahon, A. E. & Gotto, A. M. (1974) Pseudohomozygous type II hyperlipoproteinaemia. *Journal of Pediatrics*, **85**, 639–643.

Morris, J. N., Kagan, A., Pattison, D. C., Gardner, M. J. & Raffle, P. A. B. (1966) Incidence and prediction of ischaemic heart disease in London busmen. *Lancet*, **2**, 553–559.

Myant, N. B. & Slack, J. (1973) Type II hyperlipoproteinaemia. In *Clinics in Endocrinology and Metabolism*, Vol. 2 (1), Ch. 5, pp. 81–109. London: W. B. Saunders Co. Ltd.

National Heart Foundation of New Zealand (1971) Coronary heart disease: a New Zealand report. *National Heart Foundation of New Zealand*. Dunedin: J. McIndoe.

Patterson, D. & Slack, J. (1972) Lipid abnormalities in male and female survivors of myocardial infarction and their first degree relatives. *Lancet*, **1**, 393–399.

Pesonen, E., Norio, R. & Sarna, S. (1975) Thickenings in the coronary arteries in infancy as an indication of genetic factors in coronary heart disease. *Circulation*, **51**, 218–225.

Reiser, R. (1971) Control of adult serum cholesterol by the nutrition of the suckling: a progress report. *Circulation*, **63**, Suppl. 11, 11–3.

Rifkind, B. M. & Levy, R. I. (1974) Does hypolipidemic therapy prevent coronary heart disease? Cardiovascular drug therapy. In *Cardiovascular Clinics*, Vol. 6 (2), pp. 1–9. Philadephia: F. A. Davis Co.

Salt, H. B., Wolff, O. H., Nestadt, A. N. & Lloyd, J. K. (1960) Control of lipaemia in children with diabetes mellitus. *Lancet*, **1**, 71–75.

Segall, M. M., Fosbrooke, A. S., Lloyd, J. K. & Wolff, O. H. (1970a) Treatment of familial hypercholesterolaemia in children. *Lancet*, **1**, 641–644.

Segall, M. M., Fosbrooke, A. S., Lloyd, J. K. & Wolff, O. H. (1970b) Carbohydrate-induced hypertriglyceridaemia in a child. *Archives of Disease in Childhood*, **45**, 73–79.

Seidel, D., Agostini, B. & Muller, P. (1972) Structure of an abnormal lipoprotein (LP-X) characterising obstructive jaundice. *Biochimica et biophysica acta*, **260**, 146–152.

Slack, J. (1969) Risks of ischaemic heart disease in familial hyperlipoproteinaemic states. *Lancet*, **2**, 1380–1382.

Stamler, J. (1971) Acute myocardial infarction—progress in primary prevention. *British Heart Journal*, **33**, Suppl. 145–164.

Starzl, T. E., Chase, H. P., Putnam, C. W. & Nora, J. J. (1974) Follow-up of patient with portacaval shunt for the treatment of hyperlipidemia. *Lancet*, **2**, 714–715.

Stone, M. C. & Thorpe, J. M. (1966) A new technique for the investigation of the low-density lipoproteins in health and disease. *Clinica chimica acta*, **14**, 812–830.

Stone, N. J., Levy, R. I., Fredrickson, D. S. & Verter, J. (1974) Coronary artery disease in 116 kindred with familial type II hyperlipoproteinaemia. *Circulation*, **49**, 476–488.

Strong, J. P. & McGill, H. C. (1969) The pediatric aspects of atherosclerosis. *Journal of Atherosclerosis Research*, **9**, 251–265.

Tanner, J. M. & Whitehouse, R. H. (1975) Revised standards for triceps and subscapular skinfolds in British children. *Archives of Disease in Childhood*, **50**, 142–145.

Tsang, R. C., Fallat, R. W. & Glueck, C. J. (1974) Cholesterol at birth and age 1: comparison of normal and hypercholesterolemic neonates. *Pediatrics*, **53**, 458–470.

Uppal, S. C. (1974) *Coronary Heart Disease, Risk Pattern in Dutch Youth.* Leiden: New Rhine Publishers.

Vlodaver, Z., Kahn, H. A. & Neufeld, H. N. (1969) The coronary arteries in early life in three different ethnic groups. *Circulation*, **39**, 541–550.

West, R. J. & Lloyd, J. K. (1973) Use of cholestyramine in treatment of children with familial hypercholesterolaemia. *Archives of Disease in Childhood*, **48**, 370–374.

West, R. J. & Lloyd, J. K. (1975) Effect of cholestyramine on intestinal absorption. *Gut*, **16**, 93–98.

West, R. J., Fosbrooke, A. S. & Lloyd, J. K. (1975) Treatment of familial hypercholesterolaemia in children. *Postgraduate Medical Journal*, **51**, (Suppl. 8), 82–86.

Yamada, M. & Matsuda, I. (1970) Lipoprotein lipase in clinical and experimental nephrosis. *Clinica chimica acta*, **30**, 787–794.

Zelis, R., Mason, D. T., Braunwald, E. & Levy, R. I. (1970) Effects of hyperlipoproteinaemias and their treatment on the peripheral circulation. *Journal of Clinical Investigation*, **49**, 1007–1015.

INDEX

PRINTED BY ADLARD AND SON LTD, BARTHOLOMEW PRESS, DORKING